Esthetic Soft Tissue Management of Teeth and Implants

Esthetic Soft Tissue Management of Teeth and Implants

André P. Saadoun DDS, MS

Doctor in Odontologic Sciences, University of Paris
Associate Professor in Periodontics, University of Southern California
Diplomate of the American Academy of Periodontology
Diplomate of the International Congress of Oral Implantology
Visiting Professor, Hadassah Faculty of Dental Medicine, Jerusalem

WILEY-BLACKWELL
A John Wiley & Sons, Ltd., Publication

This edition first published 2013

Wiley-Blackwell is an imprint of John Wiley & Sons, formed by the merger of Wiley's global Scientific, Technical and Medical business with Blackwell Publishing.

Registered Office
John Wiley & Sons, Ltd, The Atrium, Southern Gate, Chichester, West Sussex, PO19 8SQ, UK

Editorial Offices
9600 Garsington Road, Oxford, OX4 2DQ, UK
The Atrium, Southern Gate, Chichester, West Sussex, PO19 8SQ, UK
2121 State Avenue, Ames, Iowa 50014-8300, USA

For details of our global editorial offices, for customer services and for information about how to apply for permission to reuse the copyright material in this book please see our website at www.wiley.com/wiley-blackwell.

Library of Congress Cataloging-in-Publication Data

Saadoun, André P.
Esthetic soft tissue management of teeth and implants / André P. Saadoun.
p. ; cm.
Includes bibliographical references and index.
ISBN 978-1-118-30115-9 (hardback)
I. Title.
[DNLM: 1. Esthetics, Dental. 2. Dental Implantation–methods. 3. Gingival Recession–prevention & control. 4. Periodontics–methods. WU 100]
617.6'93–dc23

2012025031

A catalogue record for this book is available from the British Library.

Wiley also publishes its books in a variety of electronic formats. Some content that appears in print may not be available in electronic books.

Cover images courtesy of André P. Saadoun
Cover design by Andrew Magee

Set in 11.5/13.5pt Minion by SPi Publisher Services, Pondicherry, India

1 2013

The Value of a Smile

A smile costs nothing, but gives much.

It enriches those who receive, without making poorer those who give.

It takes but a moment, but the memory of it sometimes lasts forever.

None is so rich or mighty that he can get along without it, and none is so poor, but that he can be made rich by it.

A smile creates happiness in the home, fosters good will in business, and is the countersign of friendship.

It brings rest to the weary, cheer to the discouraged, sunshine to the sad, and it is nature's best antidote for trouble.

Yet it cannot be bought, begged, borrowed, or stolen, for it is something that is of no value to anyone, until it is given away.

Some people are too tired to give you a smile;

Give them one of yours, as none needs a smile so much as he who has no more to give.

Frederick William Faber

Contents

Foreword

This volume addresses an area that should be of concern to the dental profession: the patient's smile. Dr. André Saadoun has attempted to demonstrate the importance of an esthetic smile to the patient and how this may be influenced by the soft tissue management of teeth and dental implants.

The author has analyzed the constituents of the smile and has addressed the various options that can result in the improvement of an individual's self-image by producing changes in those tissues. This carefully prepared text contains a thorough review of the literature of the past five decades and has applied those contributions to therapy in treating natural teeth as well as dental implants. It is gratifying to see that an emphasis is placed on the preservation of the natural dentition in health and function, and when the clinician has to replace hopeless teeth, the care necessary to improve the prognosis of implants. The advances in periodontal therapy are cited and described in some detail. This book should be of keen interest to all clinicians who are involved in oral health, which includes treating teeth and implants.

To date, there have been few attempts in the literature to correlate treatment of teeth and dental implants with their impact on the patient's smile.

The illustrations strengthen the editorial material and are well done. The reader will be stimulated to discuss the patient's smile with them during the examination phase of treatment. Helping the patient to understand the influence of oral treatment on improving their smile becomes a significant responsibility for the diagnostician and therapist.

This volume should partner with other texts that delve into periodontal and restorative treatment in great detail. Dr. Saadoun brings together the various specialties in dental medicine in a coherent fashion. There are many areas in the oral cavity, such as dental biotypes, that play an important role in decision-making by the dentist as one prepares to establish an esthetic smile. It is also clear that a patient's gratitude for an improved smile will benefit the therapist who has devoted great effort and time to studying and effecting this esthetic improvement.

The author should be complimented for putting the material into one volume, material that belongs on the shelf of every dentist.

D. Walter Cohen, DDS
Chancellor Emeritus
Drexel University College of Medicine
Philadelphia, PA

Acknowledgments

A Chinese proverb says: "*A teacher becomes a master, when his student becomes a teacher.*"

I will never forget all my masters, who have played an important role in my professional life, namely Professor Walter Cohen, Professor Morton Amsterdam, Professor Jay Siebert, Professor Saul Schluger, and Professor Per-Ingvar Brånemark.

I extend all my sincere appreciation and deepest gratitude to my colleagues and dearest friends who have motivated and encouraged me in making this dream come true by offering their clinical illustrations: Dr. Thierry Degorce from Tours; Dr. Stefen Koubi from Marseille; Dr. Cobi Landsberg from Tel Aviv; Dr. Masayuki Ohkawa from Tokyo; Dr. Gian Carlo Pongione from Turin; and Dr. Stephen Chu, Dr. Mark Hochman, and Professor Dennis Tarnow from New York.

I would also like to thank the following clinicians for contributing to making this book possible by kindly offering their clinical documentation: Dr. R. Amid, Dr. L. Sawdayee, and Mr. R. Lahav from Tel Aviv; Dr. S. Rocha Bernardes from Curitiba; Dr. L. Canullo from Rome; Dr. F. Chiche from Paris; Dr. M. Del Corso from Turin; Dr. M. Groisman from Rio de Janeiro; Dr. J. Kan from Loma Linda; Dr. C. Lepage from Paris; Dr. P. Margossian from Marseille; Dr. K.B. Park from Seoul; Dr. A. Peivandi from Lyon; Dr. A. Pinto from Paris; Dr. J.L. Pruvost from Paris; Dr. P. Schupbach from Zurich; Dr. M. Suzuki and Dr. M. Yamazaki from Tokyo; Dr. T. Kim, Dr. D. Cascione, and Dr. A. Knezevic from Los Angeles; Dr. T. Testori from Como; Dr. G. Tirlet from Paris; and Dr. H. Zipprich from Frankfurt.

I offer all my thanks to my dedicated secretaries: Justin Ordoyo, Laura Parkin Osman, Nicole Laitano and Rivka Benloulo, and to Eric Quach for his ideas for the cover of the book.

My final words of gratitude go to my family: my wife, Monique, and my daughters Karine and Catherine, for their patience and support during this long process of creative and challenging work; and to my grandchildren Noa, Emma, Olivia, and Alexandre.

I will always have the greatest appreciation and respect for my beloved parents, who gave me the thirst for knowledge and the passion to share it.

1

Introduction

Each one of us has a different response to beauty, to esthetics, and to art. The accepted standard of "beauty" in individuals in any society today is subject to an incredible amount of influence, and to their ethnic, racial, and environmental surroundings. It is necessary to maintain a healthy balance between perfect appearance and a philosophy of life that includes physical and psychological factors (Gürel, 2008a).

These concepts evoke an emotional response that varies on a personal level, affecting us through the filter of our civilization, our society, our own experience, and our individual lives (Touati, 2008).

A recent study shows that two patients out of three declare that they have an esthetic need. It also shows that this demand is greater amongst women than amongst men, and that all socioeconomic strata, even the poorest, are represented (Zlowodzki *et al.*, 2008).

Beauty varies with the criteria of time and fashion. Today's facial beauty is based more on "make-up" than on natural beauty. However, in our generation, among the facial criteria of beauty, a perfect smile has become a major feature and offers many advantages for the person wearing the smile. The mouth is responsible for 60–70% of the visual perception of the face (Fig. 1.1).

A harmonious smile does not just come from beautiful lips. It cannot be conceived without a perfectly healthy gingival frame and well-aligned, healthy, natural teeth. Since the smile is a vital component of a beautiful face and there is a high patient demand for beauty, demands for smile enhancement with cosmetic restorations (Figs 1.2a–c), periodontal surgery (Figs 1.3a–c), or implant restorations (Figs 1.4a, b) continue to increase. This is why it is more correct to speak today about plastic peri-implant surgery, rather than just peri-implant surgery.

Cosmetics can give an impression of beauty, but it is a fleeting one. However, the creation of a beautiful smile, which cannot be washed off at the end of the day, is a more permanent proposition. The fundamental criteria of dentogingival esthetics are perfectly established and must be a part of the esthetic culture of every clinician. Clinicians in dentistry must, therefore, engage in more than just guesswork. They must adopt a scientific approach when analyzing dentogingival esthetic criteria, to

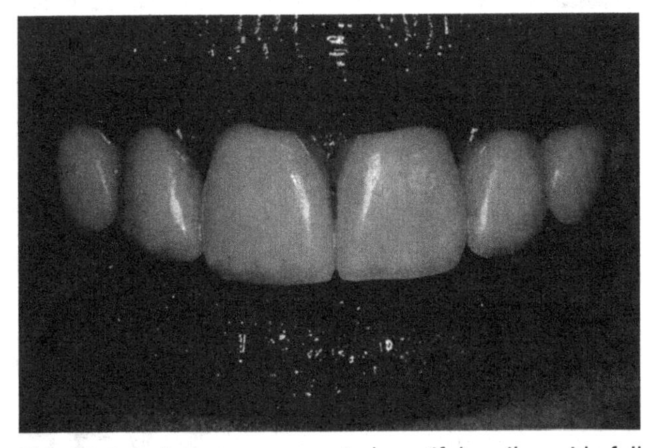

Figure 1.1 A young woman's beautiful smile, with full lips, well-aligned teeth, and a harmonious gingival contour.

Esthetic Soft Tissue Management of Teeth and Implants, First Edition. André P. Saadoun.

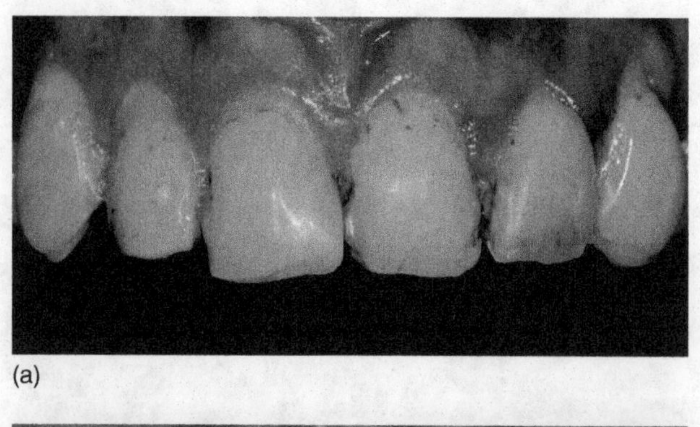
(a)

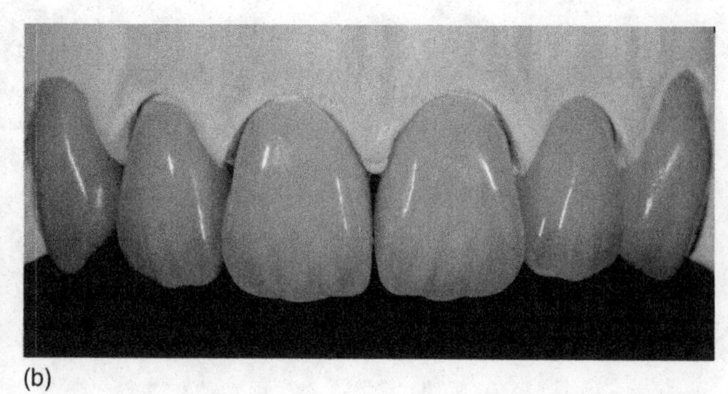
(b)

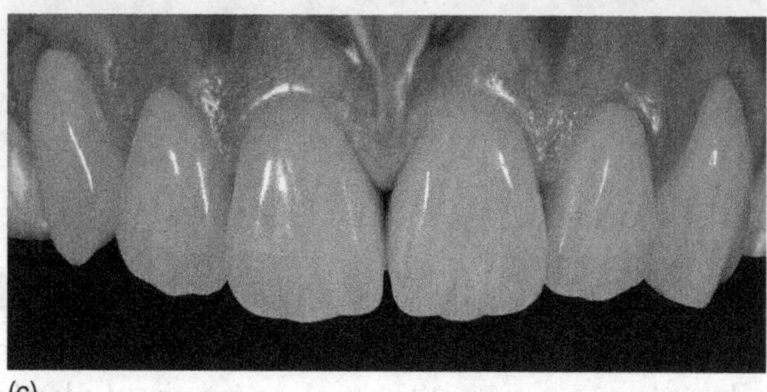
(c)

Figure 1.2 (a) Unpleasant-looking teeth with multiple decays and incisal edge abrasion. (b) A detailed view of four of the laminate veneers on the cast. (c) The laminate veneers 3 months later, with an optimal esthetic result. (Courtesy of Dr. G.C. Pongione, Rome, Italy.)

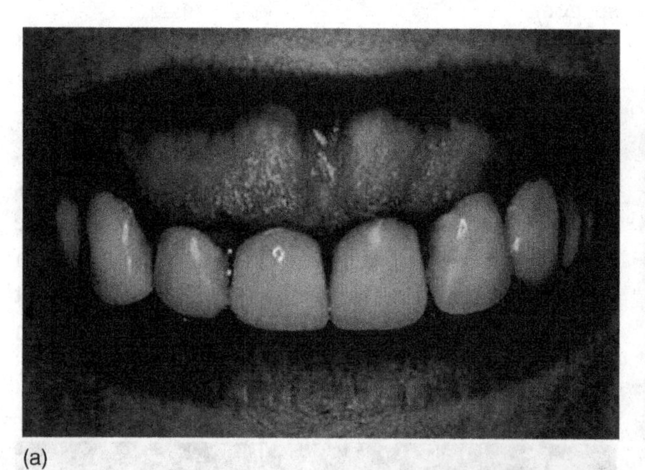
(a)

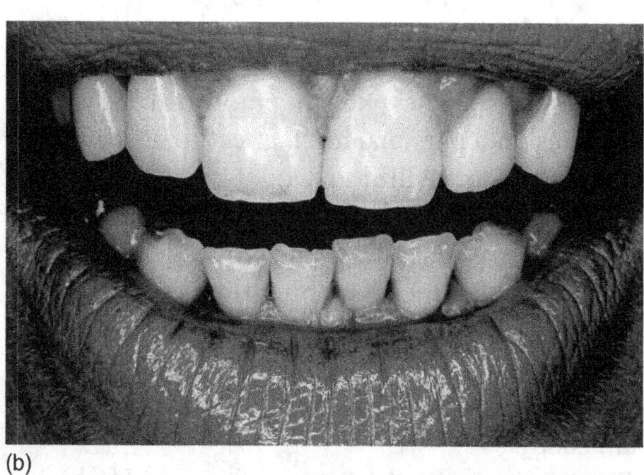
(b)

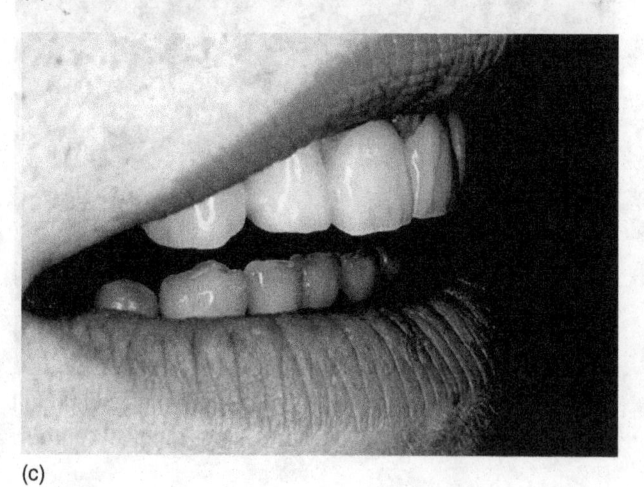
(c)

Figure 1.3 (a) The gingival smile and high lip line of a 35-year-old woman before periodontal surgery. (b) The patient's new smile, with a change in the size of the teeth after crown lengthening procedure, an elegant contour of the lips, and a limited amount of exposed gingiva. (c) A side view of the patient's new smile after full mouth periodontal surgery and prosthetic rehabilitation, with a change to the upper lip line. (Courtesy of Dr. P. Pissis, Paris, France.)

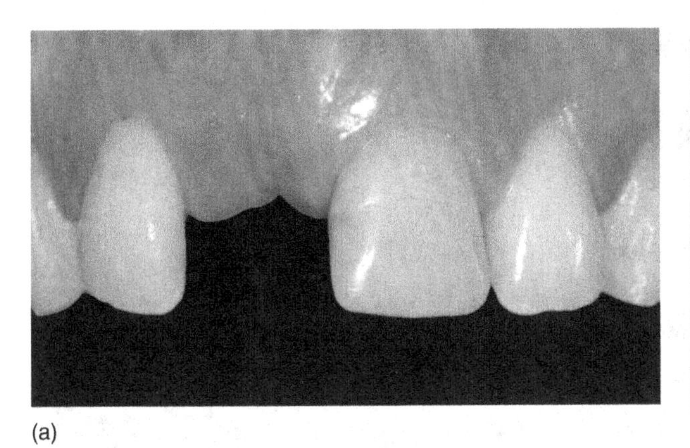

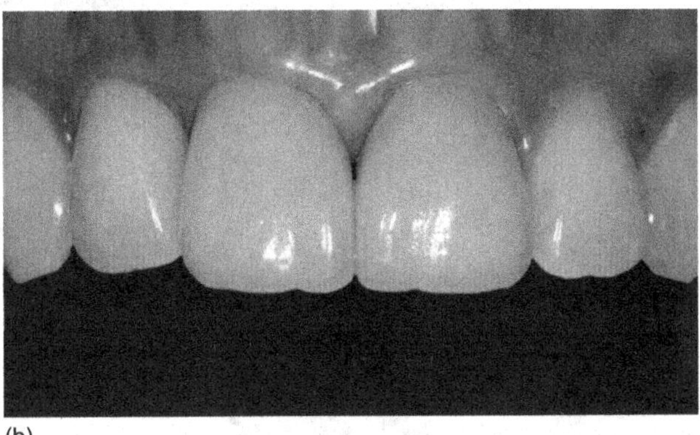

(a) (b)

Figure 1.4 (a) A woman's smile with a missing right central incisor, which was extracted 3 months ago. (b) Esthetic result after the placement of a right central implant restoration and a left incisor laminate veneer. (Courtesy of Dr. A. Pinto, Paris, France.)

establish the main alterations that are needed to their patients' smiles before proposing orthodontic, surgical, and/or restorative solutions.

The purpose of modern dentistry is to achieve the best possible result with minimal tissue invasion, thus giving the patient a beautiful smile, with a long-term, predictable result and without prejudicing the integrity of the structure of the remaining teeth. When a smile needs to be redesigned, the clinician should have the competence to evaluate and integrate this smile into the harmony of the face.

Although beauty may be the patient's only goal, and certainly the desired outcome of treatment, the objectives of orthodontics, operative dentistry, periodontal therapy, and restorative dental-implant therapy are more complex. Esthetic orthodontics has recently benefited from far more discreet appliances, such as ceramic brackets, but also by using a mini-implant or a normal implant to move teeth in an ideal relation. Esthetic restorative dentistry, which is benefiting from continual progress in the area of bonding agents, composite materials, and ceramic materials, can now provide very natural direct and indirect restorations to the anterior and posterior teeth – restorations which are indistinguishable from the natural dentition.

Periodontal therapy is leaning more and more toward tissue improvement methods, with the use of osseous, connective tissue grafts and tissue engineering, but is concerned, first and foremost, with maintaining the health of periodontal structures and correcting any gingival disharmony to achieve a balanced and esthetic gingival contour.

Implantology has revolutionized therapeutic options for every type of edentation, from a single tooth to the replacement of several teeth, and proposes increasingly esthetic solutions not only seeking to achieve good osseointegration, which is very important from a functional point of view, but also to preserve or reconstruct the harmonious peri-implant gingival morphology around the restoration, which is necessary from an esthetic point of view.

With regard to the long-term outcome of implant therapy, osseointegration is no longer the principal concern. The soft tissues and emergence profiles, the shape and shade of the restoration, must now also mirror the adjacent teeth as closely as possible. The stability of the results over time should be without question.

Nowadays, esthetic demands may take precedence over functional outcomes. Demands for "perfection" are constantly on the rise, and the standards to be achieved are getting higher and higher. In most cases, perfect results require extensive intervention, and the durability of such perfection may be unpredictable. To consistently achieve superior clinical esthetic outcomes in a significant number of cases, biology teaches us the painful lesson that patience is a virtue.

The pursuit of perfection requires a commitment on the part of the patient to surgical and prosthetic intervention that is often difficult to predict prior to initiation of care. It would be surprising to think that patients who had attended large numbers of clinical appointments to achieve excellent results had routinely understood, prior to the initiation

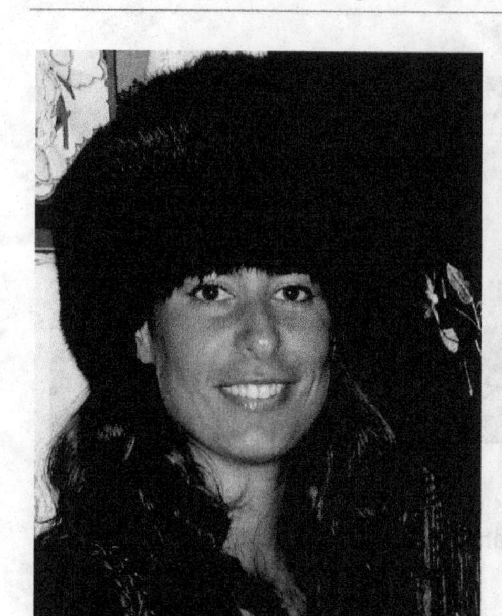
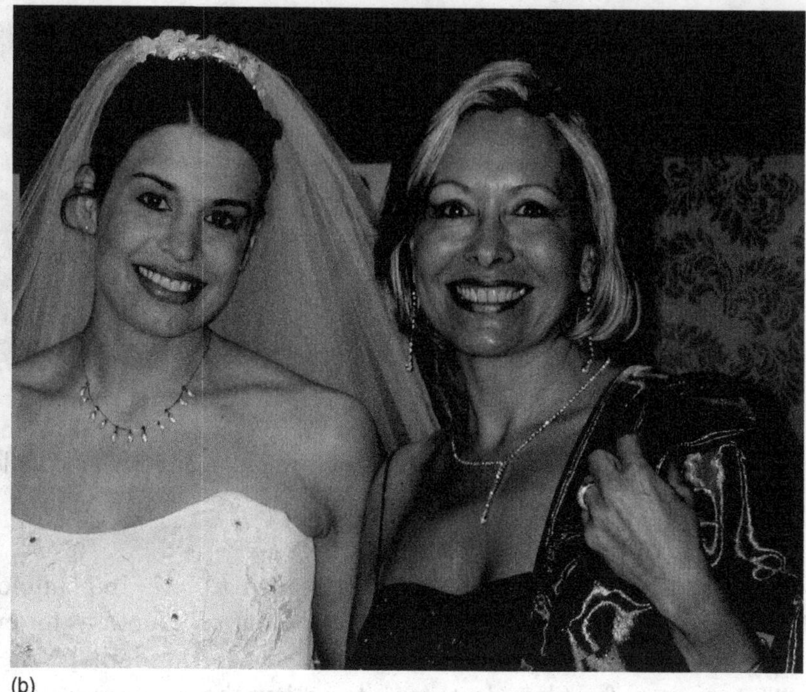

(a) (b)

Figure 1.5 (a) The smile of a 25-year-old woman. (b) The joyful smiles of a bride and her mother. (© A. Saadoun.)

of treatment, that this was what was going to be required (Eckert, 2008).

Staging certain cases and watching them develop gives time to evaluate each phase before the next step is carried forward. This in turn gives time for the body's tissues to mature, harmonize, and stabilize. While waiting for maturation of grafted tissues, good provisional restorations can often satisfy the patient during that interim period. This allows the clinician to finish the case not as quickly as possible, but as quickly as nature allows, in order to achieve the most desirable result. As clinicians, it is our duty to appreciate that each case must be approached on its own merits and that we must cater for treatment to each patient individually (Sethi, 2008).

Esthetic dentistry has the ability to change a person's life. Nowadays, a seductive smile is a precious anatomical aid to success in society. The smile is one of the most important means of communication between people. A joyful expression reveals your soul, and sometimes joy is the source of your smile, but your smile can also be the source of your joy. The esthetics and beauty of the smile are not only determined by the lips and the shape, position, and color of the teeth, but also by their existing relations with the gingiva and the overall harmony of the face (Figs 1.5a, b).

The harmony of the smile depends on esthetic criteria based on respect for the horizontal, vertical, and sagittal references. There are hundreds of languages in the world, but a smile speaks them all. According to a Chinese proverb, while laughing is selfish, the smile is a gift to others that costs nothing. A truly beautiful smile is one that lasts.

2

To smile or not to smile

The mouth acts as a mirror for the body. The link between substances in the oral cavity and other vital organs has been well documented worldwide, and oral care can have significant effects on all parts of the body (Ravins, 2008).

The perception of beauty is subject to continual change. With today's conceptual thinking and treatment planning, it is essential to incorporate an interdisciplinary approach that may include orthodontics, periodontics, operative dentistry, implant dentistry, and restorative dentistry (Gürel, 2008a).

Patients today are educated and just as concerned with feeling well as they are with looking well. Facial appeal (the attraction that a face can provoke) has an impact on health, which is defined by the World Health Organization (2006) as "a state of complete mental, physical, and social well-being and not only constituting the absence of disease or infirmity."

Esthetically oriented treatment has a significant and proven impact on the psychological balance of our patients and thus on their health (Decharrière-Hamzawi *et al.*, 2007). This esthetic demand is satisfied in various ways, with very different expectations from one patient to another, notably when talking about changes that a patient desires in the lower part of the face. The fact that this esthetic demand, across all socioeconomic strata, is greater amongst women than amongst men has been shown to be statistically significant. However, one does not have to respond to the esthetic demands of every patient, particularly if his or her wants are obviously unreasonable – or even pathological, as in the case of those with body dysmorphia (Zlowodzki *et al.*, 2008).

The clinician must adopt a scientific approach to the creation of the perfect result, employing a methodical and/or experimental strategy. This is the only way to ensure a predictable, acceptable end product.

The impact of esthetics

Our contemporary society emphasizes the importance of appearance and attaches a notion of success and well-being to beauty. Esthetics indeed plays a significant role in the psychosocial aspects that determine the nature of an individual's existence. Self-esteem remains one of the main indicators of a person's well-being (Decharrière-Hamzawi *et al.*, 2005). The medical profession must not view esthetic demands with disdain, because all imbalances in self-esteem will cause a change in health, as defined by the World Health Organization (Patzer and Faucher, 1996; Decharrière-Hamzawi *et al.*, 2007).

The impact of esthetics on behavior from infancy to adulthood (Figs 2.1a–d) has been confirmed in several publications (Savard *et al.*, 2007):

- Young babies stare at attractive faces longer than at others. As early as the infant stage, one notices a more sustained attraction to pretty faces (Bruchon-Schweitzer, 1990).
- Teachers show a preference for children who are pleasant to watch.

Esthetic Soft Tissue Management of Teeth and Implants, First Edition. André P. Saadoun.

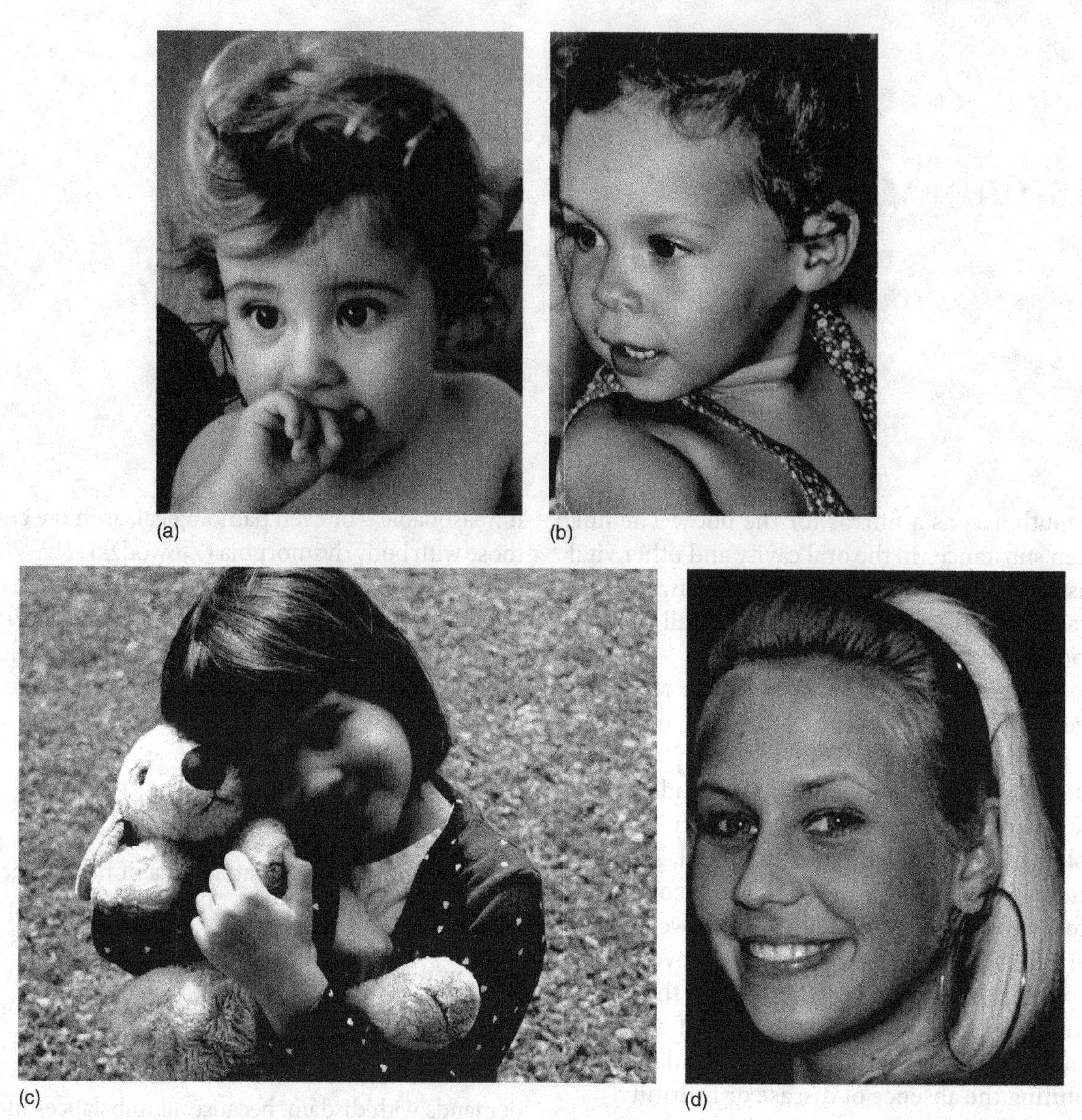

Figure 2.1 (a) A 10-month-old baby girl teething, with her fingers on her erupting teeth. (b) The smile of a 3-year-old child, with only the lower teeth showing. (c) The smile of a 4-year-old child, with the lips and some upper teeth showing. (d) An adolescent's full smile, with beautiful lips, teeth and gingiva. (© A. Saadoun.)

- Given equal ability, pupils seen as attractive earn better grades.
- The more attractive a child is, the more he or she will provoke expectations from the teacher; hence the child will benefit from a more favorable learning environment (Decharrière-Hamzawi *et al.*, 2005).
- For a good homework assignment, a bonus of 5% has been observed with respect to the average result if the appearance of a set photograph is attractive, and a decrease of 7% if it is unattractive.
- Academic failure is observed to be aggravated when a student's physical appearance is seen as unattractive by his or her peers.
- There is a link between the productivity of a business and the physical beauty of its employees.
- It seems that our brains are more attracted to people who are seen as beautiful, either in that we expect a reward or that this beauty in itself constitutes a reward (Kawabata and Zeki, 2004).
- Esthetics plays an important role in the psychosocial aspects that determine the nature of an individual's existence and the limits of that person's well-being and self-esteem.
- All imbalances in self-esteem will lead to a decrease in health, with possible repercussions at the biological level.

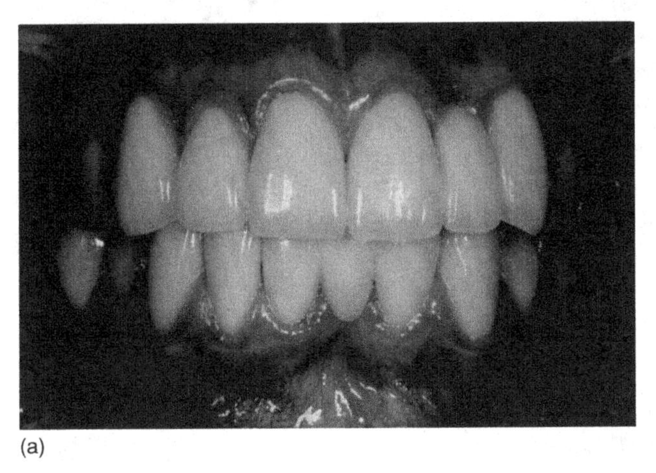

(a)

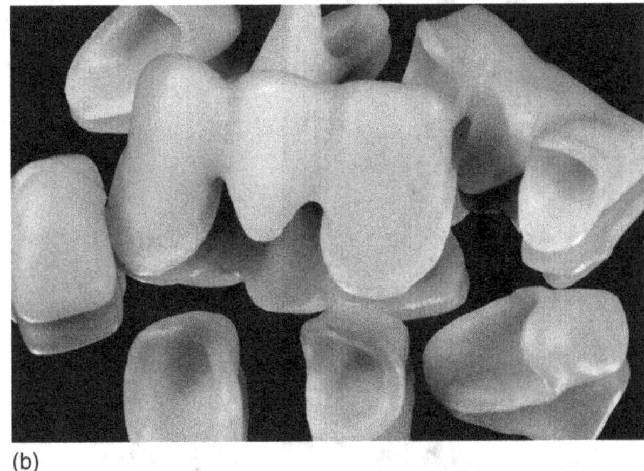

(b)

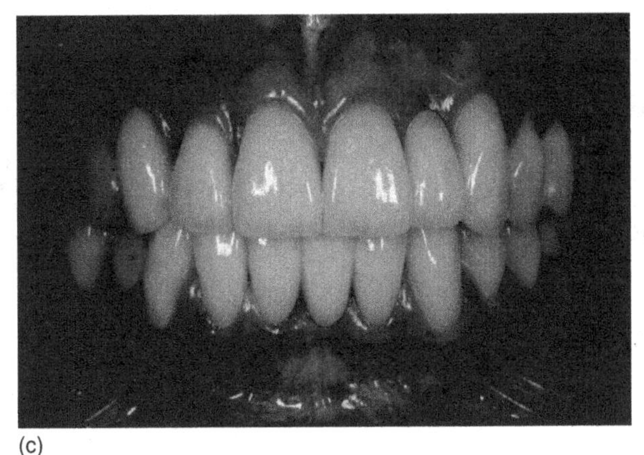

(c)

Figure 2.2 (a) An unnatural smile, with old full-mouth ceramic restoration. (b) NobelProcera™ shells of the different restorations (crowns and bridges). (c) Full-mouth restoration with ceramic, giving the patient a new smile. (Courtesy of Dr. M. Okawa, Tokyo, Japan.)

Dental esthetics

Only one out of two adults is satisfied with his or her smile, so when people say, "I need a beautiful smile," they really mean "I want a beautiful smile," and they deserve to look and feel good about themselves. Consequently, turning people's smiles into their best feature improves their perception of self-worth in life (Mechanic, 2008).

For the majority of patients, a desired change or improvement to their faces is related to their teeth; missing teeth and the whiteness of the teeth are these patients' main concerns (Figs 2.2a–c).

The majority of people seeking a consultation for esthetic dental reasons do so for social and psychological reasons:

- Changing the smile, and the lower third of the face, has a positive effect on facial features and on self-esteem (Figs 2.3a–e).
- The improvement of physical features through specialized esthetic dental therapy has a positive effect on social relations (Patzer, 1997).

Dentists, laboratory technicians, and patients have differing perceptions of what makes a smile esthetically pleasing, and their diverging opinions confirm the importance of good communication in producing a successful course of treatment. By including esthetics-specific treatments in the context of a complete treatment plan, practitioners show that they are thorough professionals, who are contributing to the improvement of the mental and social well-being, and thus the health, of their patients.

It is important to highlight the fact that such progress in dentistry could not have been made if esthetic results had not become so important to our patients as well as to our colleagues.

The desire to create more esthetically pleasing smiles was surely one of the driving forces which pushed researchers, manufacturers, clinicians, and patients to refine their criteria for what constitutes a clinical success (Miara and Touati, 2011).

The smile-related quality of life

Today, not only is there a considerable demand for esthetic dental work across all socioeconomic strata,

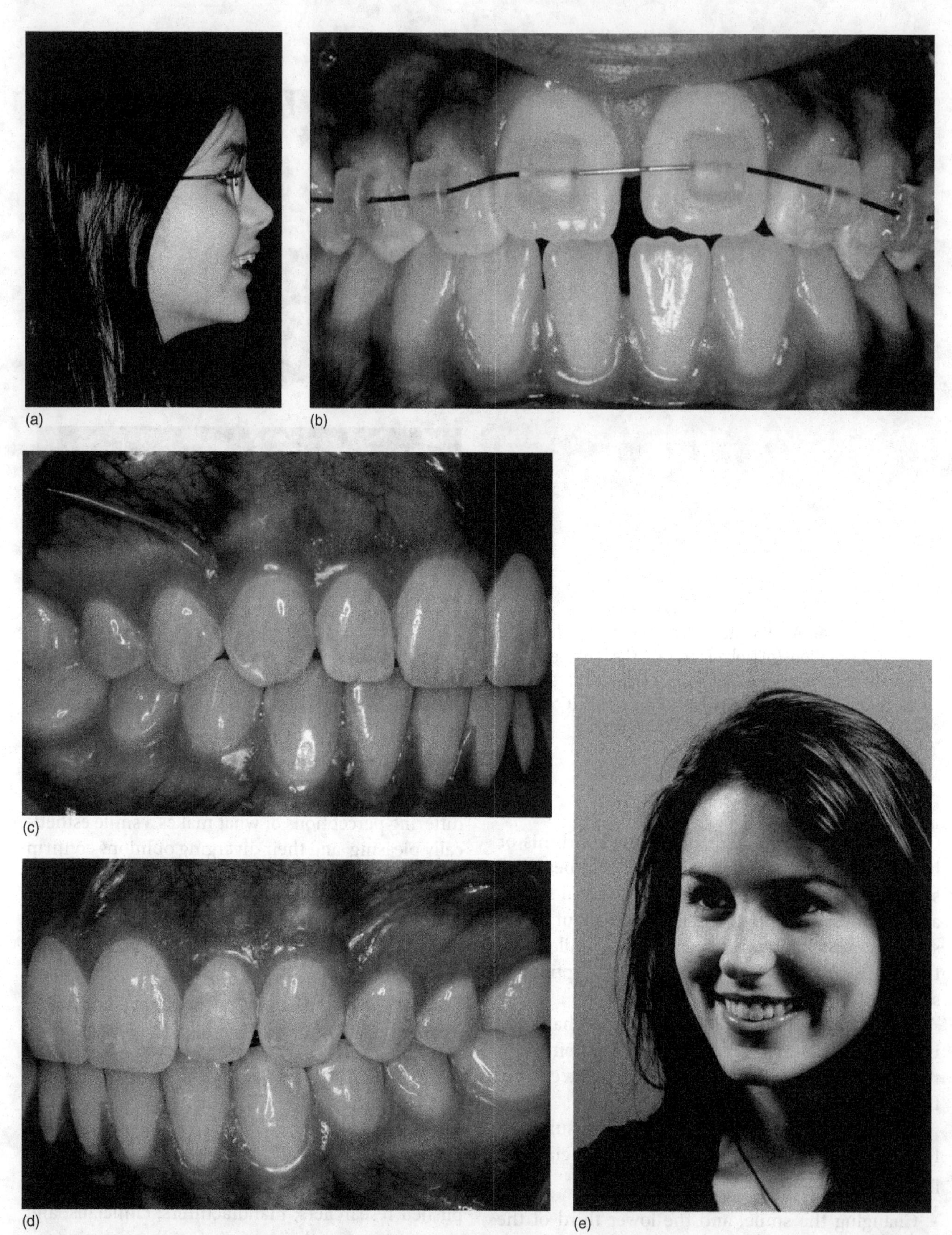

Figure 2.3 (a) The unpleasant right-side profile of a 10-year-old girl, with a short upper lip and a wide overjet. (b) A facial view showing the Class II, division I disharmonious smile, with diastema and overjet affecting the central incisors, at an early stage of orthodontic treatment. (c) The final stage of the esthetic therapy, with the teeth in a perfect occlusal relation on the right side. (d) A beautiful relationship between the teeth and the gingiva, with an excellent white esthetic score (WES) and pink esthetic score (PES) (see Chapter 4), and a perfect occlusal relation on the left side. (e) The same patient's new profile 8 years later, with a harmonious jaw relation, a symmetrical smile, and a delightful change of attitude. (Courtesy of Dr. J.L. Pruvost, Paris, France.)

but he importance of dentofacial appearance for psychosocial well-being is now widely appreciated (Neumann *et al.*, 1989). There is a correlation between having a naturally beautiful smile (Fig. 2.4a), esthetic dentistry and quality of life (Davis *et al.*, 1998; Newton *et al.*, 2004), and the notion of well-being (Singh *et al.*, 2005). Improving a smile changes the perceptions of others and contributes to improving self-esteem (Decharrière-Hamzawi *et al.*, 2007). This is proven at all stages in life.

In a study by Patel *et al.* (2008), the smile-related quality of life was found to correlate significantly with indicators of the periodontal health of the subjects, such as the number of mobile teeth, missing teeth, and gingival recession (Figs 2.4b, c) in the esthetic zone.

Periodontal health and smiling patterns were likewise correlated:

- The more teeth with probing depths between 4 and 6 mm that the subjects had, the less widely they opened their mouths when they smiled; the more hypermobile teeth they had, the less open their smiles were, and the more they were covering their mouths when they smiled.
- In the esthetic zone, the more sites of gingival recession that the subjects had, the fewer teeth they showed when they smiled.
- The periodontal health of the subjects affected their smiling patterns and their quality of life.
- Poor periodontal health (longer teeth, a gingival appearance, and bad breath) might prevent adults from expressing positive emotions which, in turn, could impact their self-image as well as their social interactions.
- This might be improved through the treatment of periodontitis and effective oral hygiene maintenance.

In the anterior esthetic zone, the replacement of missing teeth with implants significantly improves the quality of life related to oral health, especially amongst women (Ponsi *et al.*, 2011). Therefore, periodontal health, quality of life, and smiling patterns are all positively related.

Nowadays, the lower third of the face is vitally important in facial beauty:

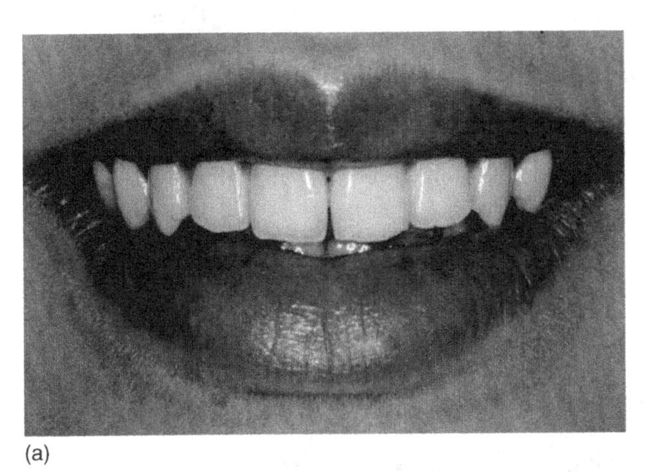
(a)

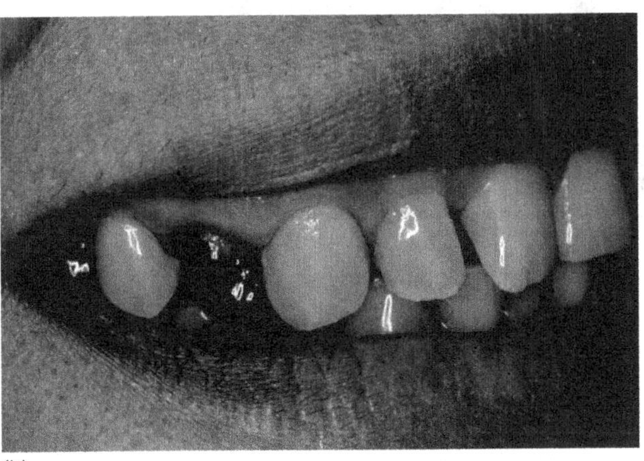
(b)

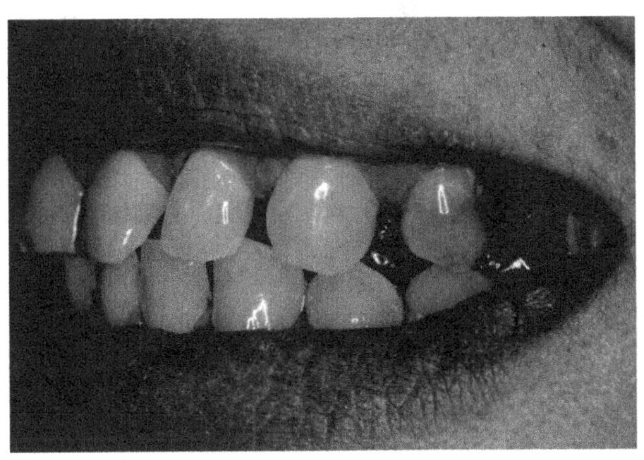
(c)

Figure 2.4 (a) A 24-year-old woman who is proud of her beautiful smile. (b) A 28-year-old woman who is reluctant to smile because of her broken teeth. (c) The patient has short teeth with diastema and bleeding gums; there are missing teeth and old amalgam restorations, and she is not wearing lipstick.

- Treatments that involve esthetic improvement of the lower third of the face seem to have positive effects on self-esteem and a more optimistic perception of life.
- Improving physical features through facial changes and, more specifically, the smile also leads to improvements in self-esteem and a change toward a more open personality (Figs 2.4d–g).

In a study by Al-Omiri *et al.* (2011), implant-supported prostheses were found to have a positive impact on participants' daily living and satisfaction with their dentition. Personality traits such as neuroticism, openness, agreeableness, and self-awareness affect patients' daily living and level of personal satisfaction.

The senior citizen's smile

Aging is accompanied by a certain number of physiological and pathological changes (Figs 2.5a, b), and even alterations that are seen as unsightly: the degeneration of the periodontium, which gives the impression of long teeth, induces teeth displacements and causes diastema, modification of the shape and length of the teeth due to wear and abrasion, disruption of tooth alignment, and a decline in lip support. With age, the maxillary teeth become less visible and the mandibular

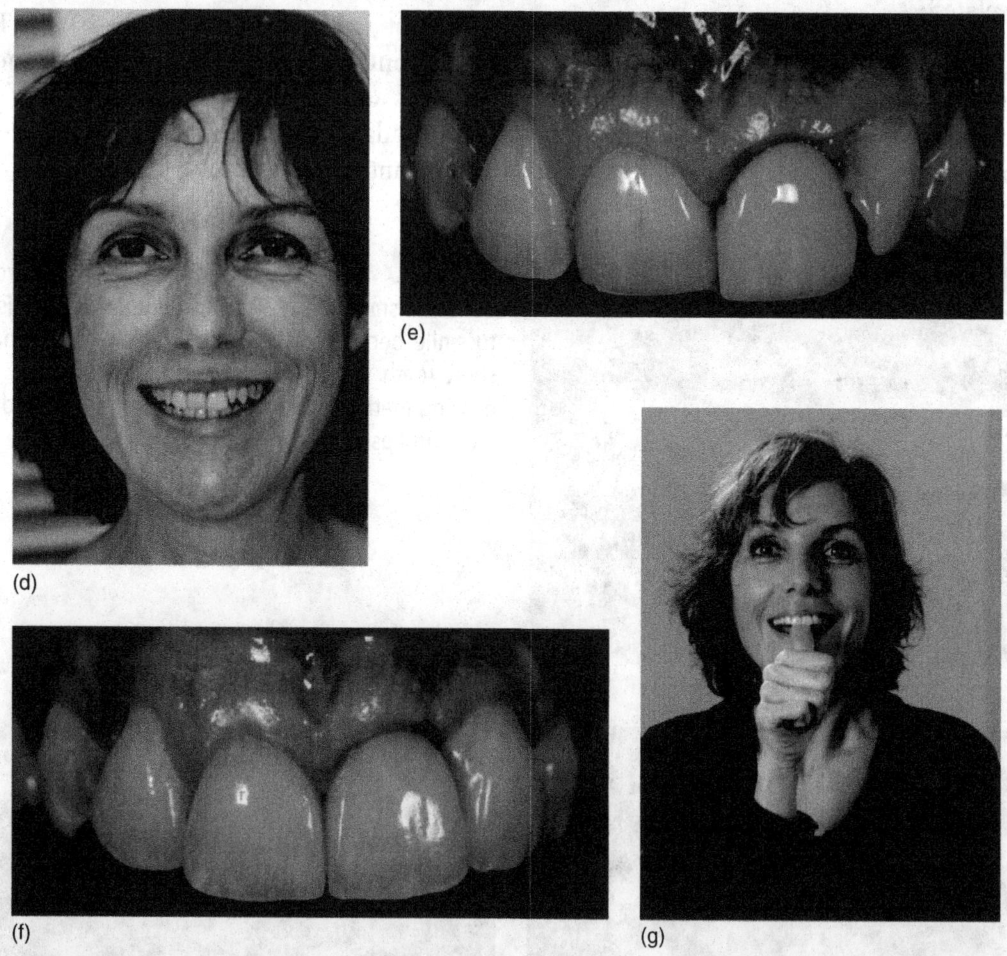

Figure 2.4 (d) The patient's depressed face at the initial consultation. (e) An old, nonfitting ceramometal restoration on the left central incisor, with gingival discoloration and a disharmonious contour. (f) A connective tissue graft (CTG) is put in place and a new ceramic restoration is undertaken after tissue maturation. (g) The blossoming face and more pleasant attitude of the patient with her new smile. (Courtesy of Dr. S. Koubi, Marseille, France.)

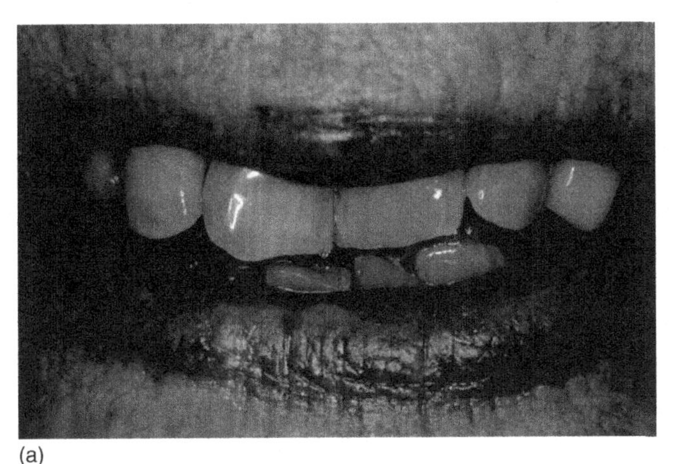
(a)

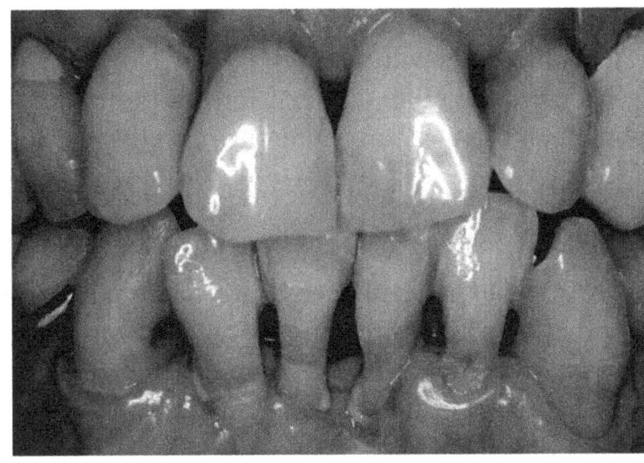
(b)

Figure 2.5 (a) A 75-year-old woman's suppressed smile. (b) She has generalized gingival recession, a disharmonious gingival contour, irregular incisal edges, diastema, long teeth, and a removable partial denture.

teeth more visible. Senior citizens are often motivated to attempt to look younger (Rignon-Bret *et al.*, 2007).

The importance of appearance and physical features for senior citizens has evolved dramatically in the past 10 years. The number and proportion of senior citizens in the population is increasing, and becoming more and more significant as the human life span in general continues to increase by 3 months every year. Nowadays, senior citizens are much more active, and their desire to look young, and to display a youthful attitude toward life, continues to increase. This "young elderly" population represents a great challenge for the clinician – and for the peri-implantologist in particular, who must achieve both function and esthetics.

In a recent study (Rignon-Bret *et al.*, 2007):

- It turned out that subjects' satisfaction with their current smiles was not well correlated with their satisfaction with their former smiles. There was a tendency to depreciate the current smile in relation to the past one.
- Overall, one out of three senior citizens wanted to change the appearance of their smile or teeth.
- The main changes desired were dental alignment (46%), tooth shape (20%), and changes to the length of the teeth (11%).
- The desire to replace missing teeth, restore oral–facial muscular support (lips, cheeks), correct gingival disharmony (gummy smile or gingival recessions), or redo existing prostheses was noted.
- Almost half of the senior citizens wanted to have their teeth whitened (47%) or had already done it.
- It is noteworthy that 82% of those surveyed were aware of orthodontic treatments and dental implants, as well as ceramic crowns (mentioned in 76% of the responses).

Several indicators seem to show an increasing demand by senior citizens for dental treatment to enhance the esthetics of the smile (Goldstein and Niessen, 1988):

- An expressed interest in esthetic treatment.
- Requests for maintenance: improvements to general appearance and to the smile have become signs of successful aging. However, studies show that the appearance of the teeth is not as important for senior citizens as it is for young people (Vallitu *et al.*, 1996; Alkhatib *et al.*, 2005).
- There is easier acceptance of treatment that enhances a person's self-image and social relations, rather than treatment that simply improves function.

- The focus of attention on the whiteness of the teeth increases with age.
- Priorities are more oriented toward tooth alignment and shape than whitening of teeth.

The behavior of senior citizens in modern society is evolving:

- Their general health needs are growing, along with their esthetic demands.
- Their demand for buccal treatment in increasing with esthetic changes in their smile.
- They are increasingly aware that a flaw in their smile can have a negative effect on their self-image and self-esteem.

Despite the increase in esthetic awareness among senior citizens, the importance that they place on the appearance of the smile could decrease with age, because their highest priority is still to take care of their general well-being and to deal with more debilitating health problems.

3

The esthetics of the face

Successful smile enhancement must begin with a facial analysis "from the outside in." An esthetically pleasing smile depends on several parameters.

The face

The face has an important influence on the perception of the esthetic quality of the smile. Several psychological studies have tested the hypothesis that the assessment of attractiveness is sensitive to facial symmetry (Thornhill and Gangestad, 1999). There is a significant difference between attractiveness and symmetry, and these parameters are not strongly related in the faces of women or men. The natural subtle asymmetry might be relatively unimportant in judging facial attractiveness (Zaidel *et al.*, 2005). Totally symmetrical faces, at least when created photographically, at times appear alien or emotionally detached because of the reduction of natural subtle asymmetry, which perhaps makes such faces appear passive and inert. Left–right facial asymmetries are discernible in beautiful models (Fig 3.1a); therefore very beautiful faces can be functionally asymmetrical (Zaidel and Cohen, 2005).

The perception of symmetry in the smile cannot be dissociated from the sagittal median line of the whole face. Focusing only on the buccal region, the symmetry of the smile depends on the midline between the maxillary incisors. By rotating one of these incisors, a visual constraint is introduced which upsets the relative symmetry of the tooth display. The asymmetry that this creates breaks the repetitious monotony of geometrical forms. Asymmetry in the tooth display or in a smiling face is not necessarily perceived as esthetically displeasing. It must be imperceptible at first glance, however, or it will produce a visual tension as the eyes are drawn more to one side of the face than to the other (Zlowodzki *et al.*, 2008).

The health and appearance of the soft tissue around the teeth are essential components of a seductive smile (Liebart *et al.*, 2011) (Figs 3.1b–f). Thus, a gummy smile may be accompanied by facial disruptions in which the lower half of the face appears to be disproportionately long, causing imbalance (Rees and La Trenta, 1989). More complex anatomical disorders can sometimes be added to morphological disruptions: Class II malocclusion, a receding chin, nasal protrusion, dentoalveolar extrusion, and maxillary endognathic deformity that warrants orthognatic surgical therapy (Ezquerra *et al.*, 1999).

The lips

In modern-day society, offering a beautiful smile means showing fully designed lips, healthy, well-aligned dentition, and a harmonious gingival contour.

The anterior esthetic zone has been defined as the area encompassed by the perimeter of the lips. The smile is a dynamic position of the lips and it varies according to the degree of contraction of the muscles, and according to the lip profile. The size of the smile varies as a function of each individual situation (Liebart *et al.*, 2011).

Esthetic Soft Tissue Management of Teeth and Implants, First Edition. André P. Saadoun.

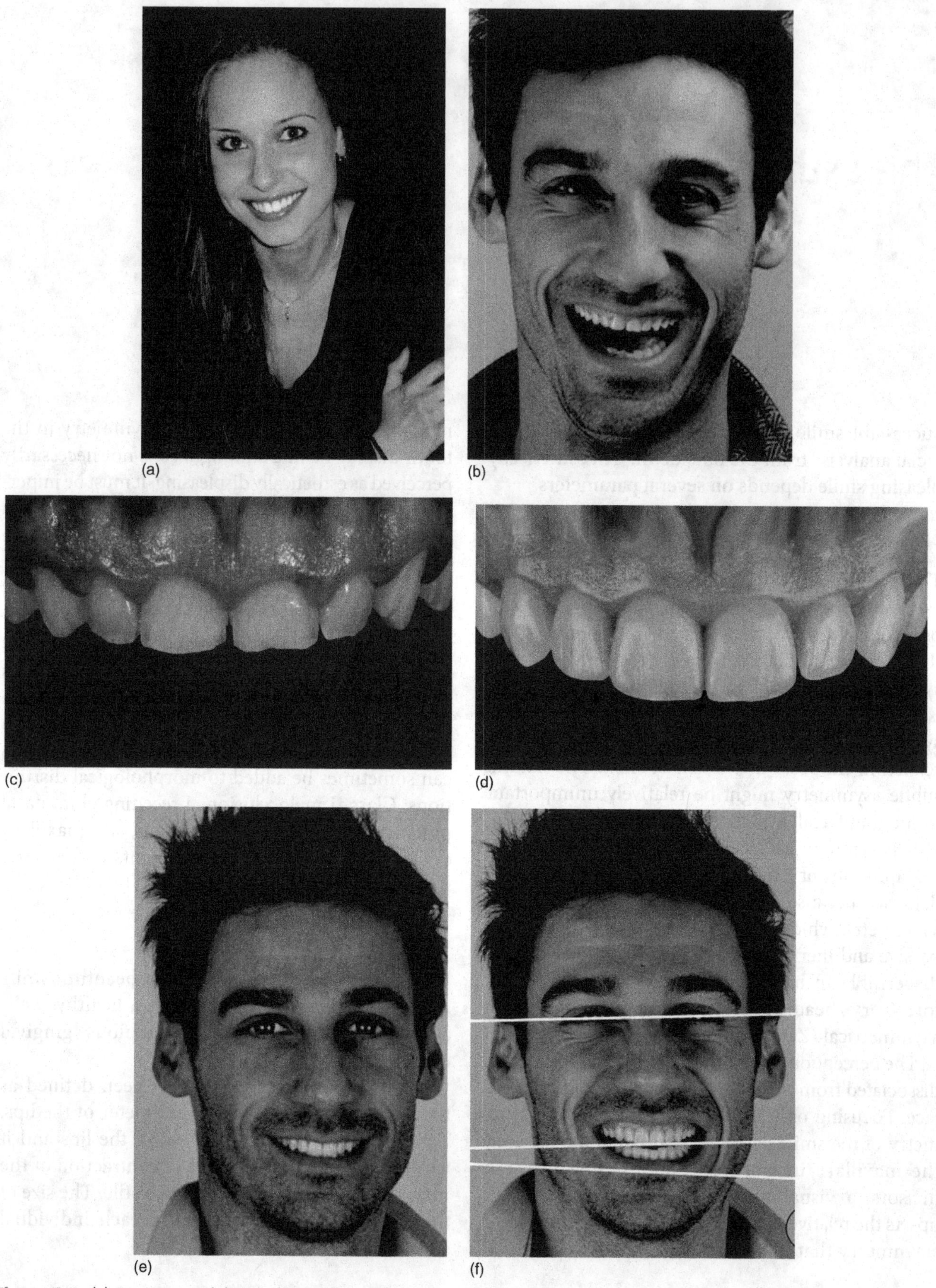

Figure 3.1 (a) A young model with a beautiful, seemingly symmetrical, face. (b) On a forced smile, the patient has an asymmetry of the lower lips, with worn maxillary and/or mandibular teeth. (c) The maxillary teeth present significant abrasion of the incisal edge because of bruxomania. (d) Laminate veneers a few weeks after cementation, with a harmonious tooth and gingival contour. (e) The new and improved smile creates a more positive attitude in the patient. (f) On an exaggerated smile, a lower left lip asymmetry still exists, as initially. (Figures (b) to (f) courtesy of Dr. S. Koubi, Marseille, France.)

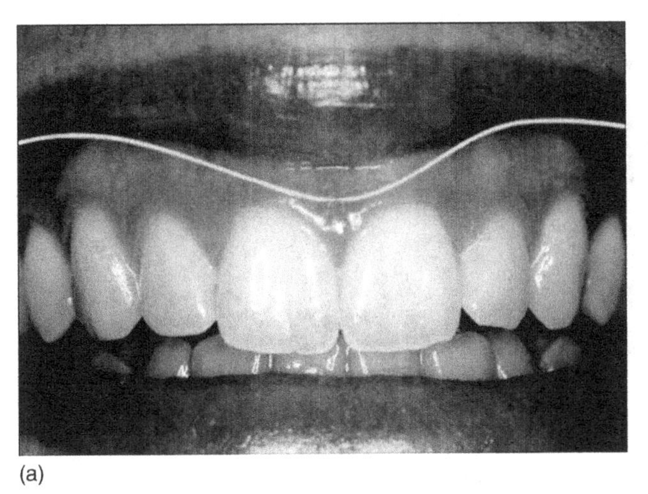
(a)

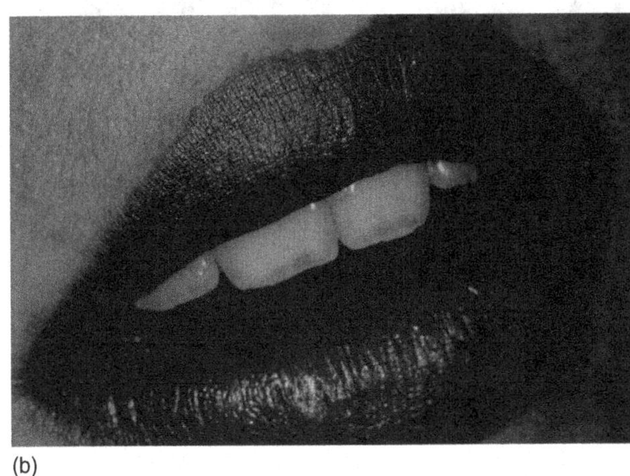
(b)

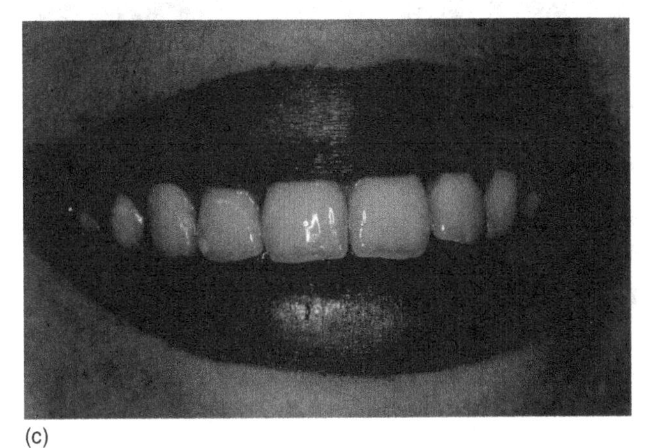
(c)

Figure 3.2 (a) In this photograph, the added line represents the imaginary upper lip line. (b) Lips during speech, showing the incisal third of the anterior maxillary teeth. (c) A forced smile, showing the gingiva on the lateral posterior areas.

The upper smile lip line, or smile line, is defined as the position of the upper lip, and the lower smile line is defined as the position of the lower lip in relation to the maxillary teeth. The anterior gingival display should follow the shape of the upper smile lip line (Fig. 3.2a).

There are different dynamic stages of smiling: the natural smile, the spontaneous smile, and the exaggerated or forced smile (Figs 3.2b, c). When smiling naturally, 40% of patients do not show their gingiva, whereas only 11% do not show gingiva when exaggerating a smile. When forcing a smile, after a spontaneous smile, 89% of patients show their marginal gingiva, depending on age, gender, and ethnicity (Barbant *et al.*, 2011b).

The relationship between the three components involved in the smile – the lips, the teeth, and the gingiva plus the alveolar bone – determines whether a particular smile has a high, medium, or low lip line (Tjan *et al.*, 1984).

The smile lip line

The smile line determines the amount of visible teeth and gingiva. It is an imaginary line on the lower edge of the upper lip, along the maxillary teeth, while smiling. The position of the smile line varies as a function of sex, age, length, the joy of expression, and the curvature of the lips (Desai *et al.*, 2009). It could also be defined as being the position of the fixed tissues (teeth or gums) in relation to the mobile tissues (the lips, and specifically the upper lip):

1. A high lip line in 10% of patients, which shows the full length of the maxillary anterior teeth and less than 2 mm of gingiva. The "high lip line smile" (Fig. 3.2d) may induce the "gummy smile": all dental surfaces are visible, as well as an excess of gingiva, which is more visible from the side than from the front. It is generally considered that a gingival smile reveals 3–6 mm of gingival tissue. Many patients with a gingival

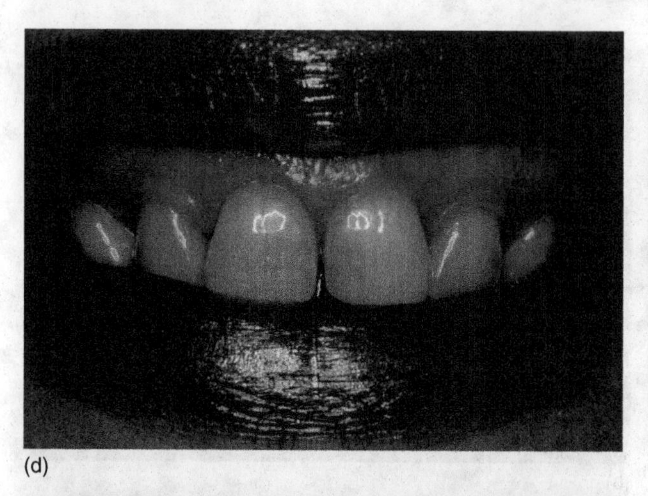
(d)

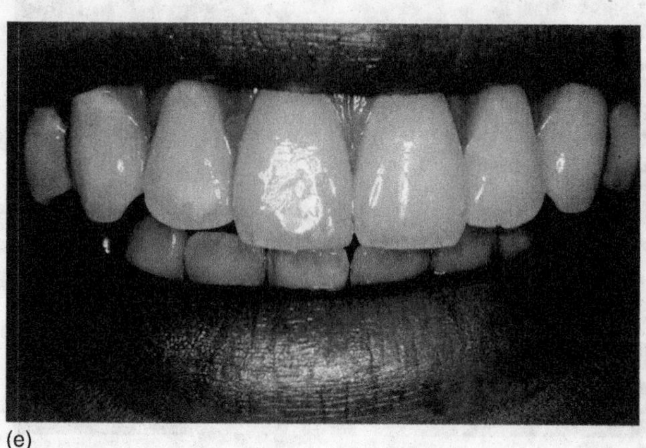
(e)

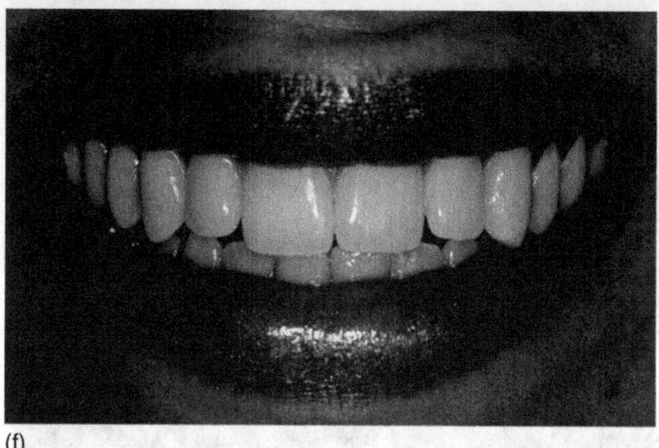
(f)

Figure 3.2 (d) A high lip line, with more than 3 mm of gingival display. (e) A medium lip line smile, showing the gingival margin and full papillae. (f) A low lip line smile, with no gingival display and only the tip of the papillae.

smile also exhibit an asymmetrical level of gingiva, which is revealed when smiling (Lowe, 2009). This situation tends to improve with age, and is observed in 10% of individuals (14% for females, 7% for males). This happens twice as often with women, to such an extent that people associate such a smile with a feminized character. Even if it does not always constitute a real esthetic criterion, it still remains the sign of a certain expression of youth. An estimated exposition of 2–3 mm is not considered as a gummy smile.

2. A medium lip line in 70% of patients, which shows 75–100% of the maxillary anterior teeth and only the interproximal papillae. The medium lip line smile (Fig. 3.2e), or ideal situation, allows all the maxillary dental surfaces to appear, as well as the interdental papillae, with up to 1 mm of exposed gingiva above the enamel crown. This gingival display, of 1 mm, is considered the most esthetic smile. According to Paris and Faucher (2003), this category represents 70% of the population (74% for females, 63% for males).
3. A low lip line in 20% of patients, which shows 25% of the maxillary anterior teeth. This interdependent relation also determines whether or not the smile is attractive, and how critical it is to undertake restoration (Garber and Salama, 1996). The low lip line smile (Fig. 3.2f), with no gingival display, could be esthetically acceptable. It is the consequence of a vertical maxillary deficiency, a long upper lip, and a hypotonic lip muscle associated with elderly patients, sometimes related to worn dentures, in which only a reduced part of the maxillary teeth are visible when smiling, the gums being totally hidden. This situation contributes to an aging appearance, sometimes prematurely, in around 20% of patients (12% for females, 30% for males), and this percentage will increase with aging.

The most harmonious smile is the one where all the buccal surfaces of the incisors are visible without excessive exposition of the gingiva or significant covering of the maxillary incisors by the lower lip (Rufenacht, 1990).

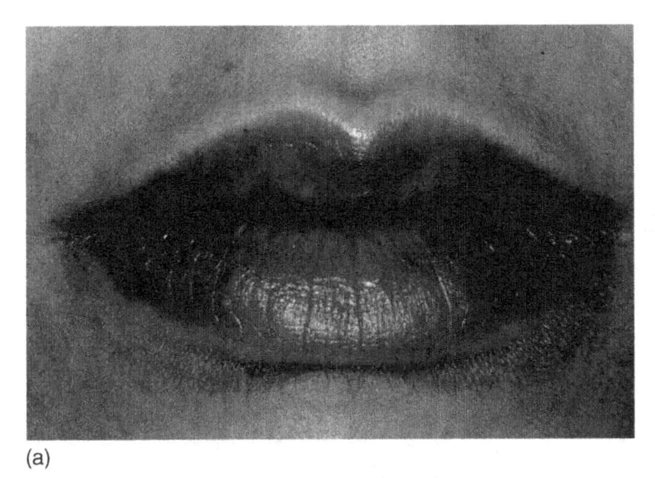
(a)

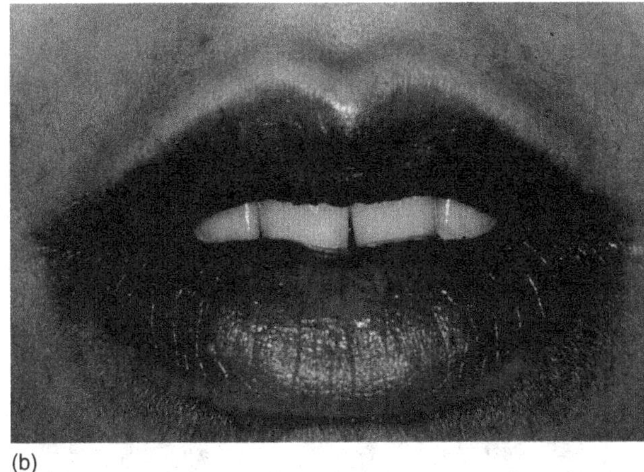
(b)

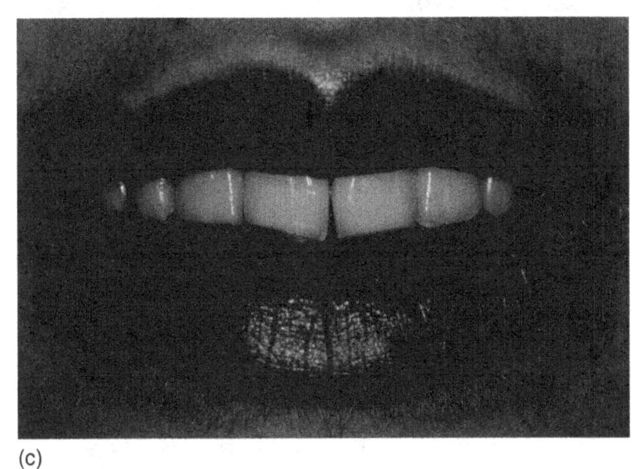
(c)

Figure 3.3 (a) Relaxed lips on a closed mouth. (b) The lip aspect while speaking. (c) The lip position for a slight smile.

The upper lip

The normal height of the upper lip, as measured between the nasal point and the lower edge of the lip, varies from 20 to 25 mm and is normally shorter in women than in men (Ezquerra *et al.*, 1999).

In the case of a gummy smile, a shortened lip (often distinctly below 20 mm and generally mobile) may be a major influence on its appearance (Paris and Faucher, 2003).

The position of the upper lip line could vary depending on the following factors:

- function – resting, speaking, or smiling (Figs 3.3a–c)
- support – dentition and edentation
- shape – thin or voluminous
- level – high, medium, or low.

The support for the lips is provided by the teeth:

- If the teeth are inclined inward, the lips look too thin (Figs 3.4a, b).
- If the teeth are inclined forward, the lips look more voluptuous (Fig. 3.4c).

1. If the lips are too thick, they can be treated with:
   - less make-up
   - orthodontic therapy, or
   - minor resective surgery.

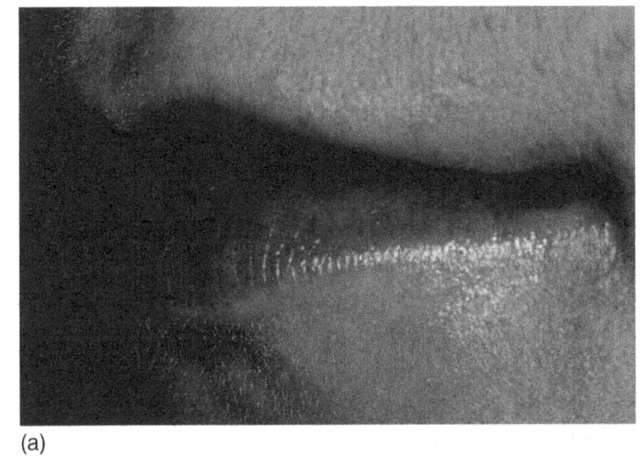
(a)

Figure 3.4 (a) A very thin upper and lower lip profile on a patient with low self-esteem.

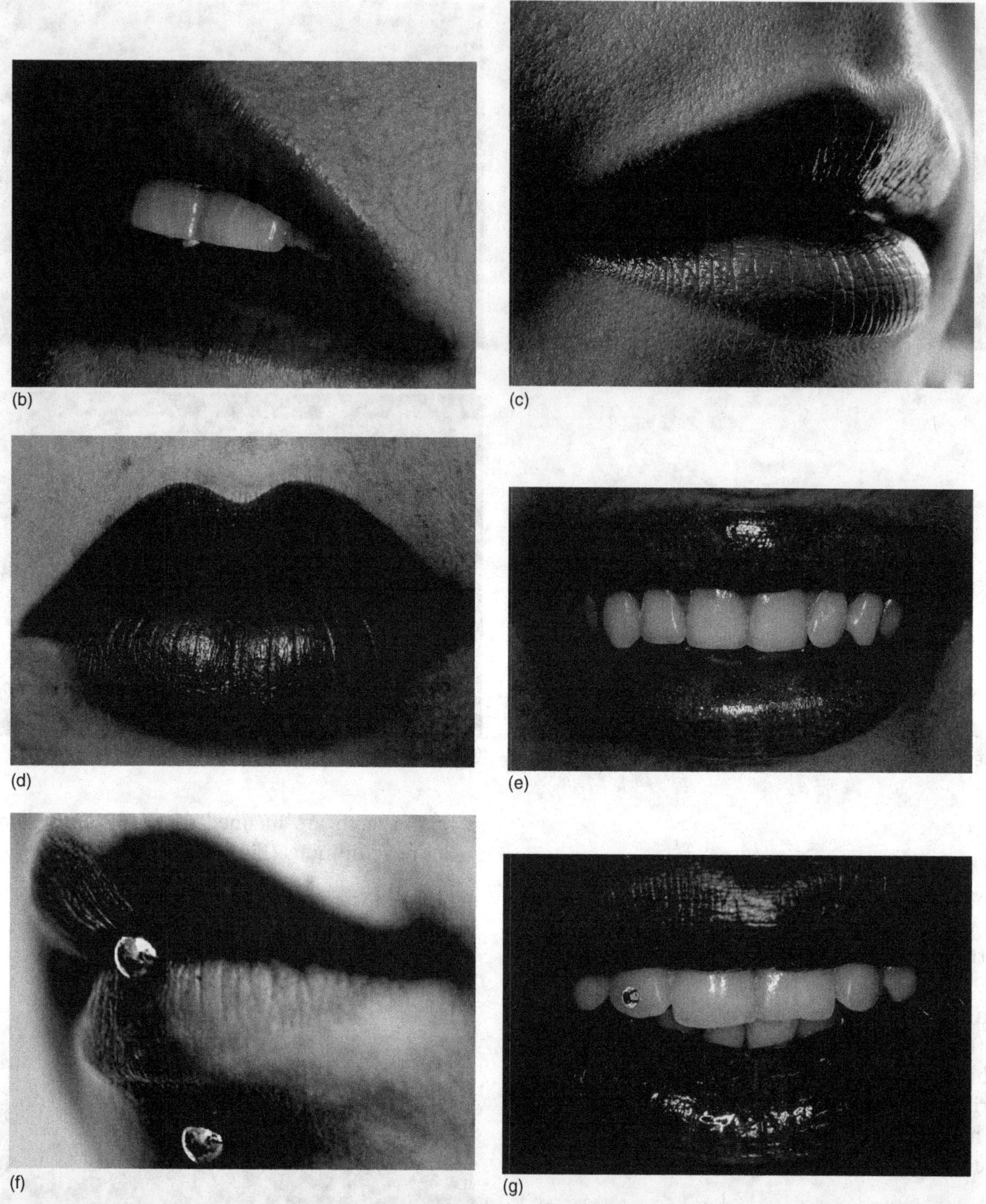

Figure 3.4 (b) Lip gloss, which enlarges the contour of the thin lips, allows a more confident smile. (c) Excessive use of lipstick enlarging the lip contour on a 15-year-old girl. (d) The lips of a professional model, with make-up to enhance her initial beauty. (e) Artificially expanding the size of the lips by means of an excessive collagen injection. (f) A lower-lip piercing an a 15-year-old girl. (g) A diamond on the right incisor, with a black beauty mark on the upper lip border.

2. Lips that are too thin could be lightly pumped up in the following ways:
   - make-up products such as pencil, lipstick, or gloss
   - excessive make-up, pigment, or tattoo (Fig. 3.4d)
   - injection of collagen or hyaluronic acid (Fig. 3.4e)
   - implantation of fat particulates and hyaluronic acid, or microsurgery, or

- accessories such as a tongue and/or lip piercing, or a beauty spot (Figs 3.4f, g).

3. When the upper lip allows too much of the maxillary gingiva to show, this may be due to:
   - a high maxillary jaw
   - a hyperfunctional upper lip or a shorter upper lip, or
   - a short distance between the nose and the upper lip.
4. These unesthetic facial morphologies could be treated by:
   - periodontal plastic surgery
   - a Botox® injection in the upper lip
   - vestibuloplasty of the upper lip
   - maxillary surgery, or orthognatic and orthodontic treatment, or
   - rhinoplasty at the tip of the nose.

For further details on this topic, see Chapter 4 ("The gingival smile").

The lower lip

In a full, optimal esthetic smile (Fig. 3.5):

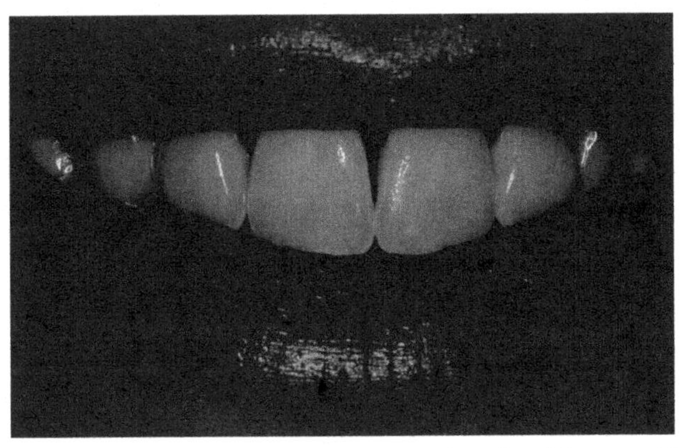

Figure 3.5 The natural esthetic smile of a 22-year-old woman, with her maxillary incisor edges following the lower-lip contour.

- The incisal edges of the upper central incisors should be above and should follow the lower lip contour.
- The lower lip should follow the contour of the maxillary teeth incisal edges.
- The edges of the lower incisors should be level with the lower lip contour.

4

The dentoalveolar gingival unit

With the growing trend in smile-enhancement therapies, more people are striving for that perfect smile. Indeed, a harmonious dentogingival junction is one that fits perfectly with the rest of the face. Not every small modification from the theoretical ideal leads to a lessening of the smile's esthetic value; such deviation may personalize the smile and keep it from becoming too monotonous. In addition, it is interesting to recall that a perfect symmetry between the two halves of the human face does not exist, and that the midline of the face and the midline of the dental arch correspond in only 70% of patients. The vertical maxillary and mandibular axes line up in only 75% of patients (Magne and Belser, 2003).

The vertical dimension of the dentogingival junction, consisting of the sulcus depth, the junctional epithelium (JE), and the connective tissue attachment (CTA), is physiologically predetermined and constant. The level of this "biological width" is dependent on the location of the crest of the alveolar bone (Figs 4.1a, b) and includes only

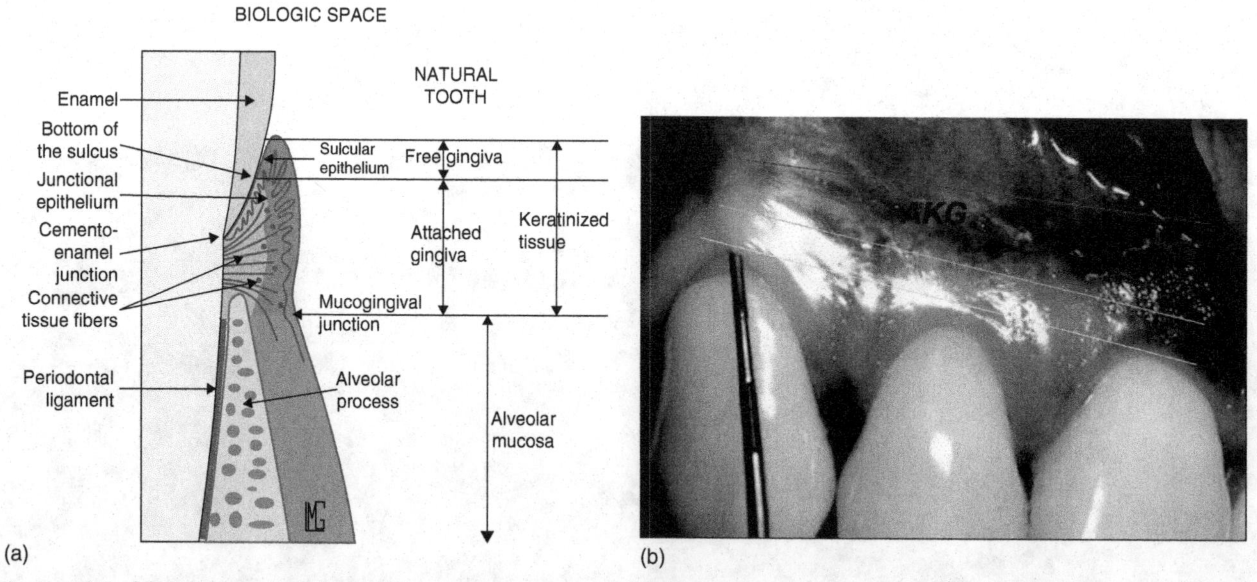

Figure 4.1 (a) A diagram of the different components of the dentoalveolar gingival unit. (Courtesy of Dr. M. Legall.) (b) Fully keratinized gingiva from the FGM to the MGJ, and defining the amount of attached keratinized gingiva with the probe.

Esthetic Soft Tissue Management of Teeth and Implants, First Edition. André P. Saadoun.

the JE and CTA. Changing the level of the alveolar bone moves the entire dentogingival junction at an apical or coronal level (Landolt and Blatz, 2008).

The composition of an esthetic and functional dentoalveolar gingival unit (DAGU) or periodontal restorative interface (PRI) must take into account the periodontal health of the bone, the gingiva, the interdental papillae (the pink esthetic score, or PES), the teeth (the white esthetic score, or WES), and the biological space (JE+CTA).

The gingiva

The esthetics of the anterior maxillary region of the dentition depends largely on the appearance of the gingival tissues surrounding the teeth. Traditionally, the physiological gingival architecture has been described as having a scalloped contour (Prichard, 1961) around the four surfaces of the tooth, in accordance with the course of the cemento-enamel junction (CEJ) (Schroeder, 1991) and is thus concave apically in the free surfaces and convex at the tip of the papilla.

Esthetic considerations

The gingival margins of the maxillary anterior dentition should be at their correct level. Asymmetrical gingival tissues can significantly affect the harmonious appearance of both natural or prosthetic dentition. The zenith is defined as the most apical point of the gingival marginal scallop (Figs 4.2a–c). The proper placement of the gingival zenith should be at the peak of the parabolic curvature of the gingival margin, which for the central incisors, canines, and premolars should specifically be located slightly distal to the middle of the long axis on these teeth. This produces the subtle inclination of the distal root that is paramount for the foundation of a beautiful smile. The zenith for the lateral incisors is located at the midline of the long axis of the tooth.

The gingival margin of lateral incisor teeth can range from being at the same level or 0.5–2.0 mm coronal to the zeniths of the central incisor and the canine teeth (Feigenbaum, 1991). The height of the

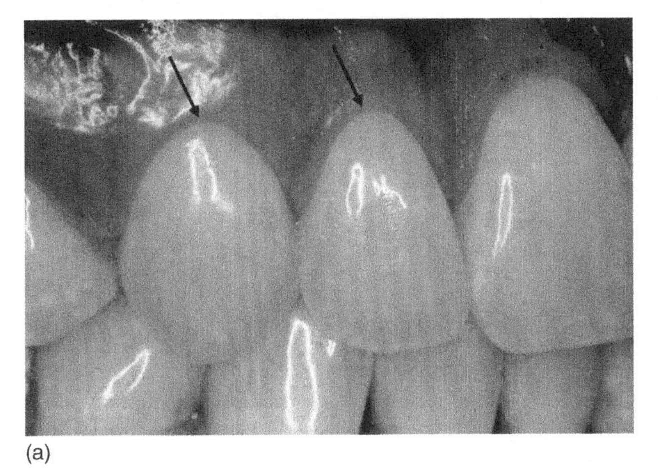

(a)

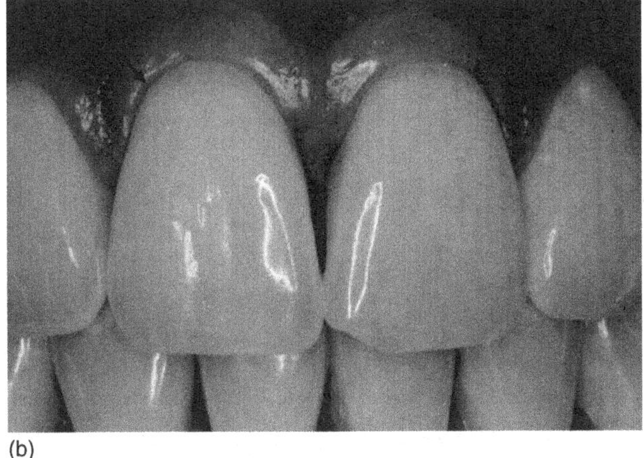

(b)

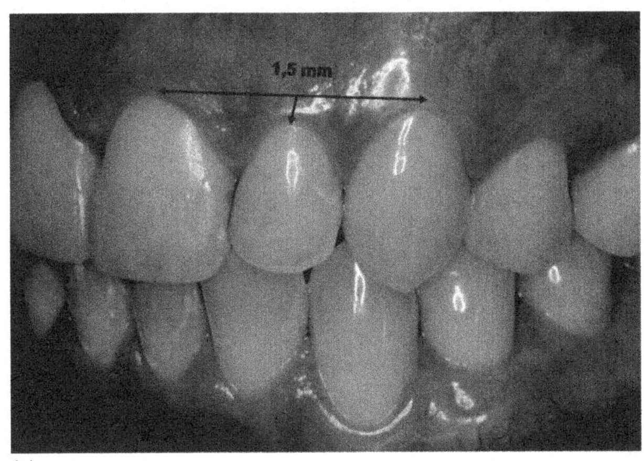

(c)

Figure 4.2 (a) The gingival zenith does not exist on the lateral incisor, but it is limited and is slightly distal on the cuspid. (b) The gingival zenith on the central incisor is located distal to the midline. (c) The gingival level of the lateral incisor is below the line joining the adjacent teeth and could vary from one side to the other.

gingival margin for the lateral incisors should be 1 mm shorter than the gingival margins of the adjacent teeth (Kurtzman and Silverstein, 2008). In other words, the gingival margin of the lateral incisor should be 1 mm coronal to the line connecting the gingival margins of the central incisor and the canine.

The gingival zenith of the canine is at the same level or slightly more apical to the gingival zenith of the central incisors. When the patient is looking straight ahead, the gingival zenith of the lateral incisor is typically below (81.1%) or on the gingival line joining the cuspid and the central incisor zenith point (15%).

More recently, it has been found that the heights of the gingival tissues over the maxillary central incisors should be slightly higher (1 mm apically) than the heights of the tissues over the maxillary lateral incisors. The heights of the maxillary canines should be at the same level apically as the central incisors, or slightly more apical. The gingival zeniths should be located at the distolabial line angles, thus creating a "raised eyebrow" over the central incisors. A directional gingival contour asymmetry has been demonstrated, with the right side higher than the left side (Charruel *et al.*, 2008).

A recent study (Mattos and Santana, 2008) has also shown that the gingival zenith is not universally displaced toward the distal aspect. The frequency and magnitude of distal displacement is dependent on the crown tooth position and its root orientation. It is more pronounced in central incisors than in lateral incisors, in which, in turn, it is more prominent than in canines. In other words, the distal position of the zenith was very frequent on the central incisor, frequent on the lateral incisor, and rare on the canine.

Consideration of these findings may improve clinical management of the dentogingival complex (DGC) and enhance periodontal surgical procedures, as well as conventional or implant restorative measures in the anterior maxillary dentition.

The gingival biotype

The gingiva can present a range of characteristics:

- Frame: harmony or disharmony, in relation to tooth eruption on the ridge (Figs 4.3a–c).

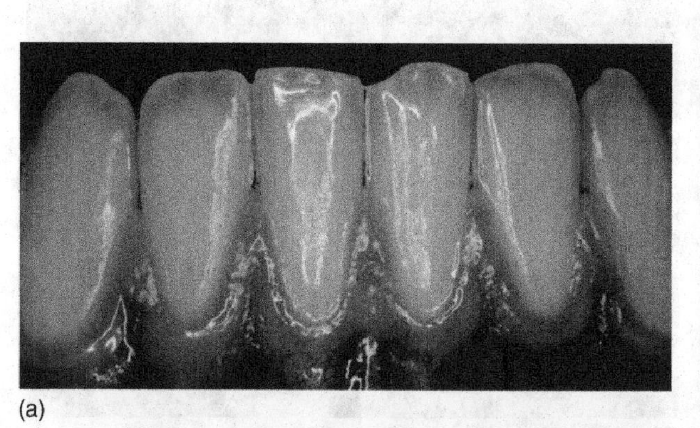

(a)

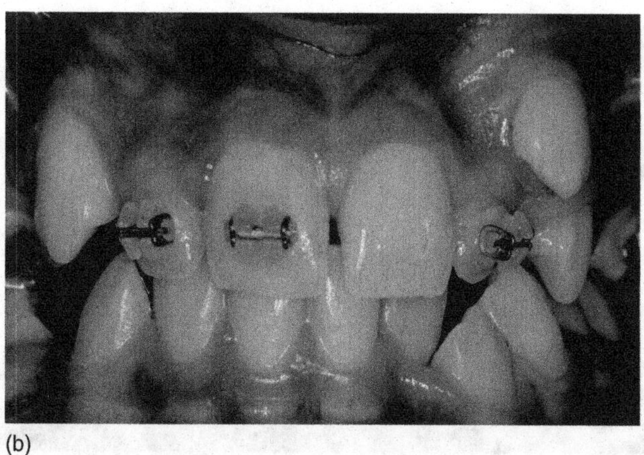

(b)

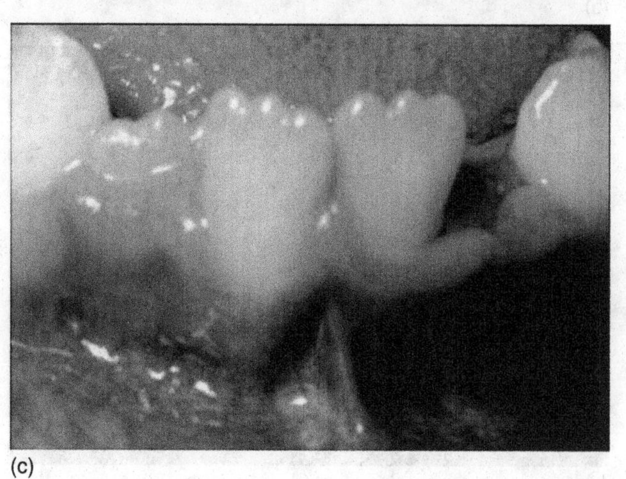

(c)

Figure 4.3 (a) The gingival contour on the lower anterior teeth, in harmony and without any inflammation. (b) Gingival and dental disharmony before orthodontic treatment. (c) The right mandibular incisor is erupting buccally with less keratinized gingiva and the left one lingually with an excess amount of keratinized gingiva.

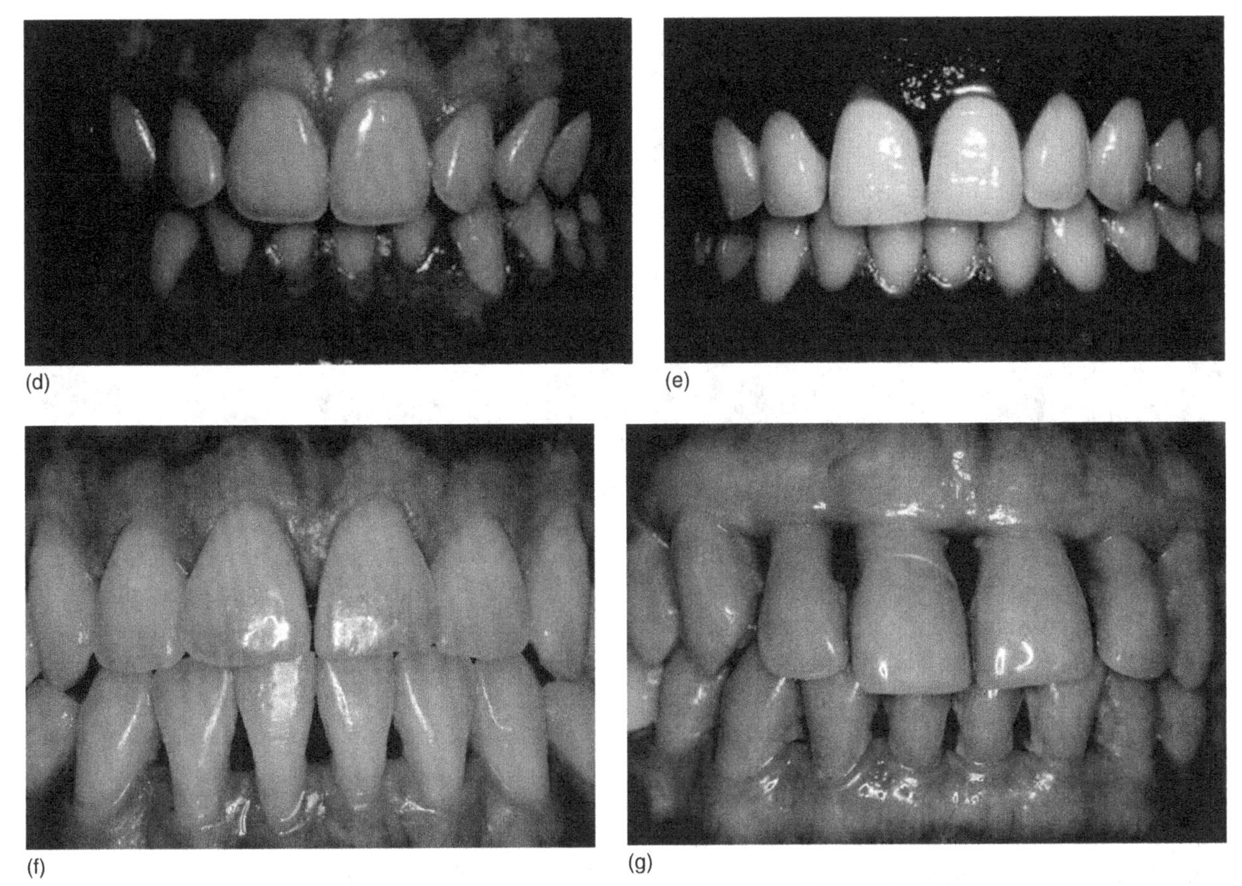

Figure 4.3 (d) Pink attached gingiva on a blond Caucasian patient. (e) Pigmented attached gingiva on a black African patient. (f) Noninflamed gingiva with a healthy gingival surface texture. (g) Inflamed gingiva induced by biofilm and calculus.

- Color: pink or pigmented, in relation to ethnicity (Figs 4.3d, e).
- Texture: normal or inflamed, in relation to oral hygiene (Figs 4.3f, g).
- Biotype: thick, medium, or thin, in relation tothe cortical bone plate (Weisgold and Coslet, 1977).

1. *Type I: the thick, flat biotype* (Fig. 4.4a). This type corresponds to a thick periodontium, with a flat form and a large quantity of keratinized gingiva, where the thickness of the attached gingiva is greater than 2 mm and the width is 5–6 mm or more, with thick marginal bone. In thick periodontal biotypes, periodontal changes may manifest themselves in the form of chronic gingival inflammation. This biotype is characterized by:
   - minimal disparity between the location of the gingival margin and the peak of the papilla
   - a flatter, thicker underlying osseous form
   - denser, more fibrotic soft tissue

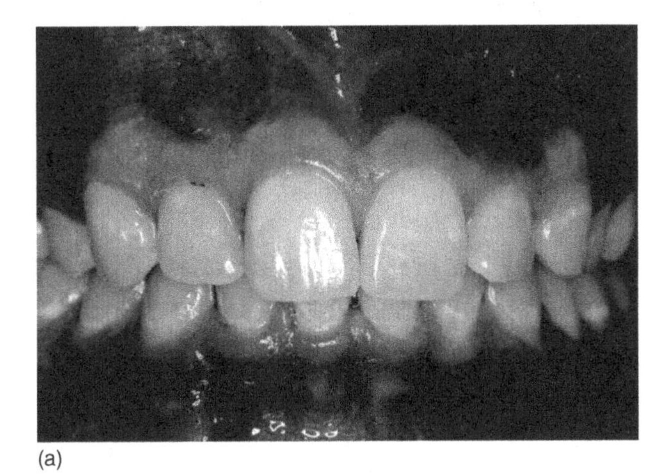

Figure 4.4 (a) The thick, flat gingival biotype.

   - a larger amount of keratinized attached gingiva, and
   - a square tooth shape.

   In thick biotypes, gingival recession is rare and bone loss is slow; but bone defects and an unfavorable bone contour occur more often.

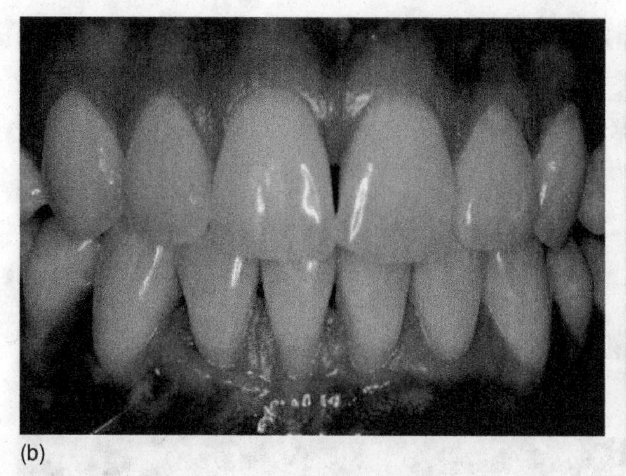

(b)

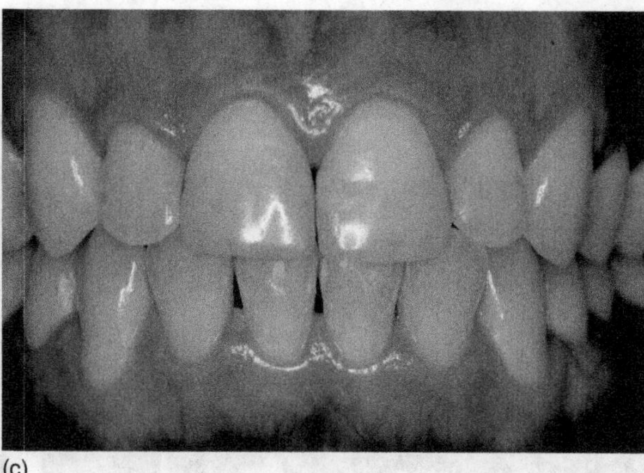

(c)

Figure 4.4 (b) The thin, scalloped biotype. (c) The medium gingival biotype.

Subsequently, this may result in periodontal pockets, root caries, tooth mobility due to the loss of clinical attachment apparatus, and tooth loss.

2. *Type II: the thin, scalloped biotype* (Fig. 4.4b). This type corresponds to a thin periodontium, with a scalloped form and a small quantity of keratinized gingiva, where the thickness of the attached gingiva is less than 2 mm and the width is 3.5–5.0, mm with thin marginal bone. In thin periodontal biotypes, postoperative periodontal changes may lead to resorption of the alveolar crest and subsequent gingival recession. This biotype is characterized by:
   - a distinct disparity between the location of the gingival margin and the peak of the papilla
   - a scalloped osseous form, and often dehiscence and fenestration
   - delicate, friable soft tissue
   - a minimal amount of keratinized attached gingiva, and
   - a triangular tooth shape.

   In thin biotypes, gingival retraction is more frequent and bone resorption is quicker. However, if cleaning of the area is adequate, bone loss and gingival recession can be avoided. On the other hand, if cleaning is inadequate or excessive, gingival inflammation persists, bone resorption is faster, and gingival recession increases.
3. *Type III: the medium biotype* (Fig. 4.4c). The medium biotype is an average of the thick and thin biotypes with ovoid teeth on women and rectangular on men.
   The Maynard and Wilson classification put more emphasis on the medium biotype in describing the relationship between the thickness of bone and gingiva.

Another biotype classification has been proposed by Maynard and Wilson (1980) and is based on classification of the gingiva/alveolar same thickness (Figs 4.4d, e).

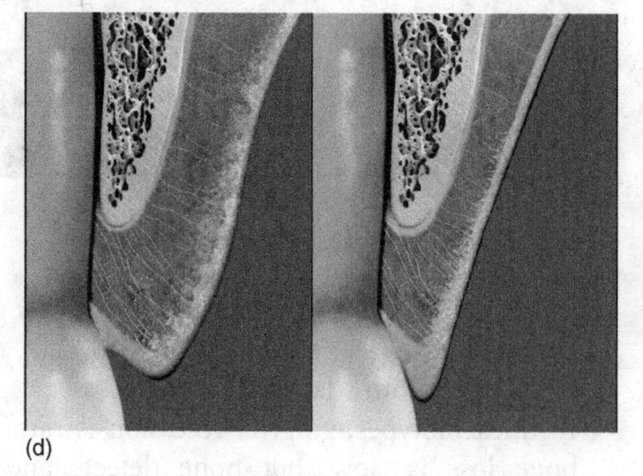

(d)

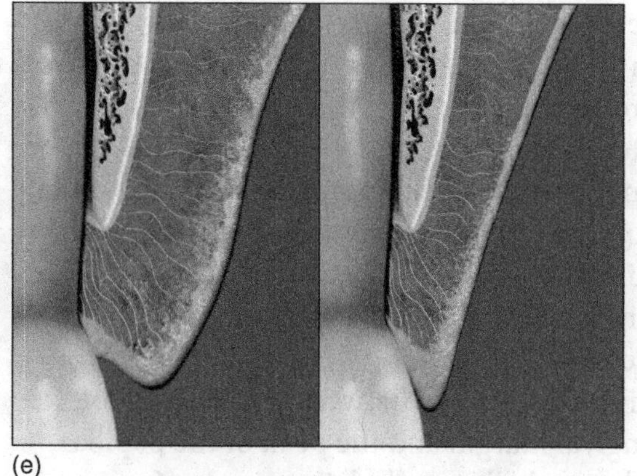

(e)

Figure 4.4 (d) Type I, thick gingiva/thick biotype; Type II, thin gingiva/medium biotype. (e) Type III, thick gingiva/medium biotype; Type IV, thin gingiva/thin biotype. (Courtesy of Dr. S. Rocha Bernardes, Curitiba, Brazil.)

Table 4.1 Bone and gingival biotypes

Type I	Thick bone	Thick gingiva/Thick bone
Type II	Thick bone	Thin gingiva/Medium bone
Type III	Thin bone	Thick gingiva/Medium bone
Type IV	Thin bone	Thin gingiva/Thin bone

The bone biotypes I, II, and III correspond to thick and medium periodontium, and only type IV corresponds to thin periodontium. This classification could be interesting in establishing the planning of implant treatment and in evaluation of the esthetic results (Table 4.1).

The presence of an adequate zone of keratinized mucosa was thought to be necessary for the maintenance of gingival health and to prevent the progression of periodontal disease. Lang and Loë (1972) suggested a width of at least 2 mm of keratinized mucosa, of which 1 mm was to be attached.

Subsequently, several authors have challenged this concept, and have shown that gingival health can be maintained with hardly any attached gingiva but with good hygiene (Miyasato *et al.*, 1977; Kennedy *et al.*, 1985).

Restoration on natural teeth has supra-, juxta-, or intrasulcular cervical limits and, in general, the gingival profile dictates the prosthetic emergence profile.

Subgingival restorations around teeth tend to recede over time (Valderhaug, 1980) and this phenomenon has been confirmed by Stetler and Bissada (1987), who reported that a narrow zone of keratinized mucosa in teeth with subgingival restorations is associated with a higher chance of gingival inflammation; this can be extrapolated to implant crown restorations. Thus, it is especially important to have a keratinized tissue zone adjacent to dental implants, because the implant restoration is always located beneath the oral mucosa margin in the esthetic zone, and it should conceal the subgingival part of the abutment. Together with its double submerged and emergent architecture, the abutment/implant restoration contributes to the shaping and formation of the peri-implant mucosa at the level of its scalloped marginal contour and the interdental papillae in harmony with the adjacent teeth (Warrer *et al.*, 1995; Saadoun and Touati, 2007; Bouri *et al.*, 2008).

Although the medium and thick biotypes account for 70% of cases, the more extreme thin biotypes, which make up about 15% of cases, are the most frequently described because of the specific challenges that they represent (Jansen and Weisgold, 1995).

The gingival thickness is related to the gingival height and the thickness of the buccal plate (Chang *et al.*, 2003). The initial thickness of the gingival tissues at the crest may be considered as a significant influence on marginal bone stability around implants within the first year of functioning after implant placement (Chang *et al.*, 1999).

The thicker the buccal plate, the less bone resorption takes place. The thicker the gingiva, the less gingival recession occurs (Schropp *et al.*, 1999). Any marginal bone remodeling around the teeth will result in:

- no gingival variation or marginal soft tissue deformity on a thick, flat biotype, but
- some gingival recession and marginal soft tissue deformity on a thin, scalloped biotype.

For background, see Saadoun *et al.* (1999) and Rompen *et al.* (2003).

In a study by Chung *et al.* (2006), implants placed in areas that lacked keratinized gingiva had a higher susceptibility to tissue breakdown due to plaque accumulation. Despite similar plaque levels, implants placed in nonkeratinized areas showed earlier loss of attachment.

Bouri *et al.* (2008) reported that implants with a narrow zone of keratinized tissue had a significantly higher chance of probing and/or bleeding (89% versus 31%) and significantly higher mean alveolar bone loss than implants with a wider zone of keratinized mucosa.

The dimensions of the peri-implant mucosa at 1 year were related to the peri-implant biotype in the maxillary anterior region (Kan *et al.*, 2003a):

- Thick biotype – the probe was not visible through the gingival margin (Fig. 4.4f).
- Thin biotype – the probe was visible through the gingival margin (Fig. 4.4g).

Since the above study was conducted, different techniques have been made available to measure soft tissue thickness; namely, visual inspection, transgingival probing (Fig. 4.4h), probe transparency,

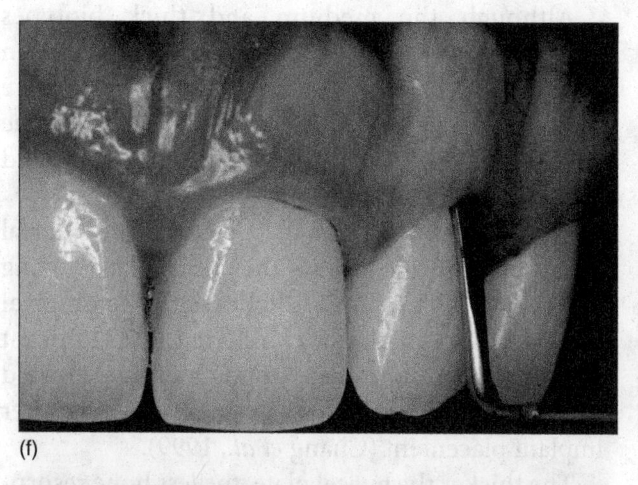

(f)

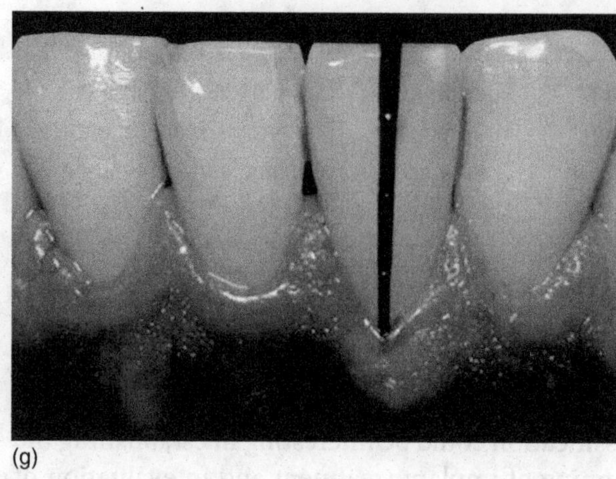

(g)

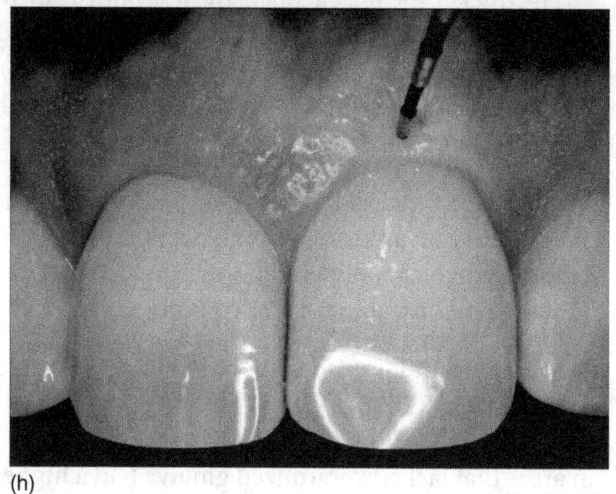

(h)

Figure 4.4 (f) The thickness of the marginal tissue hides the instrument in the sulcus. (g) The probe appears through the thin marginal tissue. (h) Transgingival probing, measuring soft tissue thickness.

ultrasonic devices, and cone beam CT imaging (Kao *et al.*, 2008; Fu *et al.*, 2011).

The thickness of the soft tissue around the teeth depends on the eruption on the ridge (see Figs 4.3b, c). However, in the maxillary anterior region with non-submerged immediate implant placement, mucosal recession between 3 and 4 years was significantly related to the buccal position implant placement rather than the tissue biotype (Chen *et al.* 2007).

In the maxillary and mandibulary anterior regions, between 19 and 50 months the thin tissue biotype showed greater peri-implant mucosal recession than the thick tissue biotype, though this was not statistically significant (Evans and Chen, 2008).

In maxillary incisors with flapless immediate implant placement post extraction, mucosal recession of more than 1 mm occurred in 24% of sites with the thin tissue biotype, compared to 10.5% of sites with the thick tissue biotype (Chen and Evans, 2009).

Therefore, the stability of the marginal gingiva depends on two anatomical parameters:

- the presence of hard tissue underlying the peri-implant gingiva, and
- the thickness of the peri-implant gingiva.

Bone resorption on thin biotypes is greater than on thick biotypes, and there is significantly more peri-implant bone loss at sites with thin tissue compared to those with thick tissue. Consequently, there is a direct correlation between the thickness of the peri-implant soft tissue and the peri-implant bone loss (Linkevicius *et al.*, 2009).

Furthermore, Nisapakultorn *et al.* (2010) found that in the maxillary incisors, the facial marginal mucosal level was significantly associated with the peri-implant tissue biotype: a thin biotype was significantly associated with an increased risk of facial marginal mucosal recession.

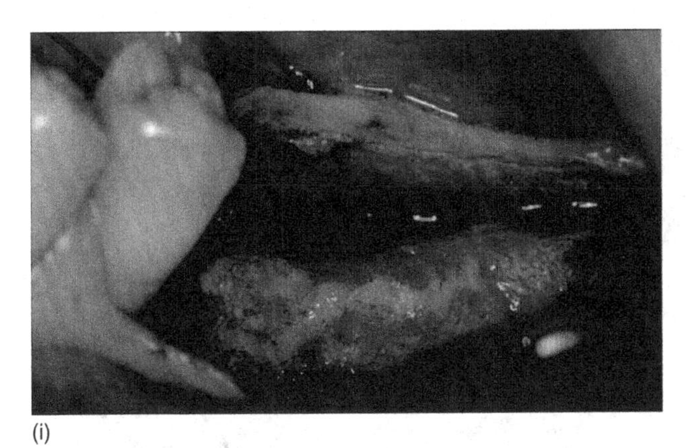

(i)

Figure 4.4 (i) Evaluation of the gingival thickness after flap elevation.

The thickness of the soft tissue influences the crestal bone change around implants (Fig. 4.4i):

- If the tissue thickness is 2.0 mm or less, crestal bone loss of up to 1.45 mm can be expected despite a supracrestal position of the implant/abutment interface.
- If the tissue thickness is 2.5 mm or more, crestal bone loss of up to 0.26 mm can be expected.
- Significant marginal bone recession could be avoided if the implant/abutment junction was positioned approximately 2 mm above the bone level; a negligible amount of bone loss, of around 0.2 mm, would then occur.

In the evaluation of marginal bone loss, the measurement of gingival thickness should be mandatory. Therefore, it is recommended that bone-level implant placement be avoided if a thin biotype is present at an implant site, or if it is necessary to change the biotype from thin to thick. In a study by Linkevicius *et al.* (2009), mean peri-implant bone loss at 1 year was found to be inversely correlated with peri-implant mucosal thickness:

- thin peri-implant mucosa, < 2 mm
- medium peri-implant mucosa, 2.1–3.0 mm
- thick peri-implant mucosa, > 3.1 mm.

Consequently, it is important to consider the influence of soft tissue thickness on crestal bone changes around implants along with the patient's biotype before any implant placement, especially in the esthetic zone (Linkevicius *et al.*, 2009).

The ideal esthetic is often difficult to achieve because the patient's clinical parameters can vary considerably, depending on the remaining hard and soft tissue in the implant site (Garber, 2010). A thick biotype presents a low risk of marginal discoloration. This risk is higher with a thin biotype, and it becomes necessary to increase its thickness to prevent marginal coloration and/or gingival recession (Leziy and Miller, 2008b). There are favorable and unfavorable factors that should be taken into consideration, and these will be described in more detail in Chapter 6 (see "Peri-implant risk factors").

The implant survival rate is not affected by the quality and quantity of the peri-implant keratinized tissue. However, a certain amount of height and thickness is important to maintain esthetic and soft tissue health around the implant – especially around an implant with a rough surface, where the adhesion of the connective tissue is fragile in comparison to the dental collagen fibers, which are inserted securely into the root cementum (Rompen, 2011).

The gingival smile

When smiling, a "gummy smile" is an excessive gum display with short clinical teeth, which reveals a more significant amount of the surface of the gingiva (Foley *et al.*, 2003). In general, it is acceptable for up to 2–3 mm of gingival tissue to be displayed upon a full smile (Garber and Salama, 2000). However, such a situation is not systematically negative, as such people often produce very pretty smiles if certain rules of harmony are respected.

An exposition of more than 3 mm of gingival tissue leads to an excessive gingival display, or a "gummy smile." However, there are other smiles with a gingival display of more than 3 mm that need to be corrected, because they are particularly unattractive (Kokich *et al.*, 1999).

Patients with a significant display of gingiva as a result of genetic factors (i.e., a skeletal deformity such as a thick alveolar buccal bone, altered passive eruption, and a short upper lip) or due to medication (anti-epileptic, antihypertensive, or immunosuppressant drugs) represent a very important challenge for the dental clinician in terms of treatment planning, because of the multifactorial etiologic factors, as well as the psychological and human relations implications associated with the appearance of the face (Nowzari and Rich, 2008).

A classification of maxillary vertical gingival evaluation has been proposed by Garber and Salama (1996), on the basis of the height of the exposed gingiva:

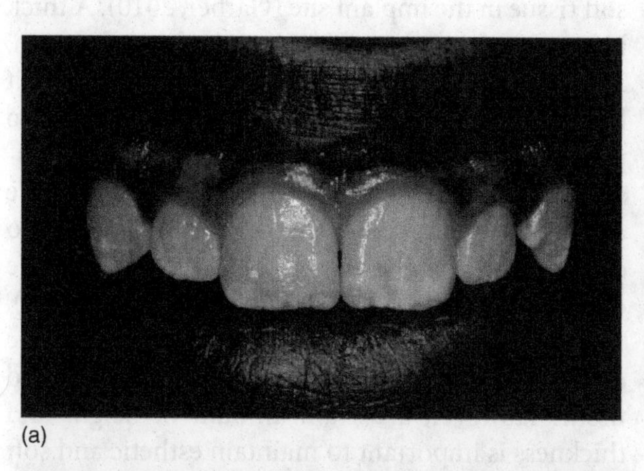

(a)

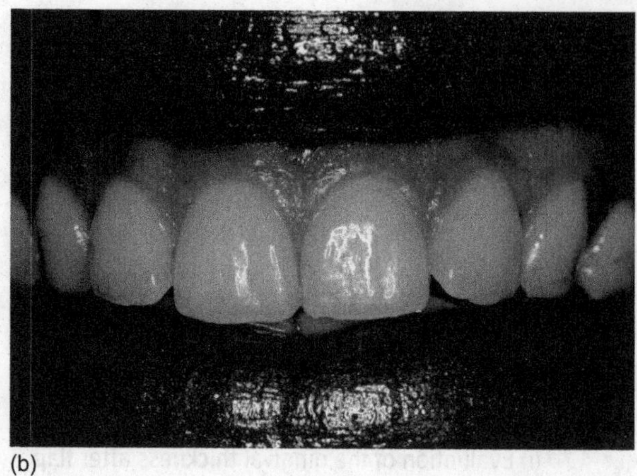

(b)

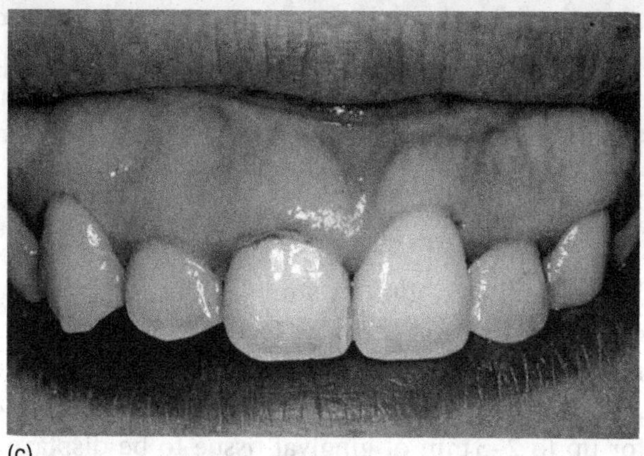

(c)

Figure 4.5 (a) A high lip line, with 2 mm of gingiva showing (Degree I). (b) A gingival smile, with > 5 mm of gingival display, but not unesthetic (Degree II). (c) An excessive gum display > 8 mm, giving an unesthetic gummy smile (Degree III).

- degree I, 2–4 mm of exposed gingiva (Fig. 4.5a)
- degree II, 4–8 mm of exposed gingiva (Fig. 4.5b)
- degree III, > 8 mm of exposed gingiva (Fig. 4.5c).

Various therapeutic protocols, depending on the height of the exposed gingiva or the excessive amount of vertical bone, are described in Table 4.2.

Although gingival exposure is generally the result of several factors, four primary etiologies can be noted for the gingival smile (Foley *et al.*, 2003; Barbant *et al.*, 2011a).

Osseous etiology: basal, alveolar, or combined

The skeletal abnormality leads to vertical maxillary hypertrophy (up to 8 mm), which is sometimes aggravated by the upper pro alveoli. The main characteristics of this abnormality are as follows (Figs 4.6a–f):

- excessive maxillary vertical growth;
- excessive growth of the maxillary alveolar bone
- malocclusion, with dental maxillary disharmony and dental malpositions
- augmentation of the lower half of the face

Table 4.2 Different therapeutic protocols depending on the exposed height of the gingiva

Degree	Gingival exposure (mm)	Therapeutic protocol
I	2–4	Orthodontic ingression with mini-implants
		Orthodontic treatment and periodontal surgery
		Periodontal surgery and restorative treatment
II	4–8	Periodontal surgery and restorative treatment
		Orthognatic surgery (depending on the root length and the clinical crown: root ratio)
III	> 8	Orthognatic surgery with or without periodontal surgery and restorative treatment

Data from Attal and Tirlet (2011).

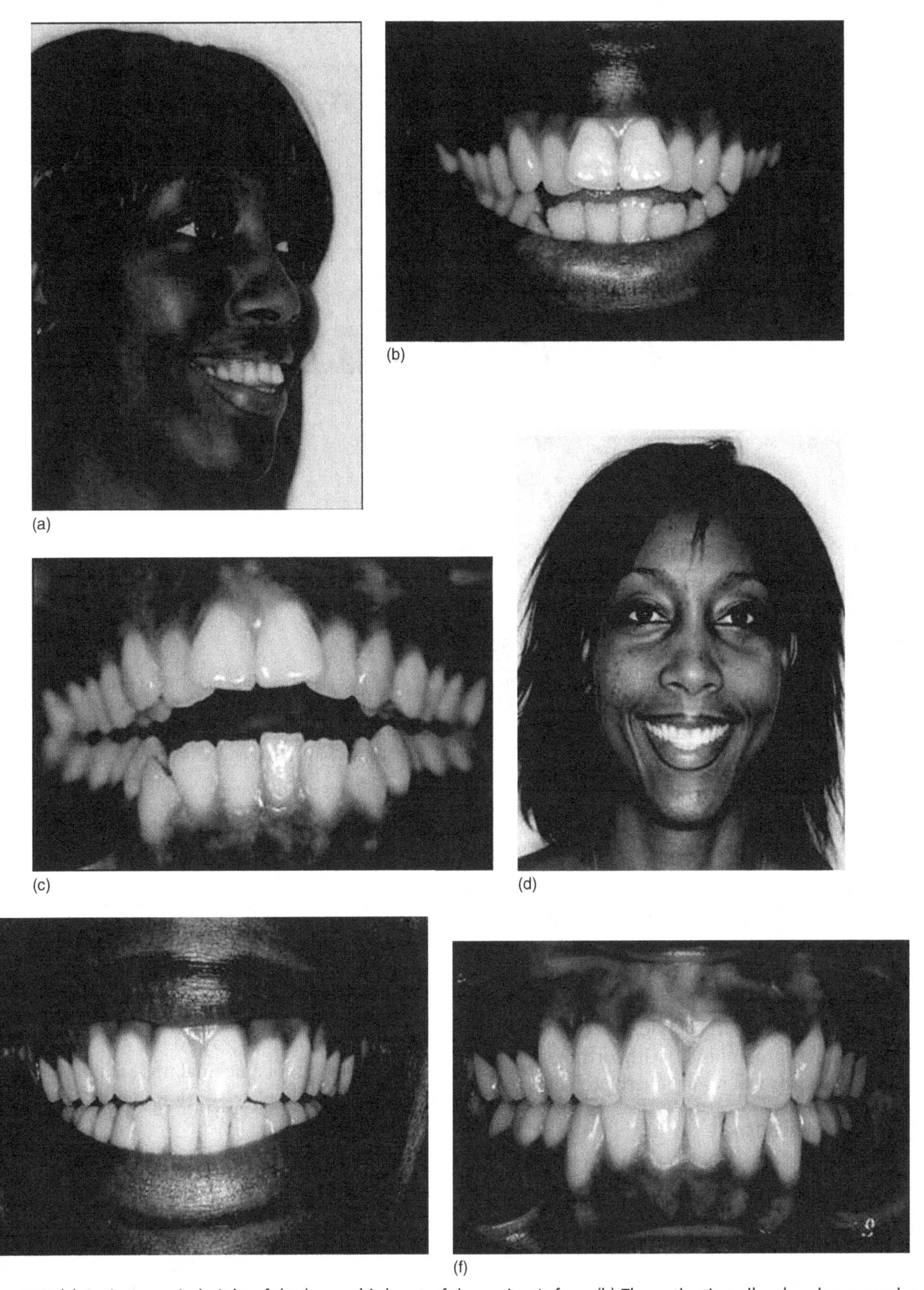

Figure 4.6 (a) An increase in height of the lower third part of the patient's face. (b) The patient's smile, showing excessive gingiva and a maxillary overjet. (c) Class II, division 1, with a large open bite. (d) The patient's face 3 years later, with a decrease in the height of the lower third part of the face after extraction of the four first premolars and orthodontic therapy. (e) The patient's beautiful smile after therapy, with a normal amount of gingiva. (f) The correct occlusal relation and tooth position after orthodontic therapy. (Figures (a),(d),(e),(f) courtesy of Dr. P. Curiel.)

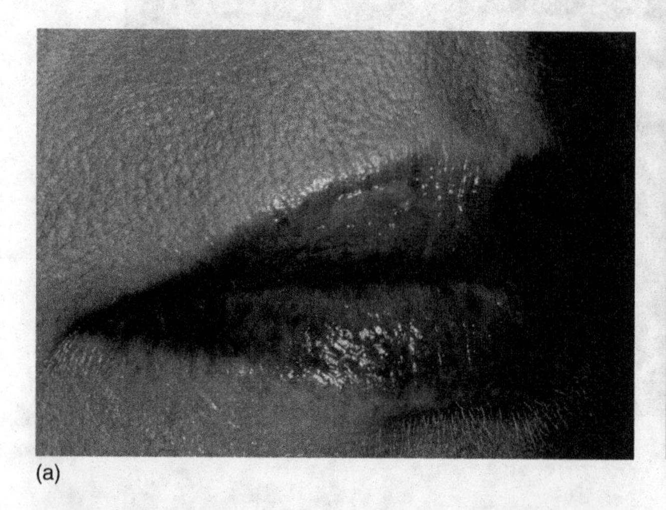

(a)

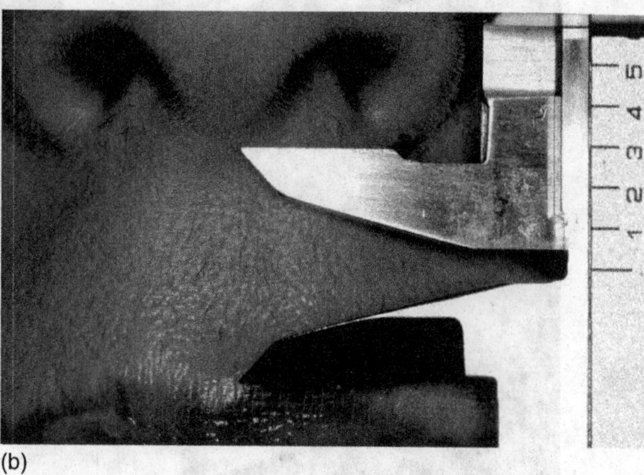

(b)

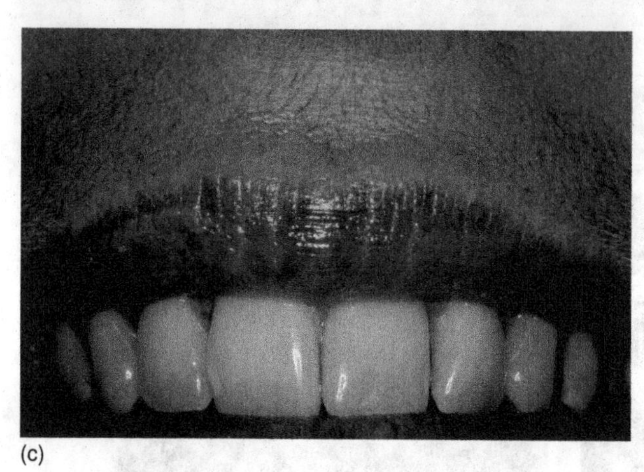

(c)

Figure 4.7 (a) Beautiful lips, with a normal upper lip height. (b) Measuring the vertical height between the nose and the tip of the upper lip. (c) The patient's beautiful smile, without showing the gingival margin.

- incompetence of the lips, and
- a convex profile and a Class II angle malocclusion.

In general, the patient's profile is highly convex and presents an augmentation of the lower half of the face, an incompetence of the lips, and a Class II angle malocclusion at rest, and at different dynamic stages of the smile (Cheng-Yi *et al.*, 2008; Toca *et al.*, 2008). Orthodontic treatment with the extraction of all the first premolars, combined with orthognatic surgery if necessary, will resolve these problems.

Muscular etiology

There is usually a short tonicity and/or a hypertonicity of the upper lip with lifting or "elevator" muscles, causing an exaggerated labial elevation. The characteristics of this abnormality are listed below:

- Hypertonicity of the upper lip (Figs 4.7a–c):
  - normal maxillary height
  - a normal length of the upper lip, between 20 and 25 mm
  - 2 mm of incisal edge showing at rest, with the full anterior teeth exposed on smiling (Figs 4.7a–c).
  - Hyperfunction of the elevator muscle of the upper lip, showing teeth and gingiva on a forced smile (Vig and Brundo, 1978; Peck *et al.*, 1992; Ezquerra *et al.*, 1999; Van der Geld *et al.*, 2008).
- Short upper lip (Figs 4.7d–f):
  - the length of a normal upper lip is 20–25 mm
  - the length of a short upper lip is less than 20 mm
  - the upper teeth are visible with the lips at rest, and
  - the lip length decreases by an average of 4 mm between the lips at rest and a spontaneous or forced smile showing the full teeth length and excess display of gingiva (Paris and Faucher, 2003).
- Symmetry or asymmetry of the upper lip (Van der Geld *et al.*, 2008) (Figs 4.7g, h).

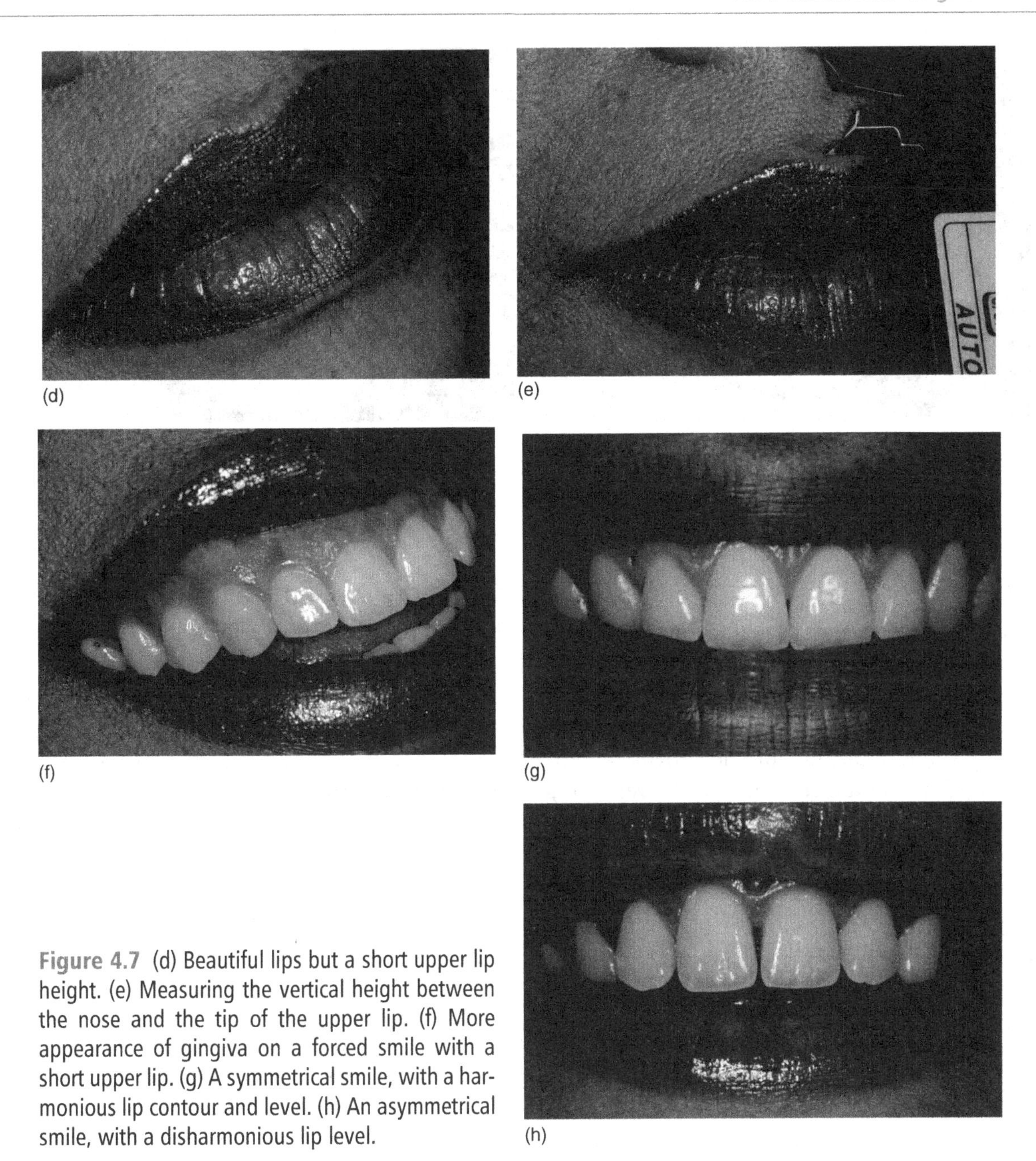

Figure 4.7 (d) Beautiful lips but a short upper lip height. (e) Measuring the vertical height between the nose and the tip of the upper lip. (f) More appearance of gingiva on a forced smile with a short upper lip. (g) A symmetrical smile, with a harmonious lip contour and level. (h) An asymmetrical smile, with a disharmonious lip level.

This clinical situation is more evident on natural and forced smiles (Vig and Brundo, 1978).

Various treatments for muscular etiology have been proposed, such as the following:

- Surgical techniques to reposition the upper lip in a more coronal position, limiting the retraction of the elevator muscle:
  - an elliptic incision in the depth of the vestibule
  - myectomy of the elevator muscle (Litton and Fournier, 1979; Miskinyar, 1983; Rosenblatt and Simon, 2006; Fairbairn, 2010), or
  - rhinoplasty associated with resection of the lowering muscle of the nasal septum (Cachay and Velásquez, 1992).
- Injection of Type A botulism toxin (Botox®) and/or hyaluronic acid (Figs 4.8a, b):
  - limits the hypertonicity of the elevator muscle of the upper lip
  - the site of the injection is 10.4 mm from the lateral edge of the nose, and
  - the site of the injection is 32.4 mm above the smile line at rest (Polo, 2005; Toca *et al.*, 2008).

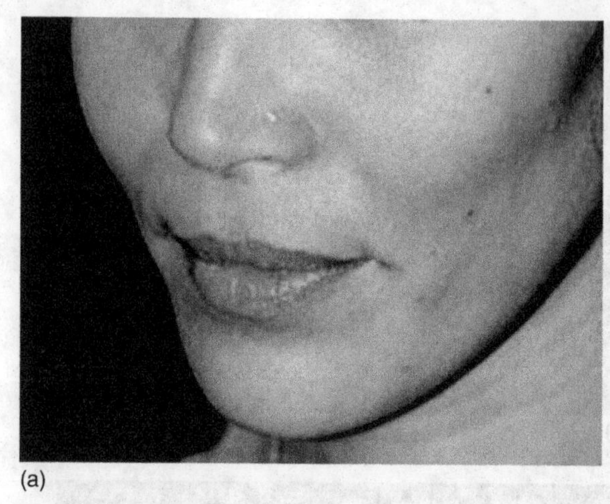

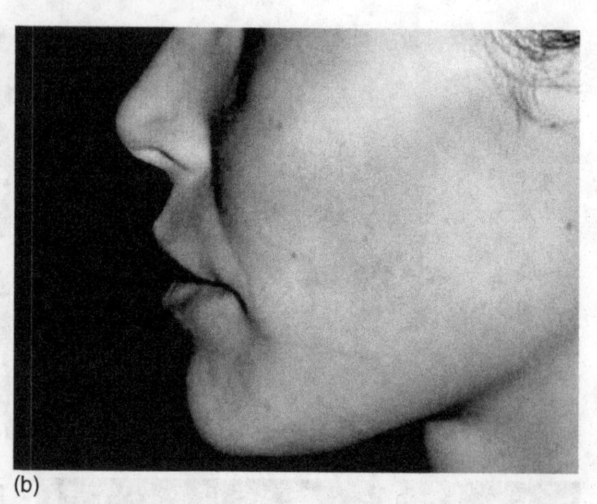

(a) (b)

Figure 4.8 (a) A profile view of a young woman, showing the missing midline tip of the upper lip. (b) Restoration of the volume of the upper lip by means of an injection of hyaluronic acid. (Courtesy of Dr. C. Lepage, Paris, France.)

Dental etiology

Short clinical crowns are usually found because of size abnormalities with small teeth, crowns shortened by parafunctional wear (abrasion, bulimia, anorexia), or incomplete eruption of teeth. It is the most important indication of the crown lengthening procedure, combined with laminate veneering if necessary. Clinical situations in which an excess of gingiva combined with short teeth can be found are as follows (Coslet *et al.*, 1977; Foley *et al.*, 2003; Fradeani and Barducci, 2008; Gürel, 2008b):

- an unusually short natural tooth length (Figs 4.9a)
- shorter teeth due to bruxomania or anorexia and/or bulimia (Fig. 4.9b), or
- shorter teeth due to delayed passive eruption (Figs 4.9c–e).

Delayed altered passive eruption

Natural teeth eruption refers to total teeth eruption with a normal relationship between the bone crest and the cemento-enamel junction (see the section on "Natural passive eruption"). Altered passive eruption refers to incomplete natural or delayed eruption, or their absence, in individuals for unknown reasons, and leads to a more coronally positioned gingival margin that may be associated with a normal or coronally displaced bone level (Figs 4.10a–d) (Coslet *et al.*, 1977; Kurtzman and Silverstein, 2008). These individuals have square-shaped clinical crowns with no natural proportion, and tend to display excessive gingival tissue upon smiling. A classification of natural passive eruption and delayed passive eruption (Table 4.3) has been described by several authors (Gargiulo *et al.*, 1961; McGuire and Levine, 1997; Gürel, 2008b; Kao *et al.*,

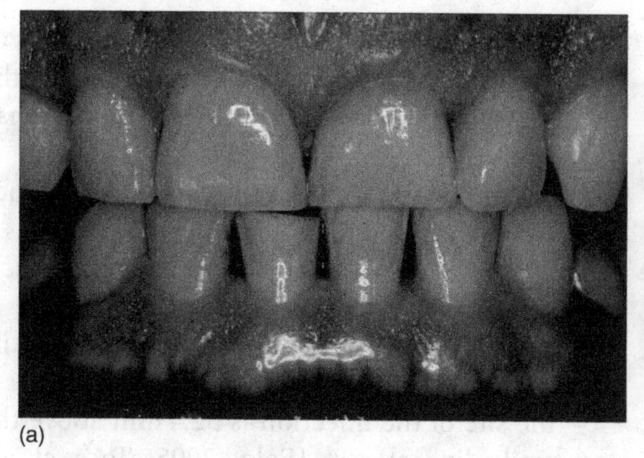

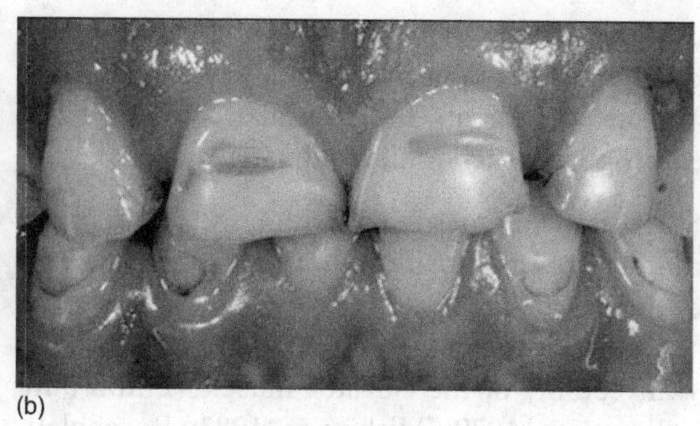

(a) (b)

Figure 4.9 (a) Maxillary and mandibular short teeth because of abrasion, at the initial consultation. (b) The teeth are worn and short because of bulimia and anorexia.

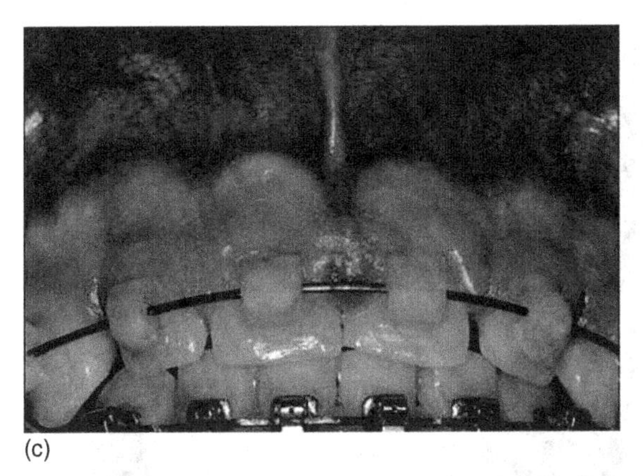
(c)

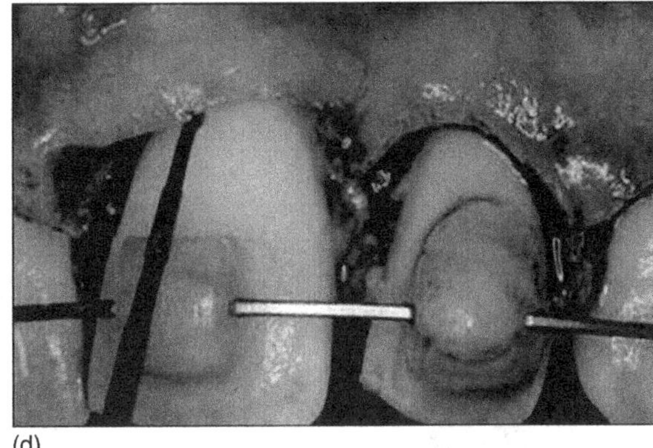
(d)

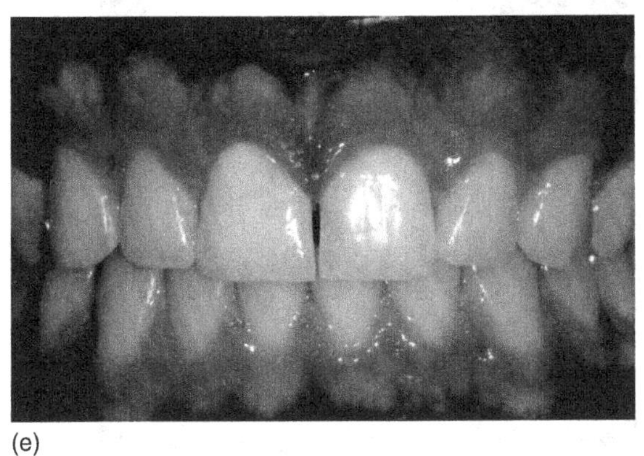
(e)

Figure 4.9 (c) Delayed passive eruption at an early stage of orthodontics. (d) Crown lengthening procedures to reestablish the normal relation between the BC and the CEJ. (e) The final result after periodontal and completion of orthodontic therapy.

2008; Monnet-Corti and Borghetti, 2008; Silderberg *et al.*, 2009).

The following three clinical parameters will allow us to distinguish a natural teeth eruption Type I-A or Type II-A from delayed (altered) passive eruption Type I-B or Type II-B (Coslet *et al.*, 1977; Goubron *et al.*, 2011):

- The quantity of keratinized gingiva is measured from the free gingival margin (FGM) to the mucogingival line, and is present in excessive (Type I-B) or limited (Type II-B) quantities.
- The distance obtained by sounding from the bone crest to the gingival margin is less than 1 mm.
- The alveolar bone crest is located at the teeth's cemento-enamel junction.

Summary

In conclusion, the gingival smile can result from various abnormalities (skeletal, muscular, dental, and physiological), and often a combination of several factors. Once the diagnosis of a gingival smile has been established on the smile at rest and the spontaneous smile, it is necessary to determine the cause. Since the gingival smile is of multifactorial origin, each particular etiology cannot be treated successfully until in-depth esthetic and etiologic diagnostics have been carried out (Nowzari and Rich, 2008). Once the correct treatment has begun, it will involve a multidisciplinary therapeutic plan – which is often quite complex – combining orthognatic orthodontics, osseous and perio-plastic surgery, and restorative treatments (Barbant *et al.*, 2011a).

The gingival smile therefore constitutes a real therapeutic challenge: it demands a rigorous overall procedure in which the surgeon, after having evaluated the nature of the anatomical disorders and the often multiple etiologies, should plan the optimal therapy. The clinician should also be aware of the relationship between hard and soft tissues, in addition to the definitive restorative or natural parameters to be achieved (Bitter, 2007), and must generally propose an interdisciplinary approach to treatment aiming to rebalance the proportions of the three elements that compose the smile – the lips, the teeth, and the gums – in harmony with the face (Garber and Salama, 1996).

A detailed explanation of the dental treatment of gummy smile etiologies will be presented in Chapter 5 (see "Crown lengthening procedures").

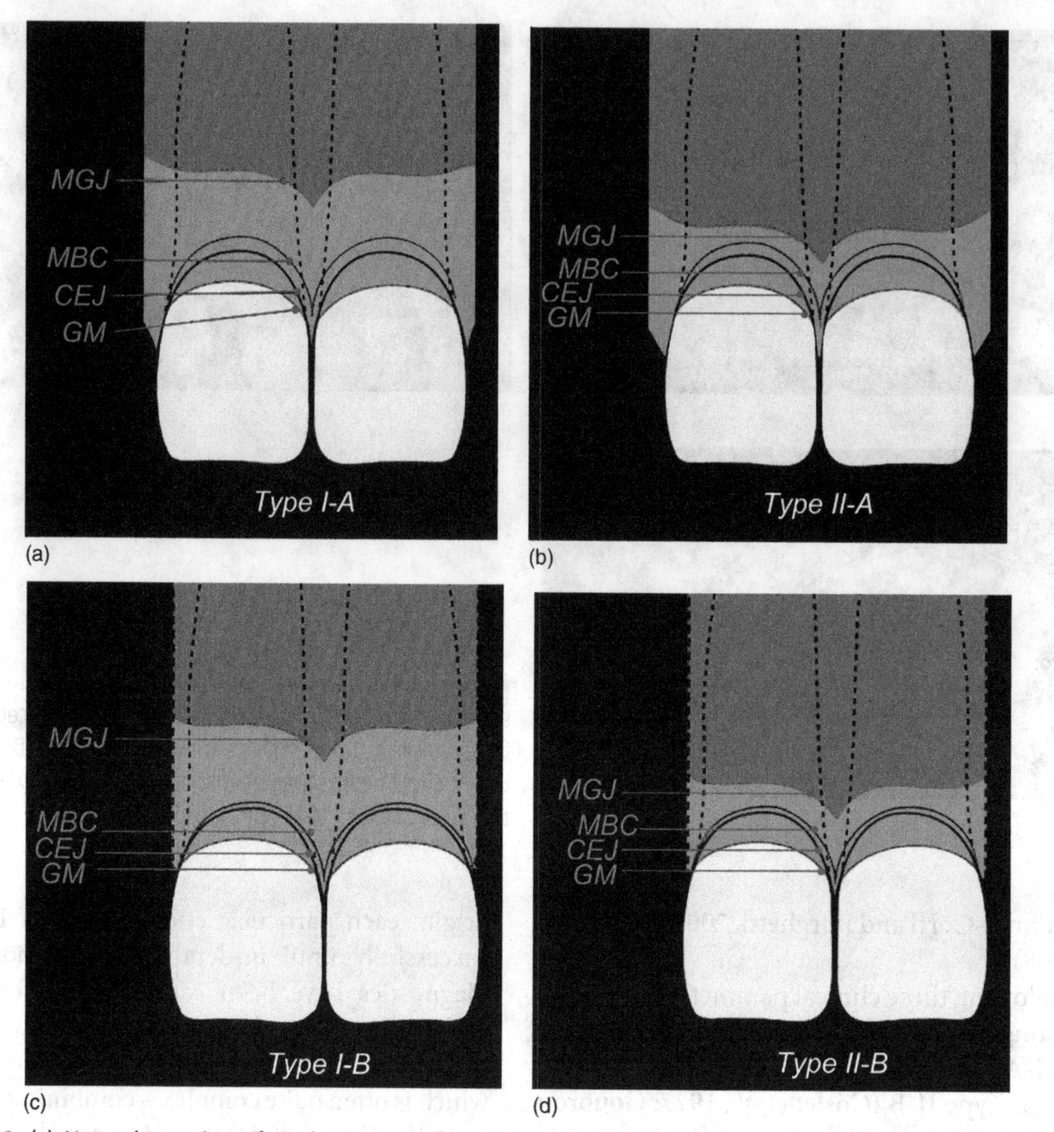

Figure 4.10 (a) Natural eruption of teeth: Type IA. (b) Natural eruption of teeth: Type IIA. (c) Delayed passive eruption: Type IB. (d) Delayed passive eruption: Type IIB. (Courtesy of Dr. G. Tirlet.)

Table 4.3 The classification of natural eruption and altered passive eruption in relation to the quantity of AKG and the relation between the CEJ and the marginal bone crest

Height of AKG and distance from CEJ to MBC	Type	Periodontal treatment
Large band of AKG: GM – MGJ > 3–5 mm > 1.5–2.0 mm between CEJ and MBC	I-A	Marginal internal bevel incision, *X* mm Gingivectomy and gingivoplasty
Limited AKG: GM – MGJ ≤ 3 mm > 1.5–2.0 mm between CEJ and MBC	II-A	Sulcular internal bevel incision Osteoectomy, apically repositioned flap
Large band of AKG: GM – MGJ > 3–5 mm < 1 mm between CEJ and MBC	I-B	Marginal internal bevel incision, *X* mm Osteoectomy, osteoplasty, or ARF
Limited AKG: GM – MGJ ≥ 3 mm < 1 mm between CEJ and MBC	II-B	Sulcular internal bevel incision Osteoectomy, osteoplasty, or ARF

AKG, attached keratinized gingiva; CEJ, cemento-enamel junction; GM, gingival margin; MBC, marginal bone crest; MGJ, mucogingival junction; ARF, apically repositioned flap.

Gingival recession

Gingival recession occurs when the location of the gingival margin is apical to the cemento-enamel junction. It results in exposed root surfaces, loss of marginal tissue, and loss of attachment, with functional and esthetic repercussions.

Gingival recession is a common clinical finding in both young and older populations, with periodontal disease resulting from poor oral hygiene and/or high standards of oral hygiene (Serino *et al.*, 1994; Dapril *et al.*, 2007). The prevalence and extent of recession increase progressively with age.

The most frequent etiologic factors associated with gingival recessions are tooth malposition, orthodontic movement beyond the alveolar plate, factitious injury, tooth mobility, iatrogenic factors related to the location of the restoration margins and periodontal treatment procedures, alveolar bone dehiscence, traumatic tooth brushing or toothbrush abrasion, and high muscle attachment with abnormal frenum (Maynard and Wilson, 1987; Saadoun, 2008).

Gingival recession has been classified by Miller (1985) (Figs 4.11a–c):

- Class I – no extension to the mucogingival junction (MGJ); no periodontal loss in the interdental bone and/or papilla.
- Class II – extension to or beyond the mucogingival junction; no periodontal loss in the interdental bone and/or papilla.
- Class III – extension to or beyond the mucogingival junction; partial periodontal loss in the interdental bone and/or papilla.

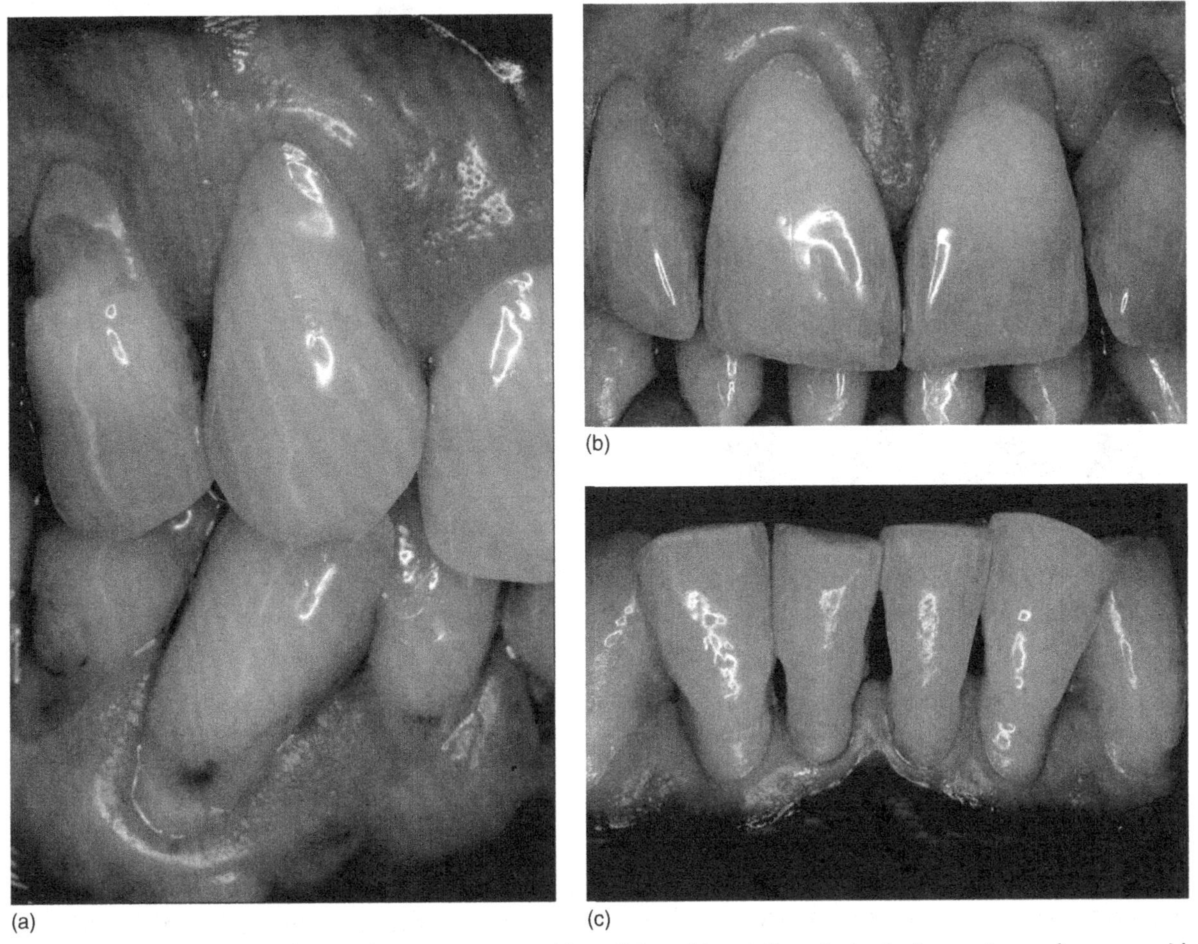

Figure 4.11 (a) Class I gingival recession on upper cuspid and bicuspid and Class II gingival recession on lower cuspid and bicuspid. (b) Class III gingival recession on upper central incisors. (c) Class IV gingival recession on the lower incisors.

- Class IV – extension to or beyond the mucogingival junction; severe periodontal loss of the mesiodistal interdental bone and/or papilla.

The prognosis of gingival coverage after periodontal surgery for single or multiple gingival recessions depends on the Miller classification and, in particular, on the height of the interproximal peak of bone to the apical teeth contact surface, adjusted to the recession and optimal stability of the graft (Holbrook and Ochsenbein, 1983) (Fig. 4.11d):

- Class I – total root coverage: 100%.
- Class II – total root coverage: 100%.
- Class III –partial root coverage: 50–75%.
- Class IV – minimum root coverage: 0–10%.

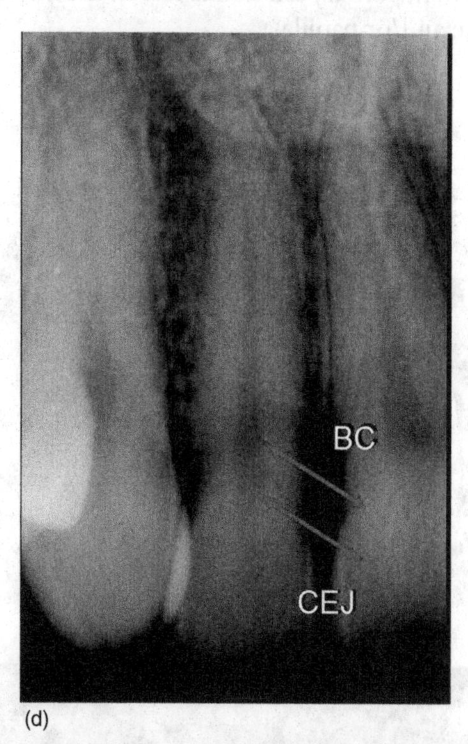

Figure 4.11 (d) The normal relationship between the adjacent CEJ line and the proximal bone crest.

Recently, a new method has been described to predetermine the root coverage in the esthetic zone: the line of root coverage (the level at which the soft tissue margin will be positioned after the healing process of the root coverage surgical technique) is predetermined by calculating the ideal vertical dimension of the interdental papillae of the tooth with marginal recession (Figs 4.11e, f). All of these gingival parameters should be taken into consideration during periodontal therapy, because complete root coverage is not always achievable in gingival recession – even with completely intact interproximal bone or attachment – if other

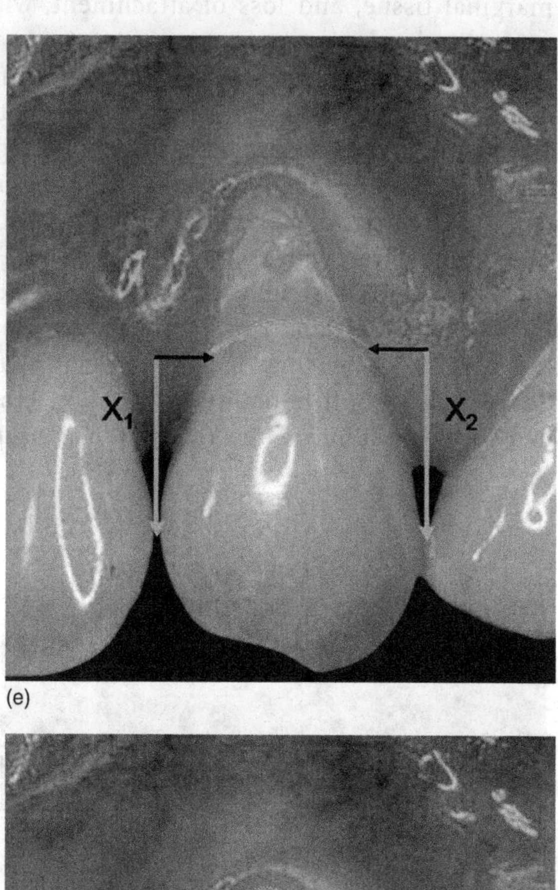

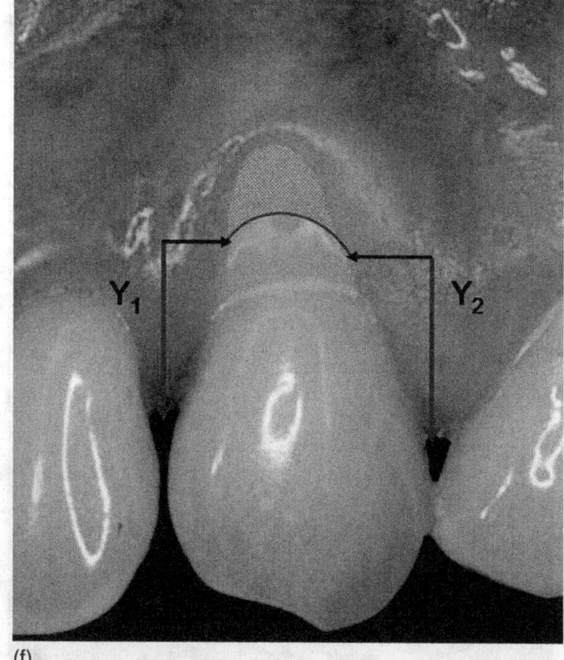

Figure 4.11 (e) The distance from the apical contact point to the recession mesiodistal line angle. (f) Transferring the mesial and distal distance from the tip of the papilla to the root surface determines the amount of root coverage (the blue shaded curve).

mitigating factors are present, such as traumatic loss of the tip of the papilla, tooth rotation, tooth extrusion with or without occlusal abrasion, or a cervical cemento-enamel defect (abrasion or abfraction) with obliteration of the cemento-enamel junction, and risk factors such as smoking (Zuchelli *et al.*, 2006).

The bone

The alveolar bone is the cornerstone of peri-implantology and also has a number of characteristics, such as (Fig. 4.12a):

- density – I, II, III, or IV (Misch, 1999)
- quantity – thickness and height
- topography – mesiodistal, buccolingual, or apico-coronal
- defects – horizontal, vertical, or combined, with or without dehiscence or fenestration on the buccal bone
- tooth relation – normal or inadequate.

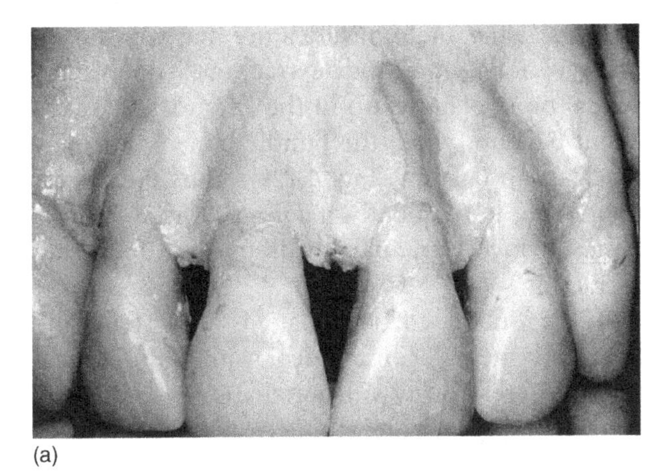

(a)

Figure 4.12 (a) On a healthy patient, the crestal bone may follow the CEJ and the underlying bone.

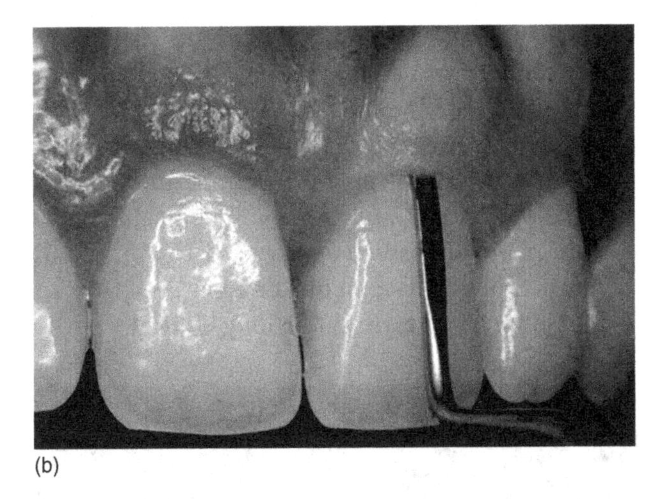

(b)

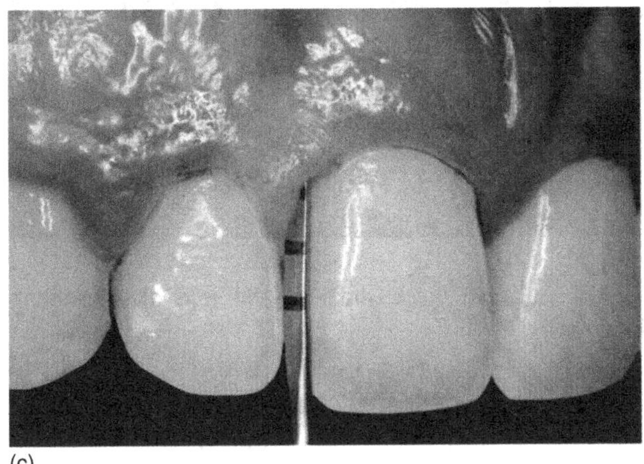

(c)

Figure 4.12 (b) Sounding the facial cortical bone. (c) Sounding the interproximal peak of bone.

In a periodontally healthy patient, the gingival margin follows the underlying osseous crest and the cemento-enamel junction. The sulcus depth is normally 1 mm and the distance from the midfacial gingival margin to the bone crest is 3 mm on the facial, while the distance from the adjacent apical contact point (ACP) to the peak of the interproximal bone is 5 mm (Garguiolo *et al.*, 1961; Tarnow *et al.*, 1992)

Bone sounding, usually performed under local anesthesia, is an important part of many surgical approaches, including crown lengthening. In an implant treatment plan, it is important to determine the level of the alveolar crest in order to decide upon the peri-implant surgical approach to be followed, and its feasibility (Figs 4.12b, c). Factors such as the thickness of the gingival tissue layer and the proximity of the alveolar bone are important considerations in crown lengthening and mucogingival procedures, and before tooth extraction, whether or not this is followed by immediate implant placement. To determine the level of the alveolar bone, a measuring instrument – a periodontal probe, or Chu's bone sounding gauge (Hu-Friedy Inc., Chicago, IL) – is used to penetrate below the gingival margin/proximal space until it reaches the underlying bone while the patient is under local anesthesia.

Pontoreiro and Carnevale (2001) have defined three osseous biotypes (Fig. 4.12d):

- Thick, with the osseous crest less than 2 mm from the cemento-enamel junction, a square tooth form, and a short clinical length.
- Medium or normal, with the osseous crest level at 2 mm from the cemento-enamel junction, an ovoid tooth form, and a medium clinical length.
- Thin, with the osseous crest level at more than 2 mm from the cemento-enamel junction, a triangular tooth form, and a long clinical length.

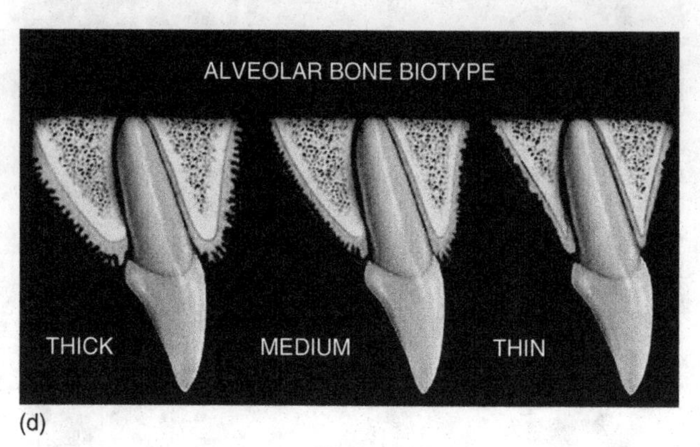

(d)

Figure 4.12 (d) Thick, medium and thin alveolar bone biotypes.

Most tooth sites (87% of cases) in the anterior maxilla have a thin facial bone wall with dehiscence and/or fenestration (Fig. 4.12e). As such, a thin bone wall may undergo a marked tridimensional

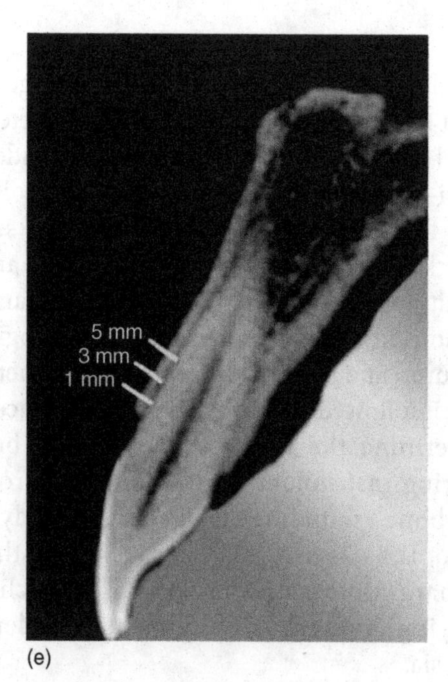

(e)

Figure 4.12 (e) The thickness of the buccal cortical plate varies depending on its vertical level.

decrease following tooth extraction. This must be taken into consideration before tooth removal, and before the planning of rehabilitation in the maxillary anterior segment of the dentition using an implant restoration. In the majority of cases, the buccal bone is thin and needs preservation and augmentation (Araújo *et al.*, 2011). The thickness of the cortical bone varies depending on its vertical level and the tooth on the arch (Table 4.4).

Table 4.4 The bone cortical thickness on maxillary anterior teeth

Bone crest apical location (mm)	Canine	Lateral incisor	Central incisor
1	0.6 ± 0.3	0.7 ± 0.3	0.6 ± 0.3
3	0.6 ± 0.4	0.7 ± 0.4	0.6 ± 0.4
5	0.6 ± 0.4	0.5 ± 0.4	0.5 ± 0.3

The alveolar process, with its corresponding volume, is the anatomical feature that we want to preserve following tooth extraction. The average buccal bone plate width in the anterior maxilla is about 0.5 mm, while the bundle bone width may reach up to 0.4 mm (Fig. 4.12f). Thus the buccal bone plate is frequently made up of only bundle bone, which gradually disappears following extraction.

If the buccal cortical plate is thin, then the bundle bone is confounded with the cortical bone. Therefore, it will automatically and completely disappear after tooth extraction (Araújo *et al.*, 2011).

As the concept of immediate implant placement becomes more widely accepted, understanding the importance of the sagittal root position through the use of cone bean computed tomography will provide vital adjunct data to treatment planning for immediate implant placement and provisionalization in the anterior maxilla. Furthermore, the proposed classification system for the sagittal root position may lead to improved interdisciplinary communication in treatment planning for implant-based therapy in the anterior maxilla.

Each sagittal root position in relation to its osseous housing is classified (Kan *et al.* 2011) as shown in Table 4.5.

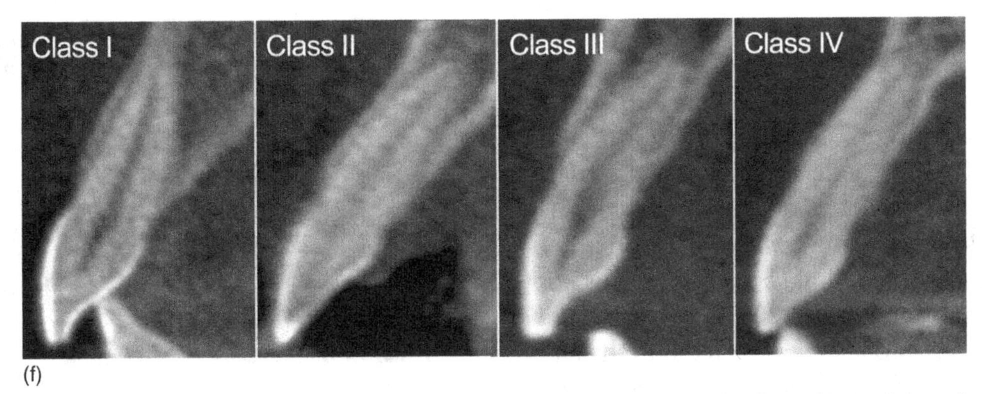

(f)

Figure 4.12 (f) The anterior maxillary root position in relation to its osseous housing: the closer the tooth is to the buccal cortical plate, the more chance there is of bone fenestration after extraction. (Courtesy of Dr. J. Kan and colleagues, Loma Linda, USA.)

Table 4.5 Classifications of each sagittal root position in relation to its osseous housing

Sagittal root position	Osseous housing relationship
Class I: 81.1%	The root is positioned against the labial cortical plate
Class II: 6.5%	The root is centered in the middle of the alveolar housing
Class III: 0.7%	The root is positioned against the palatal cortical plate
Class IV: 11.7%	At least two-thirds of the root is engaging in both cortical plates

Data from Kan *et al.* (2011).

After tooth extraction (Figs 4.13a, b), there is always (Araújo and Lindhe, 2005; Grunder *et al.*, 2005):

- removal of the circumferential and/or transeptal gingival fibers
- a loss of periodontal ligament vascularization
- no more nourishment of the bundle bone
- modeling and/or resorption of the buccal and crestal bundle bone
- a lack of transgingival fibers, with no supracrestal fibers around the implant
- marginal facial bone resorption and gingival recession
- an absence of marginal soft tissue esthetics.

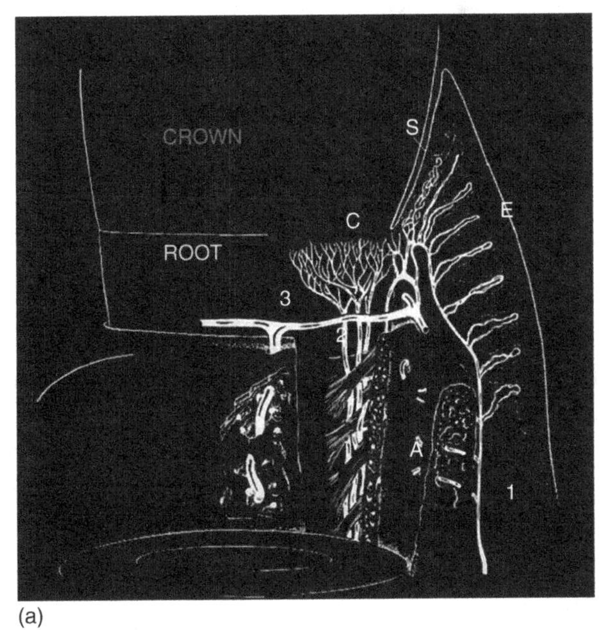

(a)

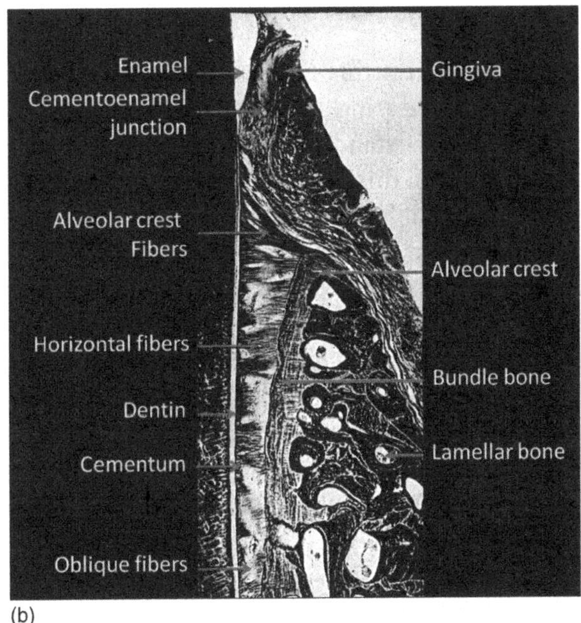

(b)

Figure 4.13 (a) A tooth still present in the alveolar socket, showing the PDL, bundle bone, and fibers. (b) A detail of the alveolar socket, the buccal cortical plate, and the gingival fibers.

In the 12 months following extraction, the buccal cortical plate loses 2–4 mm of its height and can decrease by up to 50% in width. Two-thirds of the bone resorption occurs during the first 3 months. The extent of buccal bone resorption is associated with the buccal bone width, and is twice as great when the bone thickness is < 2 mm. The association is non-linear and the 2 mm threshold accounts for this non-linearity (Araújo and Lindhe, 2005).

The extraction of one or several teeth in the anterior zone is always followed by bone resorption and a decrease of osseous volume and gingival thickness, with partial or total loss of intradental papillae (Fig. 4.13c).

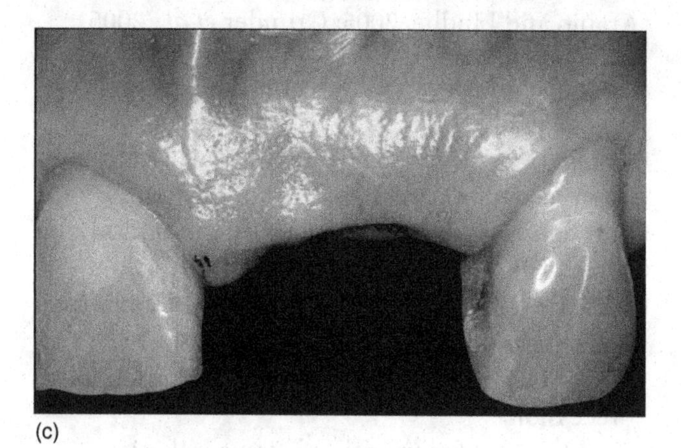

(c)

Figure 4.13 (c) The healed site 3 months after extraction, with buccal deformity.

In order to correct this tissue defect and to prevent aggravation during implant treatment, it is imperative to understand several biological factors which play a role in this process. It is recommended to use all the available procedures for bone and soft tissue regeneration, so that an optimal prosthetic integration can be obtained, one that blends in perfectly with the adjacent natural teeth (Touati, 2009).

In a study by Nevins *et al.* (2006), in comparison with the nongrafted sites, the dimensions of the alveolar process, as well as the profile of the ridge, were better preserved in Bio-Oss® grafted sites. The patient gains a significant benefit from receiving osteoconductive Bio-Oss® grafting material at the time of the extraction, with the loss of less than 20% of the buccal plate in 80% of cases.

The placement of a biomaterial in an extraction socket (Figs 4.13d–f) decreases the risk, and may modify the modeling and counteract the marginal hard and soft tissue ridge contraction that occurs following tooth removal.

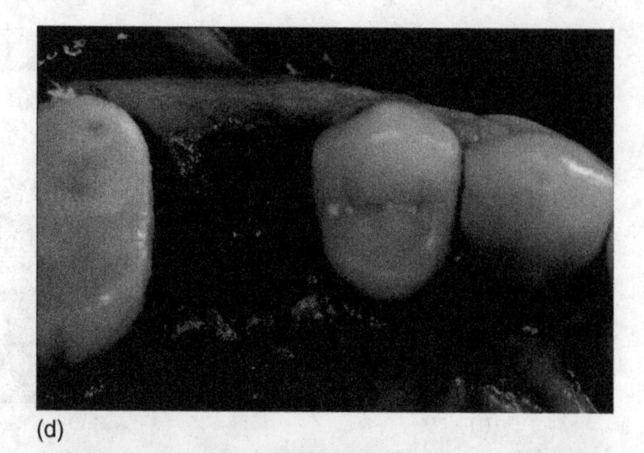

(d)

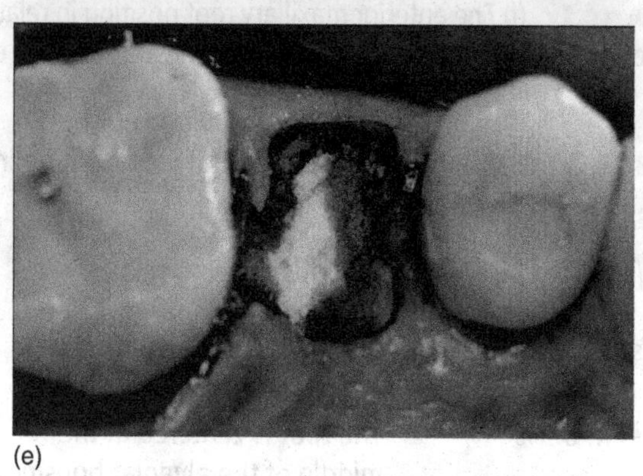

(e)

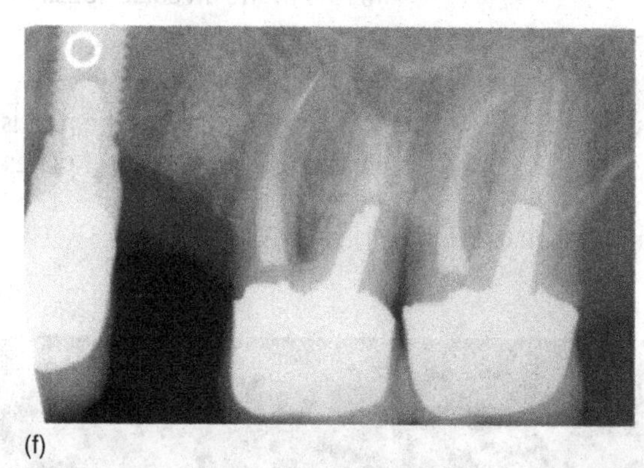

(f)

Figure 4.13 (d) The alveolar socket immediately after extraction. (e) A Bio-Oss® Collagen block in the alveolar socket. (f) An X-ray 3 months after the alveolar socket has healed, showing the Bio-Oss® graft.

The insertion of Bio-Oss® Collagen in the alveolar socket allows management of the loss of bone volume (Araújo and Lindhe, 2009):

- the resorption of the buccal cortical plate is counterbalanced
- the profile and the dimensions of the alveolar crest are preserved, and

- at the same time, new bone formation is activated inside the bone socket.

In a study by Araújo *et al.* (2006), the bone-to-implant contact that was established during the early phase of socket healing following implant installation was partly lost when the buccal bone wall underwent continued resorption. Therefore, implant placement failed to preserve the hard tissue dimensions of the ridge following tooth extraction. The buccal as well as the lingual bone walls were resorbed. In the buccal aspect, this resulted in a greater marginal loss of osseointegration in relation to the bone thickness.

It has been demonstrated that the placement of Bio-Oss® Collagen in the void between the implant and the buccal–cortical bone walls of fresh extraction sockets modifies the process of hard tissue healing, provides additional amounts of hard tissue at the entrance of the previous socket, improves the level of marginal bone-to-implant contact, and maintains the level of the soft tissue margin (Paolantonio *et al.*, 2001; Botticelli *et al.*, 2003, 2004).

Grafting the fresh extraction sites with Bio-Oss® Collagen, followed 3–4 months later by implant insertion, has shown that the amount of mineralized bone increased from about 29% (2 weeks) to about 45% (4 weeks) of the volume of the newly formed tissue (Araújo *et al.*, 2011).

A loss of bone is evident in the majority of clinical situations. Indeed, after anterior tooth extraction, the residual bone thickness is less than 1 mm. In the majority of clinical situations, the residual bone thickness is insufficient to allow for good vascularization, inducing an irreversible loss of the cortical bone. Today, it is recommended not only to try to preserve this area by means of a nontraumatic flapless extraction, but particularly to prepare the site automatically by adding a bone graft and a 2 mm thickness of soft tissue. This will allow three-dimensional augmentation of the site and the maintenance of the bone tissue in this area (Ishikawa *et al.*, 2010).

A pre-extraction buccal cortical plate evaluation (on the midfacial and proximal areas) (Figs 4.14a–c) should become a prerequisite before and after extraction, to determine the surgical and prosthetic implant treatment plan (Elian *et al.*, 2006). Upon evaluation of the surgical site, the primary goal of therapy is to preserve the favorable hard and soft tissue architecture, which is closely related to the biotype

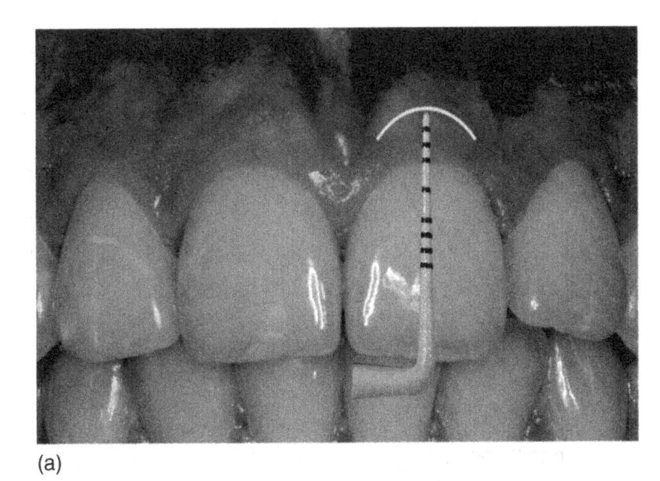

(a)

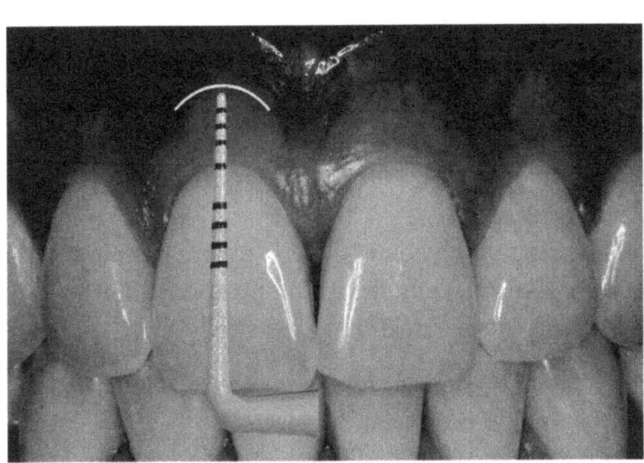

(b)

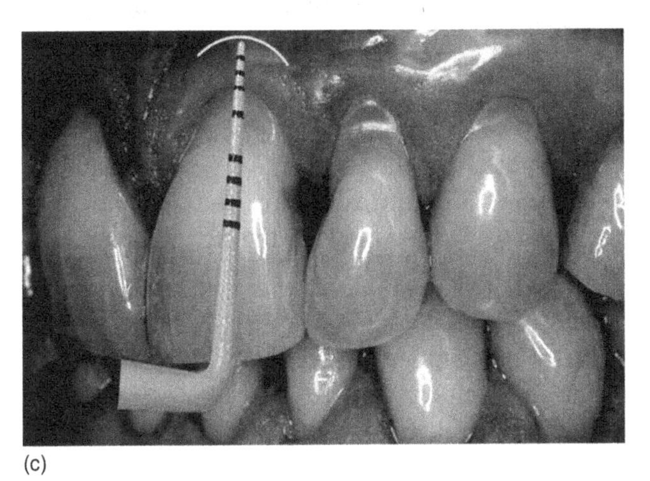

(c)

Figure 4.14 (a) A pre-extraction buccal cortical plate sounding evaluation: (a) normal bone level; (b) bone dehiscence; (c) recession and/or bone dehiscence.

and to the quality and quantity of the underlying structural alveolar bone. Several changes occur in the vertical height of peri-implant gingival and/or crestal bone after exposition and restoration with one- or two-unit dental implants. In a 3–5-year longitudinal prospective study, more gingival recession occurred

Table 4.6 Alveolar socket surgical management and implant placement timing

Classification	Alveolar socket and buccal bone quality	Implant replacement procedures	Immediate loading
Class IA	Intact with thick gingival biotype	Flapless, with immediate implant placement	Optimal
Class IB	Intact with thin gingival biotype	Immediate implant with CTG	Good
Class II	Alveolar socket with facial defect	Immediate/delayed, with GBR/CTG: SSS/NSRT	Unacceptable
Class III	No alveolar bone housing	SSS/NSRT: delayed/late implant placement	N.A.

CTG, connective tissue graft; NSRT, new socket repair technique; GBR, guided bone regeneration; SSS, socket seal surgery.

around wide-diameter versus standard-diameter implants (Small *et al.*, 2001). It is widely accepted that osseous and soft tissue remodeling occurs within 6 months.

The current alveolar socket surgical management and implant placement timing protocols (Table 4.6) following tooth extraction are as follows:

- Alveolar socket without buccal wall defect: alveolar socket preservation.
- Alveolar socket with buccal wall defect: bone crest preservation and/or augmentation.
- Absence of alveolar bone crest: alveolar socket sealing to protect the space for guided bone regeneration (GBR).

Depending on the alveolar socket morphology that remains after the extraction, the implant could be placed using the following timing regimen:

- Immediate implant placement after extraction, with temporization.
- Immediate implant placement after extraction, without temporization.
- Early delayed, 6–8 weeks after extraction: non-submerged, one stage.
- Delayed, 8–12 weeks after extraction: submerged, two stages.
- Late delayed: site development prior to or in conjunction with implant.

Immediate implantation (Figs 4.15a–e)

Immediate implant placement must respect precise indications and contraindications, and presents some advantages (Saadoun, 2002):

- Immediate implant placement indications:
  - Sufficient bone volume at the implant site.
  - An intact buccal cortical plate, for soft tissue stability.
  - An apical bone height sufficient for primary stability of the implant.
  - The existence of interproximal bone peaks between adjacent teeth, for regeneration of the papillae.
- Immediate implant placement contraindications:
  - The absence of primary stability caused by a large alveolar socket or the absence of apical bone.
  - A sensitive technique for implant anchorage.
  - The presence of significant microbacterial infectious lesions can affect the therapeutic result.
  - Acute soft tissue inflammation because of untreated periodontal disease.
  - Advanced periodontal disease, with loss of the bone surrounding the teeth.
  - Sub-optimal implant integration. As a result, it becomes necessary to delay the placement of the provisional crown.
  - An absence of soft tissue to cover the extraction site.
  - The thickness of the periodontal biotype can affect the esthetic results.
  - No correlation between the implant and the alveolar socket.
- Advantages of immediate implant placement:
  - Fewer soft tissue procedures are necessary, which indirectly limits the cervical bone resorption. This biological phenomenon is systematic

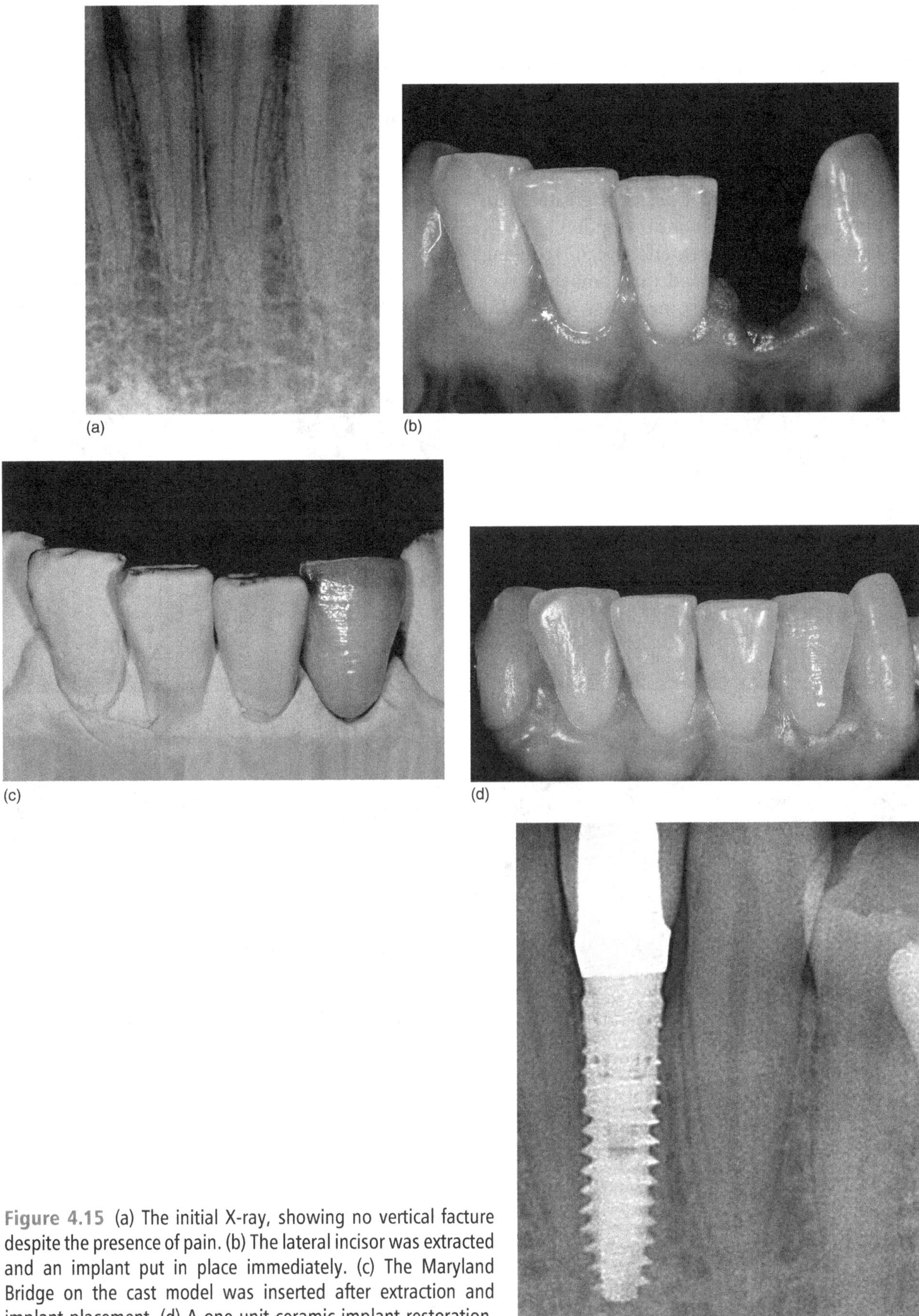

Figure 4.15 (a) The initial X-ray, showing no vertical facture despite the presence of pain. (b) The lateral incisor was extracted and an implant put in place immediately. (c) The Maryland Bridge on the cast model was inserted after extraction and implant placement. (d) A one-unit ceramic implant restoration. (e) The final X-ray, showing a perfect connection between the implant and the restoration. (Courtesy of Dr. G.C. Pongione, Rome, Italy.)

and significant during the first 3 months, and can result after in the loss of 40% of the height and 60% of the thickness of the alveolar socket.
- The immediate placement of a long resorbing allograft material in the alveolar socket, especially if the horizontal defect is greater than 2 mm, will also limit bone resorption.
- This technique is very effective in reducing the treatment time, and the number of surgical sessions that are necessary, compared with more traditional methods.
- Implant placement with primary stability greater than 35 N cm will allow immediate loading with a temporary crown.
- If the provisional crown can be placed without any functional contact, this technique provides optimal implant integration and a guided soft tissue healing/esthetic.

Delayed implantation (Figs 4.16a–g)

The tooth should be extracted delicately, to preserve all potential bone and the quantity of gingiva, and a

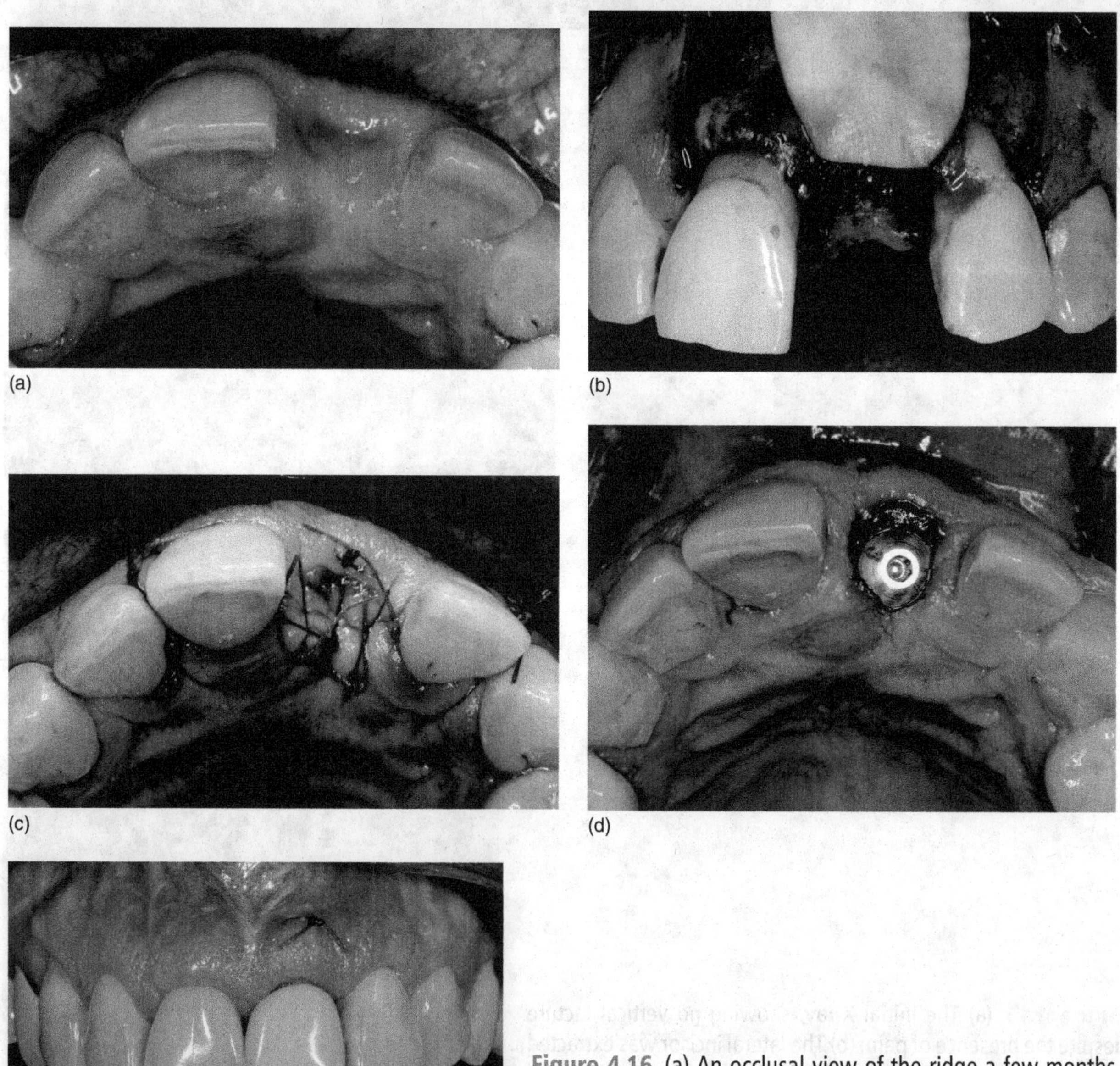

Figure 4.16 (a) An occlusal view of the ridge a few months after the extraction. (b) Delayed implant placement with a bone graft and membrane. (c) An occlusal view of the ridge at the end of the surgical session. (d) Exposition of the implant with the CTG roll flap procedure. (e) The temporary crown and buccal suture to secure the CTG.

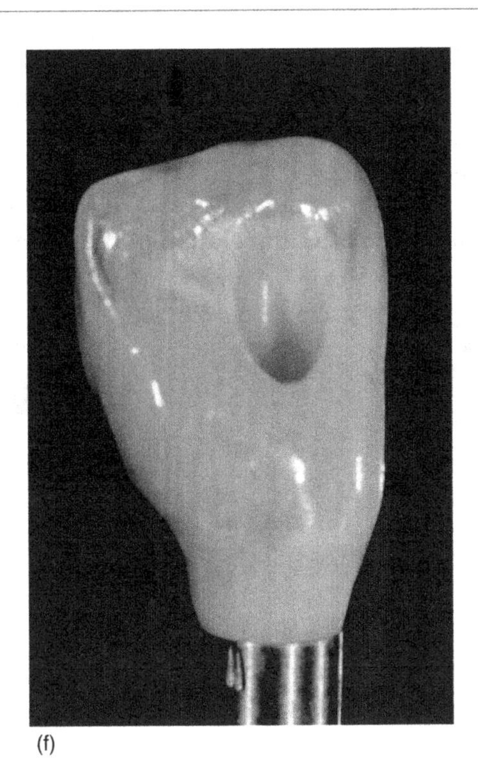

(f)

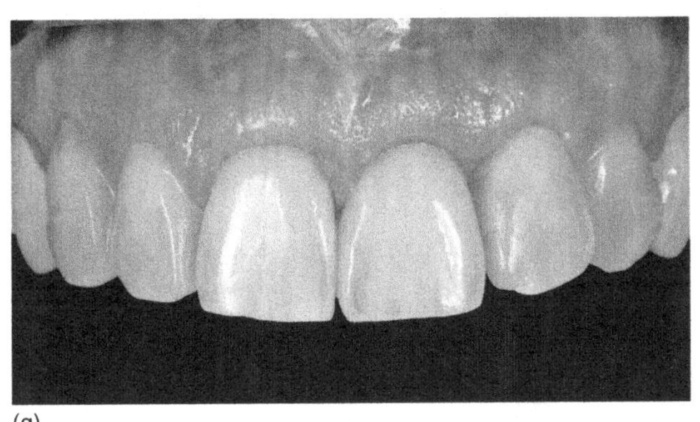

(g)

Figure 4.16 (f) A lingual view of the one-screw type final implant restoration. (g) The harmonious gingival contour of the esthetic implant ceramic restoration. (Courtesy of Dr. P. Margossian, Marseille, France.)

removable acrylic resin denture or a bonded provisional denture with a convex pontic should be inserted immediately to guide the healing of the soft tissue. With early delayed implantation, the soft tissue is mature and bone resorption is usually limited. Implantation is carried out 6–8 weeks after extraction, when the soft tissue has covered the extraction site. A roll procedure during the implant exposition phase will increase the thickness of the buccal tissue. Delayed implantation performed 8–12 weeks after extraction is preferred as a satisfactory esthetic outcome for patients with a thin gingival type.

In an esthetic zone, a flap preserving the adjacent papilla should be avoided to prevent scarring of the vertical releasing incision. An autogenous bone or xenograft covered with a resorbable membrane and a connective tissue graft can be used before, or in conjunction with, implant placement to maintain or increase buccal thickness. This prevents or limits the bone resorption and soft tissue retraction that always occur after extraction.

Delayed implant placement in a three-dimensional position performed after 6–8 weeks of soft tissue healing, combined with a simultaneous guided bone regeneration procedure, allows the rebuilding of the hard and soft tissue contours. The midterm follow-up of 2–4 years showed that the risk of mucogingival recession was low with this treatment concept (Buser *et al.*, 2008).

Late implantation or site development

Late implantation and loading is recommended in the case of a narrow or deformed anterior alveolar ridge, where the ridge morphology may not allow the correct placement of the implant and will fail to result in an esthetic outcome. Therefore, it is necessary to use a two-stage surgical approach, using guided bone regeneration with an autogenous graft and an allograft membrane, and/or a connective tissue graft before, or in conjunction with, implant placement if necessary, to recreate the overall bone and gingival contour.

A bonded provisional restoration will prevent loss of papilla height and soft tissue contour, and may also enable implant healing without micromovement, as well as decreasing patient discomfort.

Various techniques of both hard tissue (bone block or particulate) and soft tissue augmentation (epithelio-connective graft or membrane) can be used to achieve implant restorations which best mimic natural, healthy teeth and their supporting structures.

Socket seal surgery, using a subepithelial connective tissue graft placed over the bone graft in the alveolar socket, augments the quality and quantity of the soft tissue around and above the implant to be placed or exposed at the second stage, as well as having a wound-protection capacity.

The classical indication for socket seal surgery with a connective tissue graft is recommended when all of the socket walls remain intact, no recession is allowed, and/or no primary stability exists for immediate loading. Therefore:

- The implant is placed immediately after extraction, during the site development procedure, if primary stability can be achieved. After implant osseointegration, a tissue punch will be then enough to expose the implant head with a cover screw (Figs 4.17a–i).
- The implant could also be placed at the second stage, after integration of the bone in the

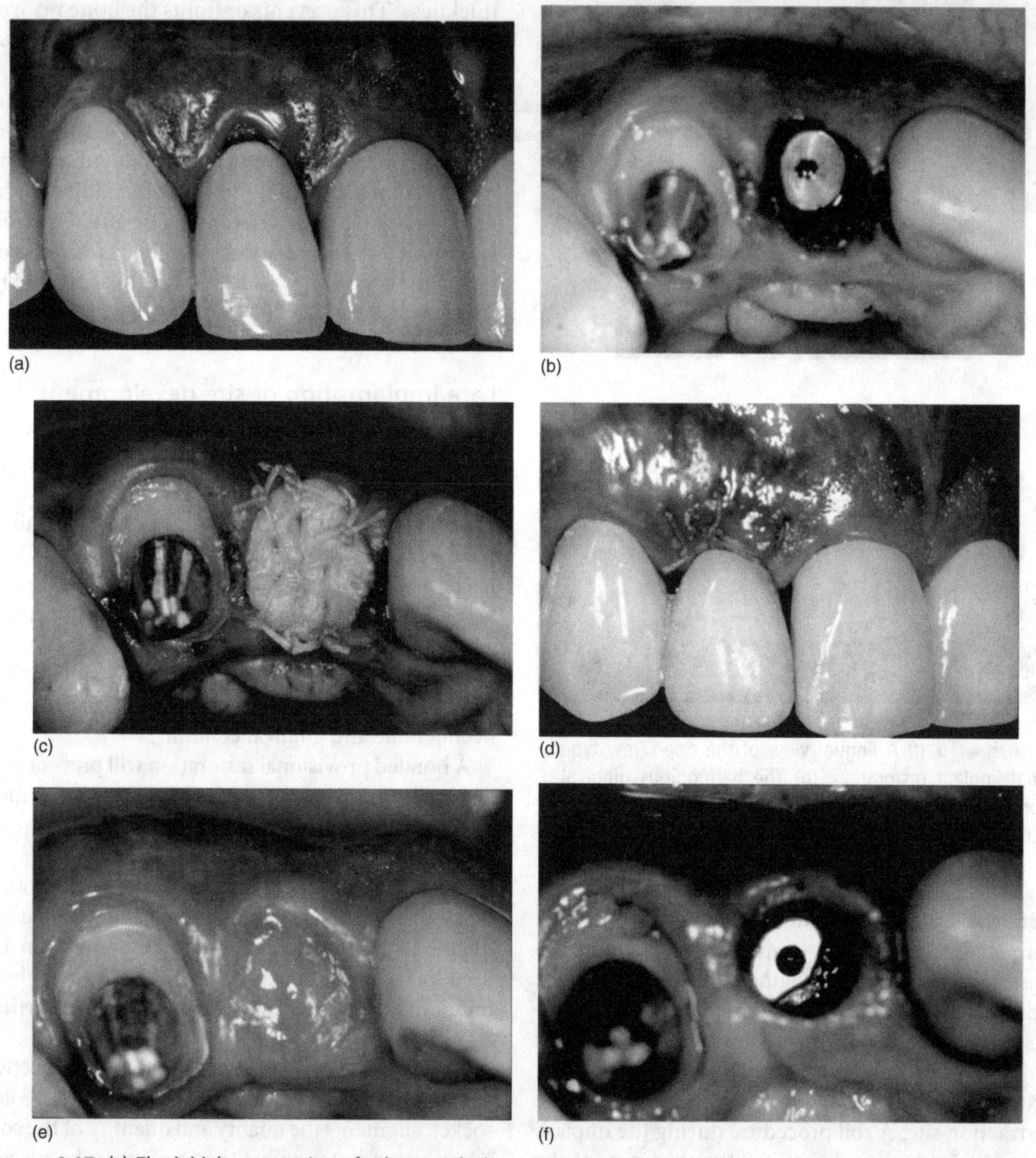

Figure 4.17 (a) The initial presentation of a loose right lateral incisor (RLI) and right cuspid (RC). (b) Immediate implant placement with a cover screw after extraction of the RLI/RC post-core. (c) Socket seal surgery on the RLI site with key suture points. (d) An immediate temporary bridge, with a crown on the RC and a pontic on the RLI. (e) Bridge removal after 6 months, showing an optimal gingival contour. (f) A slightly palatal punch was performed to expose the implant cover screw and an anatomical healing abutment was placed into the implant.

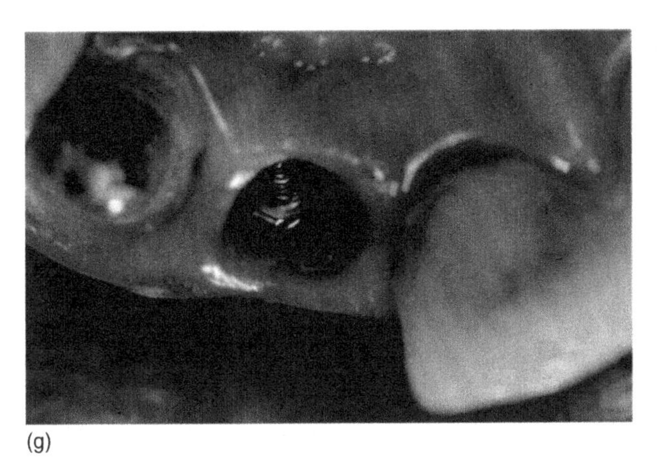

(g)

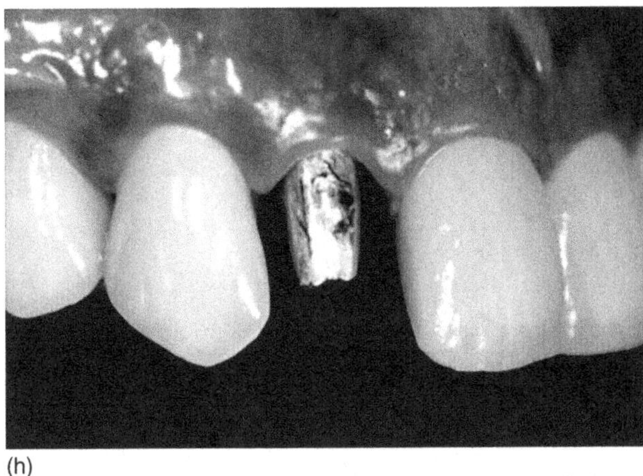

(h)

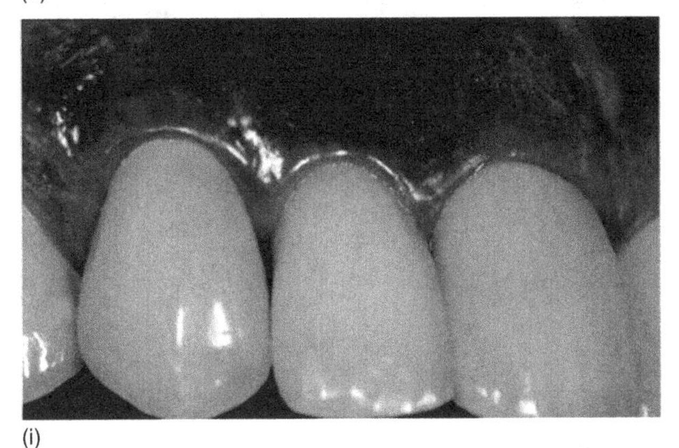

(i)

Figure 4.17 (g) The emergence profile on the RLI after removal of the healing abutment. (h) The final implant abutment and temporary crown on the cuspid. (i) Ceramic tooth restoration on the RC and ceramic implant restoration on the left cuspid at 6 months. (Courtesy of Dr. C. Landsberg, peri-implantologist, Dr. R. Amid, Restorative dentist, and Mr. R. Lahav, Tel Aviv, Israel, Laboratory technician.)

alveolar socket, if there is no apical bone for primary stability.

- Soft tissue recession is minimized by enhancing the width of the labial margins and the interproximal papillae. The soft tissue height and width are preserved, and the clinician's ability to design and sculpt the soft tissue contour around the implant restoration is enhanced to impart an optimal esthetic outcome (Landsberg, 1997, 2008).

Successful management of the extraction socket can be challenging, particularly in the esthetic zone. When the tooth is compromised with osseous and/or gingival defects, the precaution principle must prevail, given that the sequences are more numerous and the duration of treatment is longer. The implant should only be placed when the conditions are favorable and the mucosal environment is optimal. The total maturation of tissue, and especially the reformation of the papilla height, requires more time than has previously been thought (Touati, 2011). Proper management is necessary to ensure that the implant used to support a restoration will remain stable. A simple, noninvasive approach to the grafting and management of sockets when soft tissue is present but the buccal plate is compromised following tooth extraction has recently been described (Elian *et al.*, 2007).

In the new socket repair technique (NSRT), a correctly sized resorbable membrane can also be placed onto the internal walls of the extraction socket, plugged under the palatal flap, and sutured to the palatal margin to cover the defect, and the socket filled with an effective bone grafting material, eliminating the need for flap reflection and limiting the external cortical bone resorption. The implant is then placed 4–6 months later, using a tissue punch procedure (Figs 4.18a–l).

When comparing immediate implant placement and the other implant timings, there is evidence to suggest that immediate restoration and conventional loading protocols appear to have similar outcomes with respect to soft tissue alterations:

- According to Chen *et al.* (2009), immediate implant placement does not make any difference

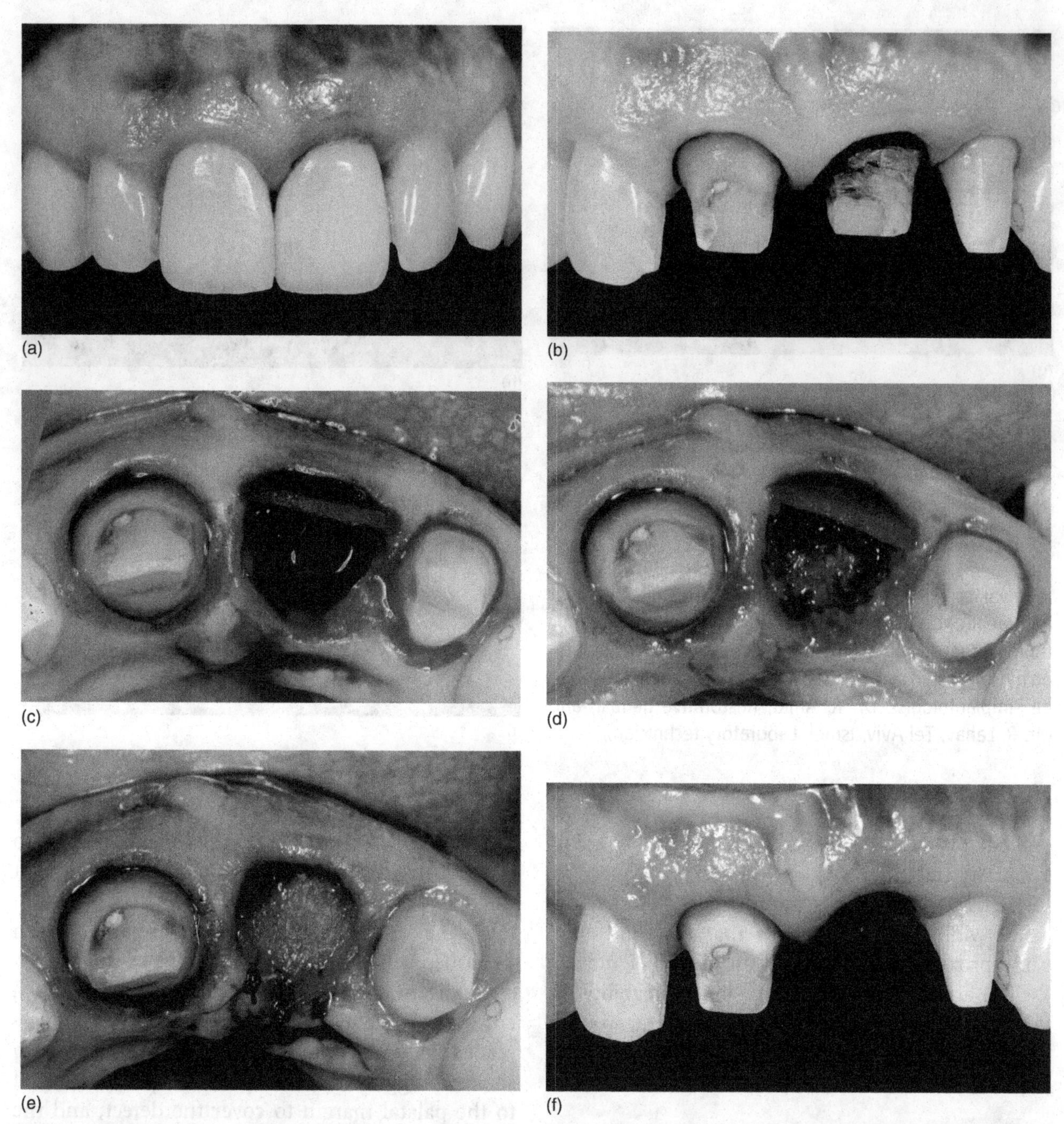

Figure 4.18 (a) An old restoration on the two central incisors, with amalgam tattoo on the AKG. (b) The important apical infection of the left central incisor was an indication for extraction. (c) An occlusal view of the alveolar socket after deep curettage and disinfection, with no absence of buccal wall. (d) A cone-shaped resorbable membrane is inserted inside the alveolar socket, against the internal wall of the buccal bone. (e) The alveolar socket is then filled with xenograft material and covered by the membrane, which is stabilized with some sutures on the palatal flap. (f) A buccal view at the end of the surgical session, showing slight coronal retraction.

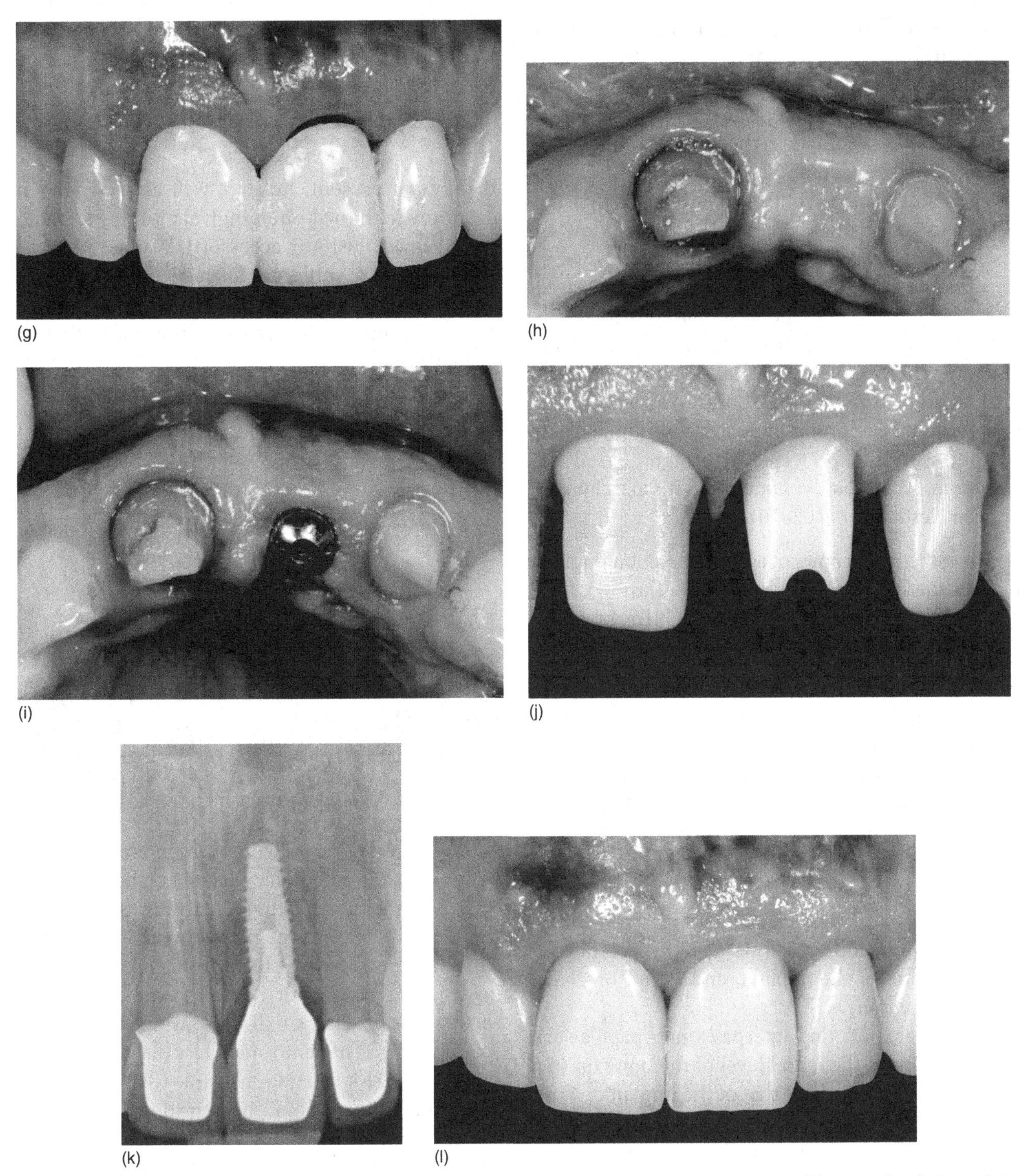

Figure 4.18 (g) A three-unit temporary bridge is cemented, with no pressure on the pontic site. (h) An occlusal view of the ridge 5 months later, with full healing of the socket graft and minimal deformation. (i) The implant is placed through a tissue punch with a healing abutment, at 6 months from the extraction/grafting time, in an optimal 3D position and angulation. (j) The ceramic shell is adjusted on the tooth and the zirconium implant abutment is screwed in 6 months after implant placement. (k) A radio-alveolar X-ray of the tooth and implant restoration. (l) The final tooth and implant restoration, with an optimal gingival contour and papilla height. (Courtesy of Dr. D. Tarnow, peri-implantologist, and Dr. S. Chu, restorative dentist, New York, USA.)

compared with delayed implant placement with regard to bone loss. Although patient-evaluated esthetic outcomes with post-extraction implants are generally favorable, there are relatively few studies that evaluate esthetic outcomes using objective parameters.

- This randomized controlled study, comparing soft tissue changes 3 and 6 months following extraction, failed to identify differences between patients treated with immediate or delayed approaches for mid-buccal or interproximal soft tissue margins, although greater decreases in ridge width were observed in sites lacking bone grafting.
- Both immediate and delayed treatment approaches appear to be appropriate following tooth extraction, with the preferred treatment based on factors other than resultant soft tissue changes (Van Kesteren *et al.*, 2010).

The esthetic outcomes of a post-extraction implant present the following characteristics (Tarnow *et al.*, 1992; Jemt, 2004; Schropp *et al.*, 2005; Darby *et al.*, 2009; Tawil, 2009):

- Tissue alterations leading to recession of the facial mucosa and papillae are common with immediate placement (Classes IA and IB).
- There is evidence that early or delayed placement (Classes II and III) is associated with a lower frequency of peri-implant gingival recession compared to immediate placement (Classes IA and IB).
- Risk indicators for recession with immediate placement include a thin tissue biotype, a buccal malposition of the implant, and a thin or damaged facial bone wall.
- The height of the interproximal papillae is dependent on the initial level of the bone on the adjacent teeth, and not that of the implant.
- The risk of papilla loss is seven times greater in delayed versus immediate implant placement. However, there is no significant difference at 1.5 years because of soft tissue remodeling.
- If the distance between the contact point and the bone crest is < 5 mm, papilla always regenerates between an implant and the adjacent tooth.
- In the case of implant placement in the esthetic anterior zone, the two-stage approach is recommended in the presence of a thin biotype, or a connective graft should be plugged buccally during immediate implant placement to change the biotype.

The teeth

If they are present, healthy, well-aligned, and in harmony with the bone/gingival biotype, teeth are the ultimate fashion accessory. Visible beautiful teeth during a smile conform to today's ideal of beauty (Fig. 4.19a). In today's society, they have become a major component of the image that we display to others.

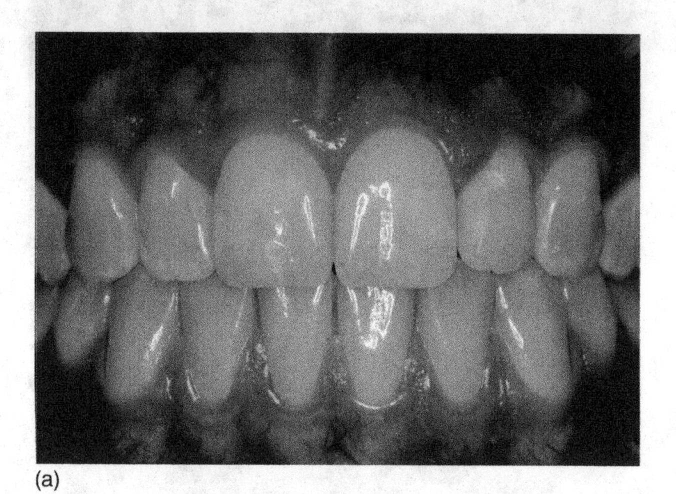

(a)

Figure 4.19 (a) A young woman's beautiful teeth.

Studies about dental composition emphasize the proportions of maxillary incisor teeth (with their width:height ratio) rather than their dimensions, the ideal proportion ranging between 75 and 80%. This differentiates long teeth from short teeth. It is evident that short teeth – even those shortened due to wear – and also small-dimensioned teeth in a worsening case of dento-maxillary disharmony, will increase the risk of a gummy smile (Robbins, 1999).

Several factors should be considered in relation to the teeth:

- morphology – triangular, ovoid, square, or rectangular (Figs 4.19b–e)
- position and orientation – ideal or malpositioned (Fig. 4.19f)
- dimensions – length and width in proportion, diameter
- the bone/gingiva relation – optimal or inadequate (Fig. 4.19g).

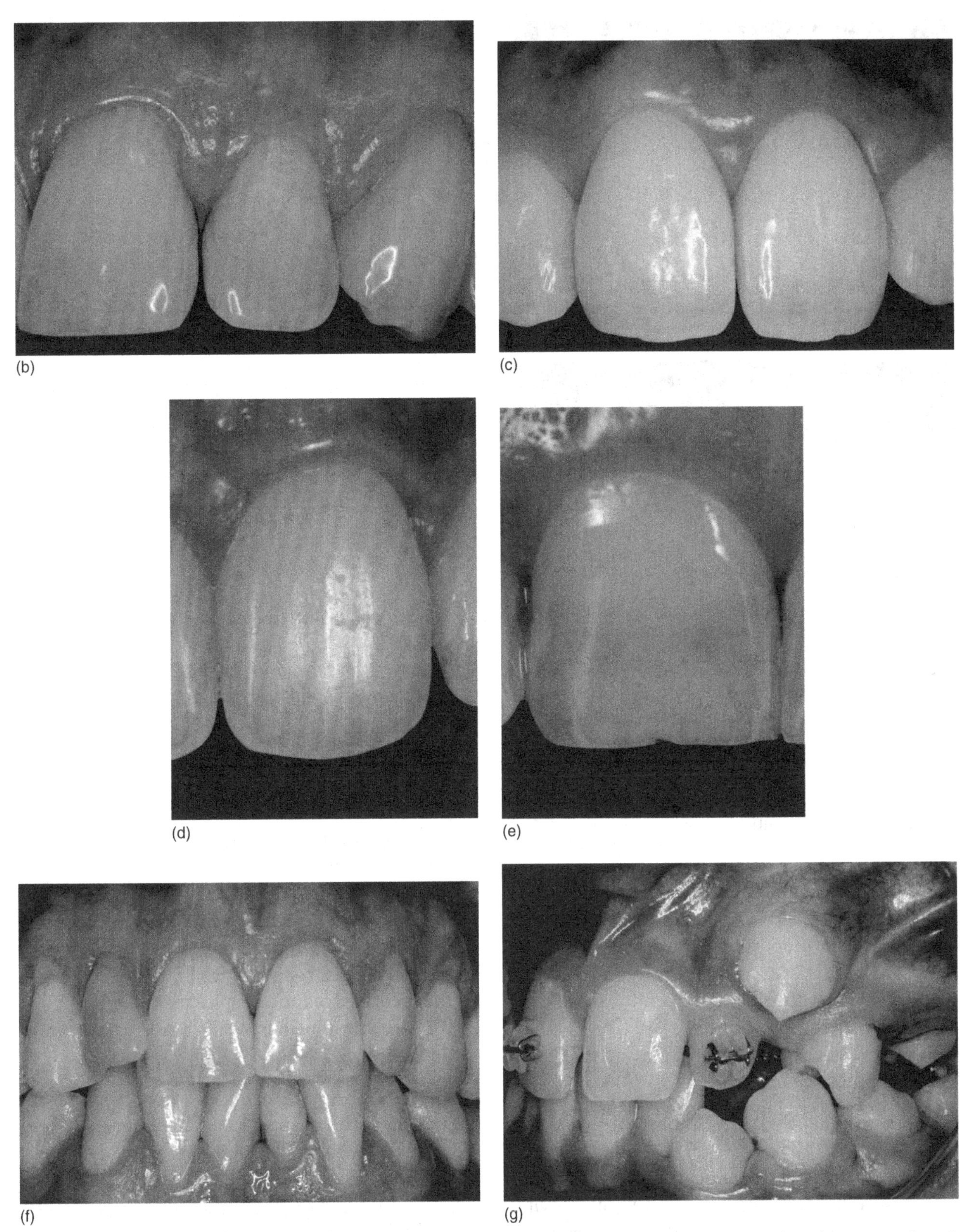

Figure 4.19 (b) Triangular teeth, related to the thin biotype. (c) Ovoid teeth, related to the medium biotype on female. (d) A rectangular tooth, related to the medium biotype on male. (e) A square tooth, related to the thick biotype. (f) Malpositioned teeth on a 40-year-old man. (g) Crowded left teeth before extraction of the first premolars.

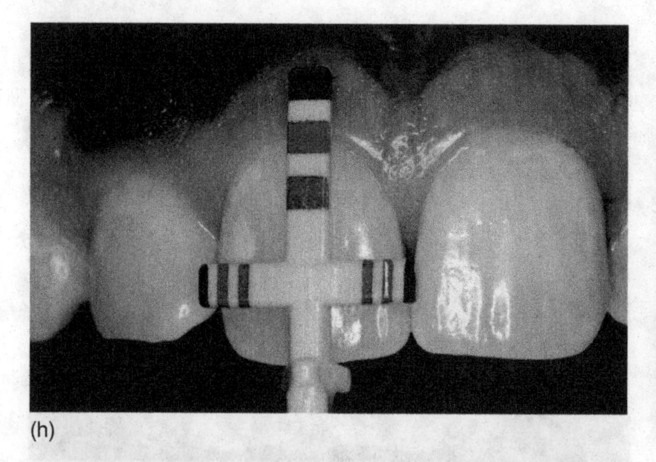

(h)

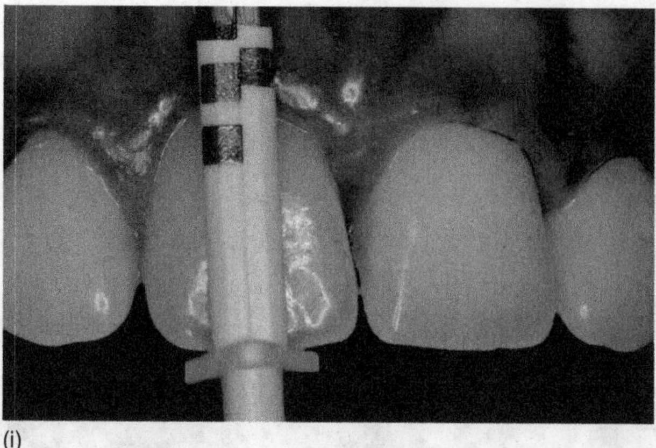

(i)

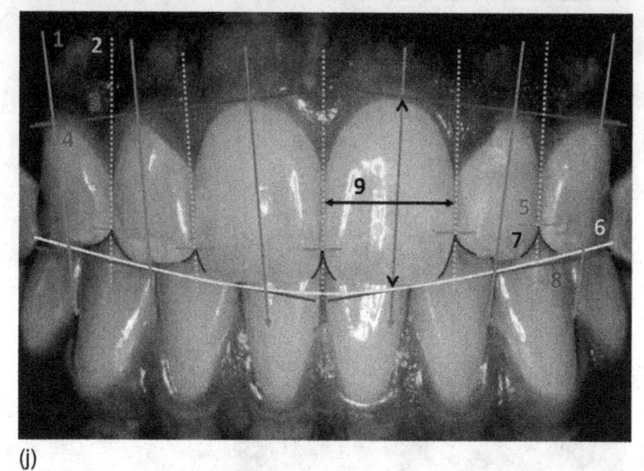

(j)

Figure 4.19 (h) Chu's T-bar, to check if the tooth is in ideal proportion. (i) The In-line Bar used for crown lengthening procedures. (j) A diagram of the ideal anterior maxillary tooth relation and position.

- contact point – high or low
- surface of contact – small or large.

Several parameters must be considered when designing an esthetic smile, including:

- the width-to-length ratio of the maxillary central incisors (0.75–0.80)
- the mesiodistal proportional width of the maxillary anterior teeth
- the position of the maxillary central incisors in the face (i.e., the "e" position)
- the relative gingival zenith position and the height contour of the gingival margin
- an assessment of gingival control (Charruel *et al.*, 2008).

Innovative esthetic measurement gauges (T-bar and In-line) introduce a means of objectively quantifying tooth size discrepancies (Figs 4.19h, i) and enabling the clinician to perform esthetic restorative dentistry with success and predictability (Chu *et al.*, 2008).

There is a well-defined anterior dental composition from the right bicuspid to the left bicuspid, based on the following criteria (Fradeani, 2004) (Fig. 4.19j):

- axial teeth inclination (1)
- tooth position – their arrangement in relation to each other (2)
- gingival outline at a harmonious level and the related zenith (3, 4)
- occlusal interdental contact areas (5)
- the curve of the tooth component of the smile, from the incisal edge to the cuspid tip (6)
- the inter-incisal edge angles (7)
- the incisal edges and cuspid tips (8)
- the tooth proportions, or the ratio between width and length (9).

Following detailed observations of natural teeth, categories of appearance attributes have been developed, with classifications assigned in each category. These definitions are comprehensive and provide a utilitarian description of all the essential features that comprise tooth appearance other than shade (Weinstein, 2008).

The width of the average maxillary central incisor has been measured at approximately 10–11 mm (Chiche and Pinault, 1994). Using the "Golden Proportion" as a guide, one can arrive at an appropriate measurement for the width and the length of the central incisor. The next consideration is that the width-to-length ratio of an esthetic maxillary central incisor is 75–80%. Thus, the 10 mm long central incisor should measure 7.5–8.0 mm mesiodistally if it is proportionally correct. The "e" position is esthetically desirable so that a patient can show 50–70% of the maxillary incisor teeth.

In a study by Chu *et al.* (2008), the central incisor, the lateral incisor, and the canine teeth were found to vary in width from 5.5 mm to 8 mm, 4.5 mm to 6 mm, and 4.5 mm to 7 mm, respectively, and nearly 90% of the patients fell within ±0.5 mm of the combined gender-normative values. An average discordance of dentition exists in a population of male and female patients. Chu *et al.* found that the mean values and normal distribution differed significantly between genders, with females consistently 0.5–1.0 mm smaller than males. The average maxillary incisal display varies according to gender, being 3.4 mm for females and 1.9 mm for males (Tucker, 2009).

Mandibular anterior teeth are more consistent in size and variability than maxillary anterior teeth, the mean discordance values being 50% and 36%, respectively, and 90% (i.e., at ±0.5 mm) and 80%, respectively. The average mandibular incisal display also varies according to gender, being 0.5 mm for females and 1.2 mm for males (Tucker, 2009).

Unlike the maxillary anterior teeth, in which gender differences exist for all tooth groups, in the study by Chu *et al.* (2008), only the mandibular canine tooth group showed a gender difference, which is a critical factor in restoration. This finding is clinically relevant in that proper tooth biometry must be diagnosed and identified for each patient before any tooth or implant restoration is attempted, in order to create an esthetically pleasing smile and functional occlusion.

Symmetry of the central incisors is critical for an esthetic smile, while symmetry of the lateral incisors and canines is not as critical (Fradeani and Barducci, 2004). Nevertheless, studies of the symmetry of the tooth display have demonstrated that a small amount of asymmetry does not destroy the harmony of the smile. This result shows the importance of a global analysis of symmetry, taking into account the entire face and not just the buccal region (Zlowodzki *et al.*, 2008).

Tooth disproportion, such as a lateral incisor shaped like a grain of rice, could easily be treated with a bonded composite or a laminate veneer (Figs 4.20a–c).

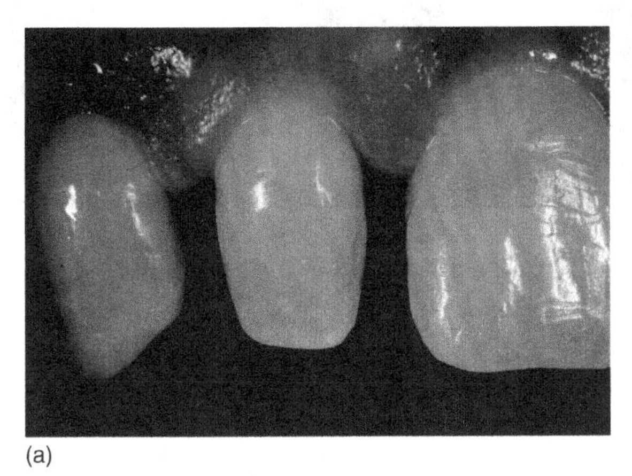

(a)

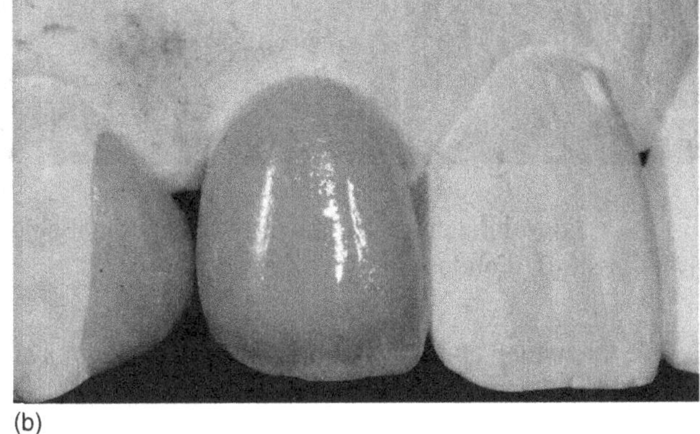

(b)

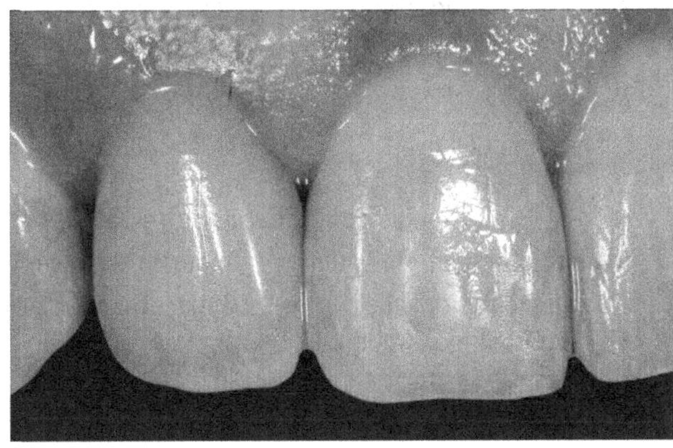

(c)

Figure 4.20 (a) A rice-shaped lateral incisor, with interproximal diastema mesially and distally. (b) A ceramic chip on the cuspid and a large laminate veneer on the lateral. (c) The esthetic result 1 month later, with excellent PES/WES, reestablishment of the tooth proportions, and a normal height of the mesiodistal papillae. (Courtesy of Dr. G.C. Pongione, Rome, Italy.)

Natural passive eruption

The period of tooth eruption is very long. It takes 10 years or more for the periodontal structure to reach dimensional stability and its final size. While the teeth are reaching their occlusion, by a natural process of active eruption, another process is running in parallel, which is the apical migration of the marginal gingiva until 2 mm of sulcular depth is obtained (Monnet-Corti and Borghetti, 2008; Toca *et al.*, 2008). According to Gargiulo *et al.* (1961), natural passive eruption can be described in four different stages (Figs 4.21a, b), depending on the junctional epithelium (Foley *et al.*, 2003; Monnet-Corti and Borghetti, 2008; Toca *et al.*, 2008; Barbant *et al.*, 2011b).

The natural apical migration of the marginal gingiva in relation to the cemento-enamel junction due to physiological/functional passive teeth eruption is defined in four stages, as shown in Table 4.7.

The interproximal bone height and the interdental implant papilla

When teeth are present, an interesting phenomenon occurs. The gingiva on the facial surface of the tooth

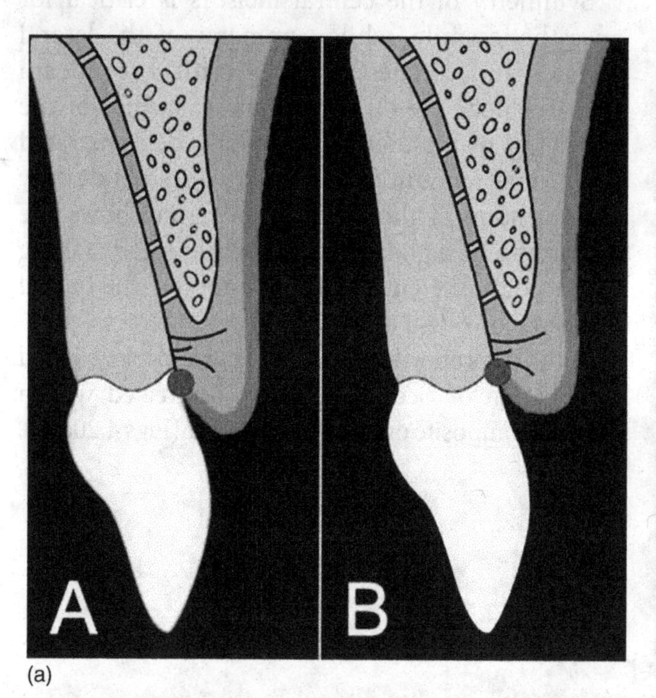

(a)

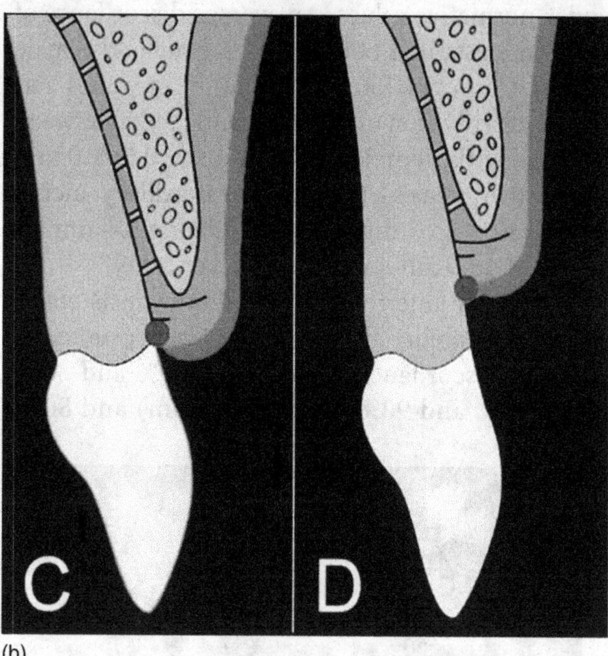

(b)

Figure 4.21 (a) Natural apical migration of the marginal gingiva: Class A-B. (b) Natural apical migration of the marginal gingiva: Class C-D. (Courtesy of Dr. G. Tirlet.)

Table 4.7 The natural apical migration of the marginal gingiva in relation to the CEJ due to physiological/functional passive teeth eruption

Class	The junctional epithelium …	Clinical crown height	Bone Level/CEJ relation
A	… is in contact with the enamel	Two-thirds of the height of the anatomical crown	Correct relation; no apical bone migration
B	… is at the CEJ level	Three-quarters of the height of the anatomical crown	Correct relation; no apical bone migration
C	… is at or below the CEJ, but totally on the root cementum	Equal to the height of the anatomical crown	Correct relation; no apical bone migration
D	… migrates apically below the CEJ, exposing more root	Greater than the height of the anatomical crown	Bone Level is more apical than the correct relation with the CEJ

Data from Gargiulo *et al.* (1961), Coslet *et al.* (1977), and Barbant *et al.* (2011a).

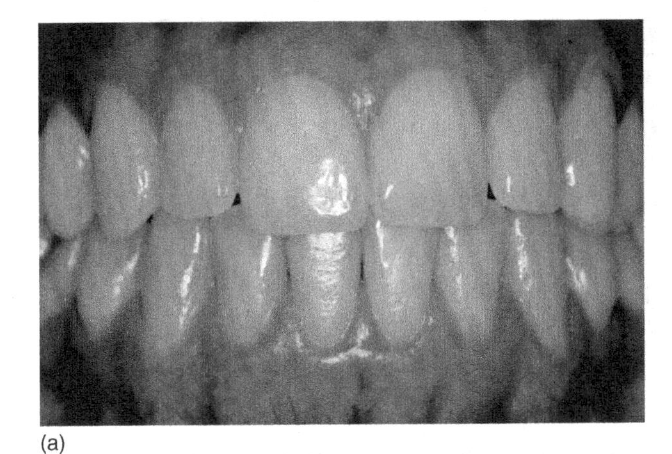

(a)

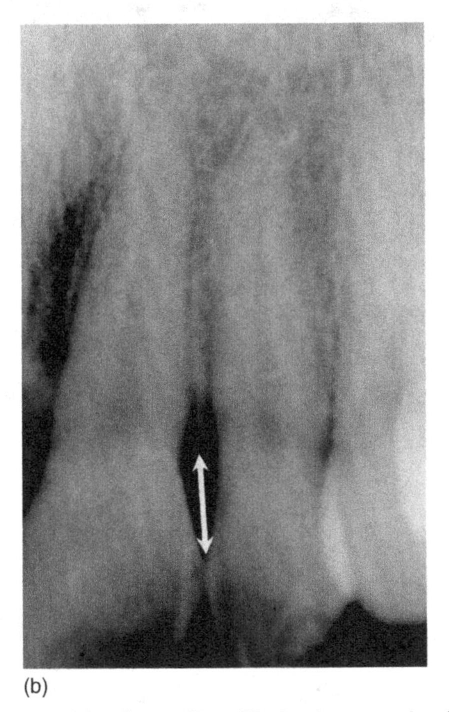

(b)

Figure 4.22 (a) All papillae fill the interproximal spaces between well-aligned teeth. (b) The interproximal crestal bone is at the correct level from the contact point and the tooth prognosis is in relation with the apical contact point and the proximal bone crest.

is positioned so that, on average, the free gingival margin is 3 mm coronal to the bone crest. However, the interproximal papilla between teeth is positioned, on average, 4.5–5.0 mm coronal to the interproximal bone crest, 1.5 mm on average more coronal to the crest of bone than the facial tissue (Figs 4.22a, b). This additional 1.5 mm, along with the 3 mm average proximal osseous scallop, results in the tip of the papilla being on average 4.5–5.0 mm coronal to the facial free gingival margin (Spear, 2008).

Table 4.8 The relationship between the IP, the ACP, and the IABC

ACP/IABC (mm)	Papilla regeneration (%)
< 5	100
5	98
6	56
7	17
8	10

IP, interproximal papilla; ACP, apical contact point; IABC, interproximal alveolar bone crest.

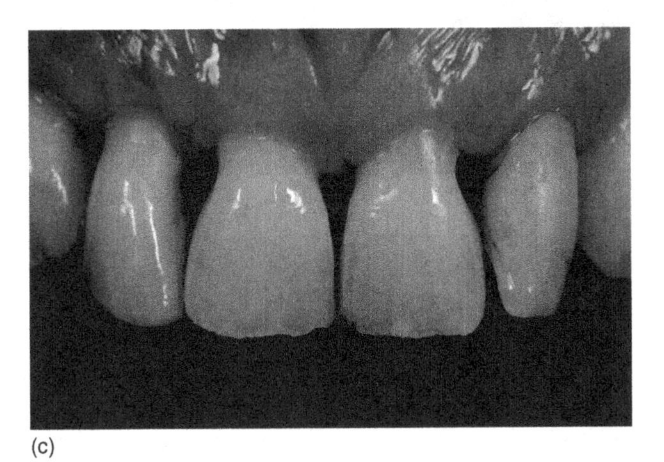

(c)

Figure 4.22 (c) The clinical aspect of the interdental spaces, with the absence of papillae and a long triangular incisor after periodontal surgery.

The interproximal dental relation

There is a relationship (Table 4.8) between the height of the papilla (IP), the apical contact point (ACP), and the interproximal alveolar bone crest (IABC). Each increase of this distance by 1 mm will decrease the potential percentage of papilla regeneration (Tarnow *et al.*, 1992).

There is also a relationship (Fig. 4.22c) between the apical contact point, the height of the papilla, the height of the interproximal alveolar bone crest (IAHB or IABC), and the tooth prognosis (Salama *et al.*, 1998):

- *Class 1 IHB.* Optimal prognosis: 2 mm from the cemento-enamel junction, or 4–5 mm from the apical contact point – at point A.

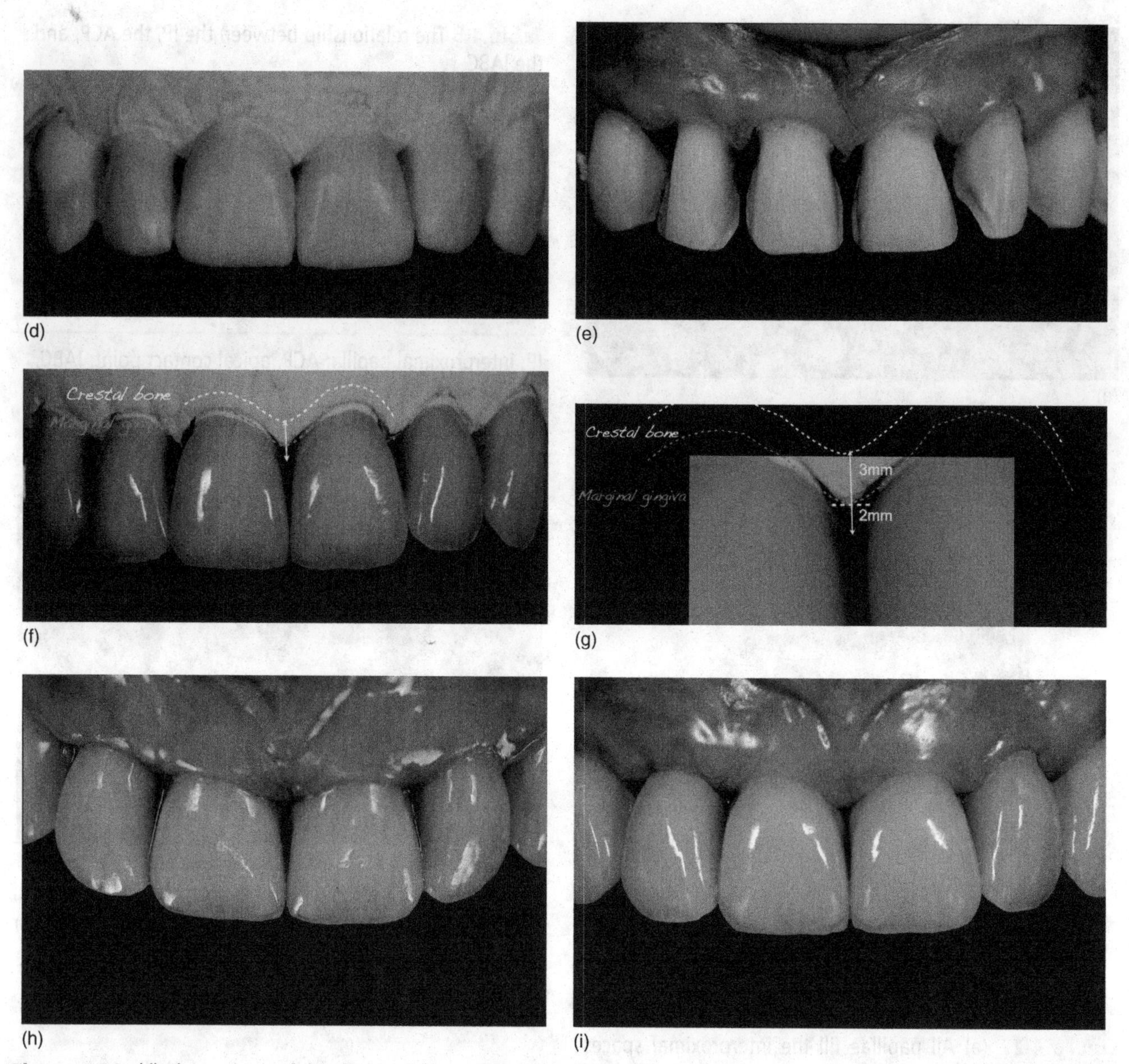

Figure 4.22 (d) The wax-up of the diagnosis cast model, closing the interproximal spaces with a harmonious teeth shape. (e) Laminate preparation, leaving homogeneous available space with palatal return on the six anterior teeth. (f) Ceramic laminate veneers on the cast model. (g) Building the apical contact surface to reestablish the normal 5 mm distance from the interdental bone crest. (h) Laminate veneers restoring contours, and the interproximal bone distance and apical contact surface at the end of the cementing session. (i) Regeneration of the gingival margin and the interproximal papillae after 8 weeks. (Figures (c)–(i) courtesy of Dr. S. Koubi, restorative dentist, Marseille, France.)

- *Class 2 IHB.* Guarded prognosis: 4 mm from the cemento-enamel junction, or 6–7 mm from point A.
- *Class 3 IHB.* Poor prognosis: >5 mm from the cemento-enamel junction, or >7 mm from point A.

The interdental papilla does not exist, or is incomplete, if:

- the interproximal bone is destroyed by periodontal disease or changes after periodontal surgery (Figs 4.22c–i)
- the tooth shape is too triangular, or the width of the lateral incisor is small (Fig 4.20a–c)
- there is adjacent root proximity
- there is excessive adjacent root divergence
- there is a large diastema (Figs 4.23a–c).

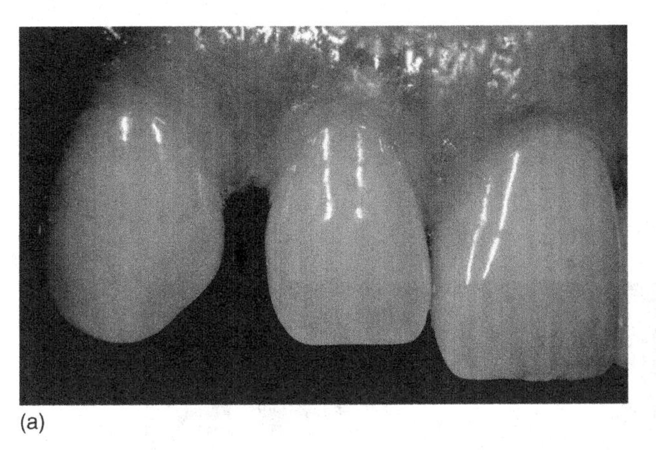
(a)

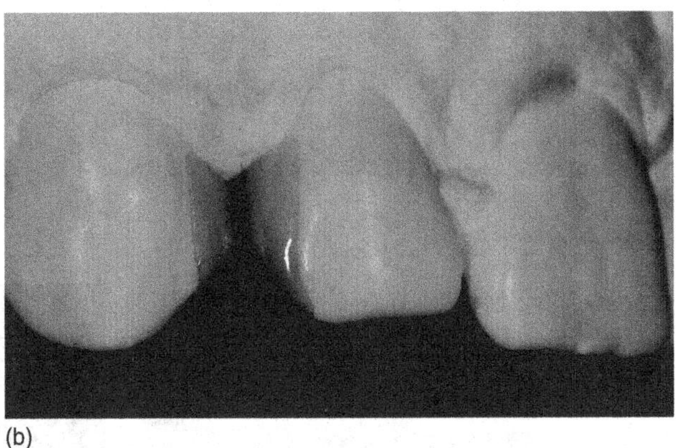
(b)

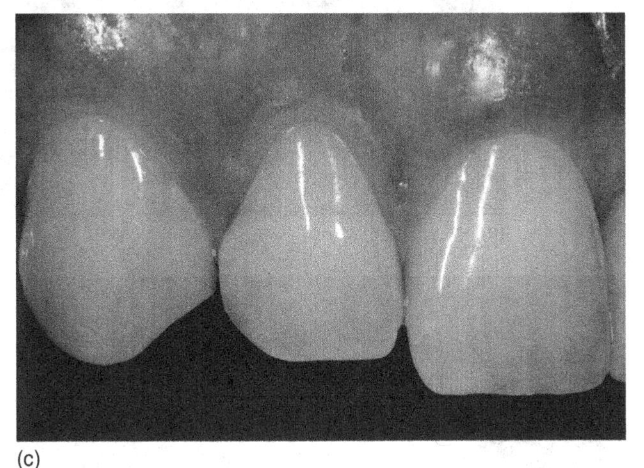
(c)

Figure 4.23 (a) A large diastema between the right cuspid and the lateral incisor. (b) A buccal view of the two adjacent ceramic chips on the mesial of the cuspid and the distal of the lateral. (c) The final esthetic outcomes, with regeneration of the papilla. (Courtesy of Dr. G.C. Pongione, Rome, Italy.)

There is a relation between the contact surfaces of teeth and the height of the interdental papilla (Tarnow, 2008) (Figs 4.24a–d):

- the contact surface gives the shape of the collar
- the smaller the contact surface, the higher is the papilla
- the larger the contact surface, the lower is the papilla
- the papilla becomes shorter from the central incisor to the canine and to the molar
- the papilla height is 40% of the tooth length from the zenith point
- the top of the papilla is 60% of the tooth length from the incisal edge.

There is also a relation between the height of the teeth contact surfaces and the height of the interdental papilla (Chu *et al.* 2008) (Figs 4.24e, f):

- the mesial and distal papillae are of about equal height
- the apical point of the contact surface area determines the height of the papilla
- the interproximal bone crest determines the height of the papilla
- the height of the surface of contact decreases from the central incisor to the molar (Figs 4.24g, h).

It appears that Tarnow *et al.*'s rule (1992) does not apply in the same way to teeth and implants (Tarnow *et al.*, 2003). The height differences measured between the inter-implant and interdental papillae can be explained by the low vascularization and specific attachment of peri-implant tissues. The periodontal ligament and bundle bone are absent at the implant level. Although known as a stress absorber, the periodontal ligament also plays a major role in the vascularization of soft tissues. This vascular plexus prevents exterior aggression and promotes healing. It is less developed at the peri-implant soft tissue level, which is thus more fragile.

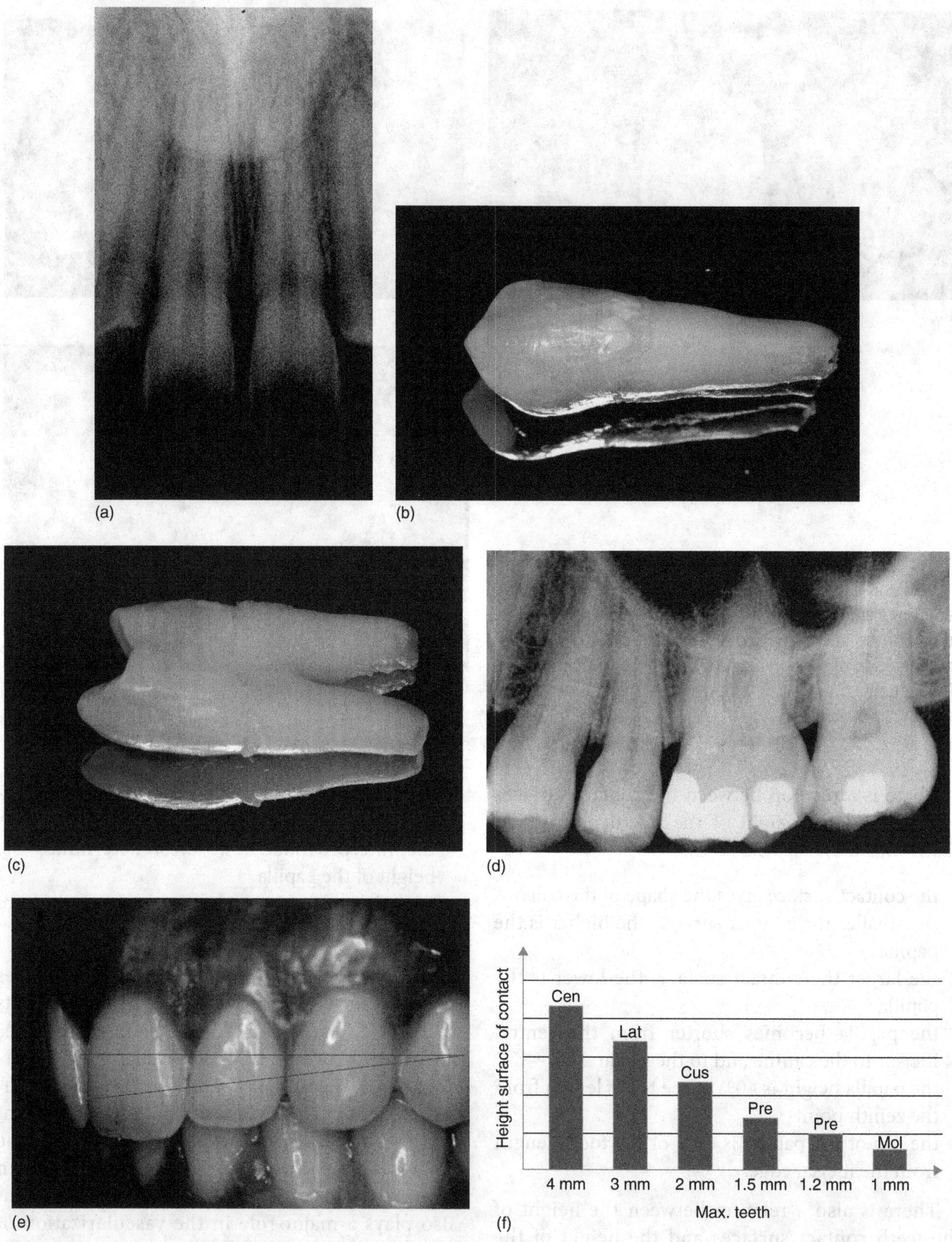

Figure 4.24 (a) The height of the papilla decreases from the anterior to the posterior areas. (b) The buccal CEJ has a more pronounced curved shape on the premolar. (c) and a flat curve on the distal proximal surface. (d) The height of the bone peak decreases from the distal of the cuspid to the molar. (e) The height of the contact surface decreases from the central to the molar. (f) The proximal contact length and height decrease from the anterior to the posterior area (according to Tarnow, 2008).

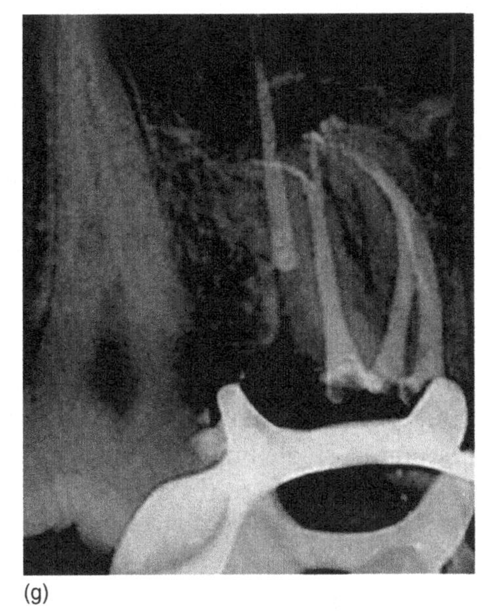

(g)

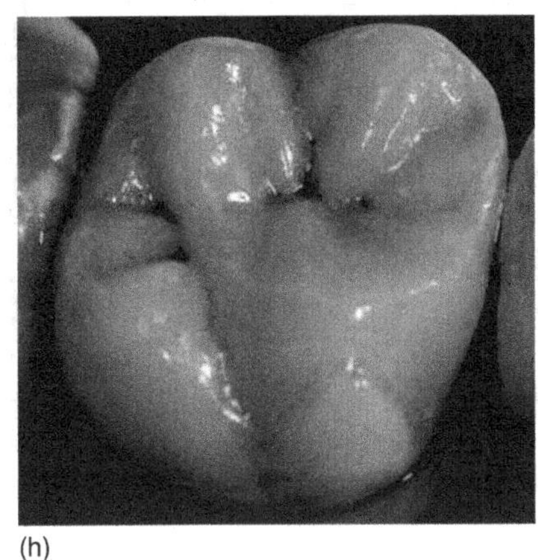

(h)

Figure 4.24 (g) An endodontic treatment X-ray on the first maxillary molar with a normal IPB height. (h) Fully cemented with adequate proximal surfaces and a good gingival contour, showing optimal interdental papillae. (Figures (g)–(h) Courtesy of Dr. G.C. Pongione, Rome, Italy.)

The interproximal implant relation

Management of the papilla differs or varies depending on the following horizontal and vertical relations: tooth adjacent to tooth, tooth adjacent to implant, implant adjacent to implant, tooth adjacent to pontic, and pontic adjacent to pontic (Esposito *et al.*, 1993; Saadoun *et al.*, 1999; Tarnow *et al.*, 2000):

- Horizontal biological criteria for implant placement (Figs 4.25a, b) are as follows:
  - from the implant to the adjacent teeth, 1.5–2.0 mm
  - between the implant and the central incisors, 2.0–2.5 mm
  - from an implant to an adjacent implant, 3–4 mm
  - between two maxillary central incisor implants, 4.0–4.5 mm.
- Vertical biological criteria for single or multiple implant restorations (Fig. 4.25c) are as follows:
  - bone crest/tooth contact point restoration, 5 mm
  - bone crest/tooth–implant contact point restoration, 4.5–5.0 mm

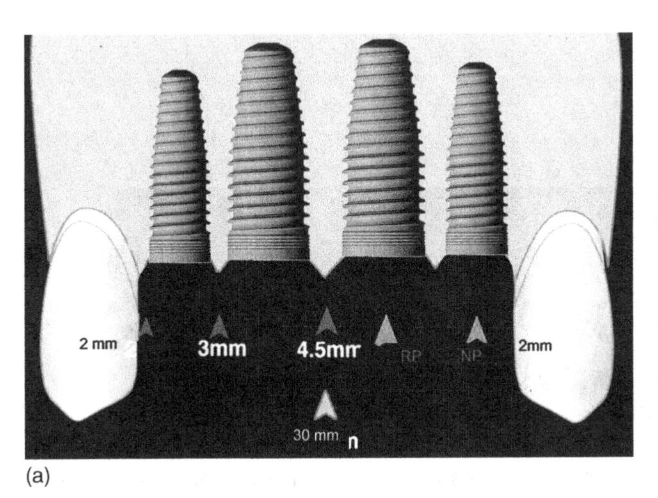

(a)

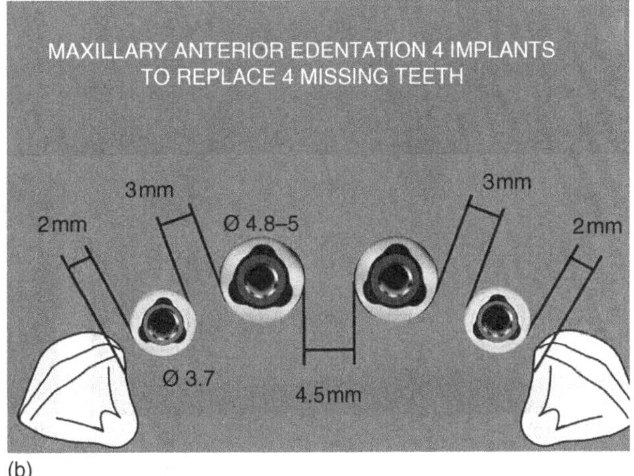

(b)

Figure 4.25 (a) The inter-implant distance between adjacent teeth and the implant. (b) Horizontal biological criteria for implant placement.

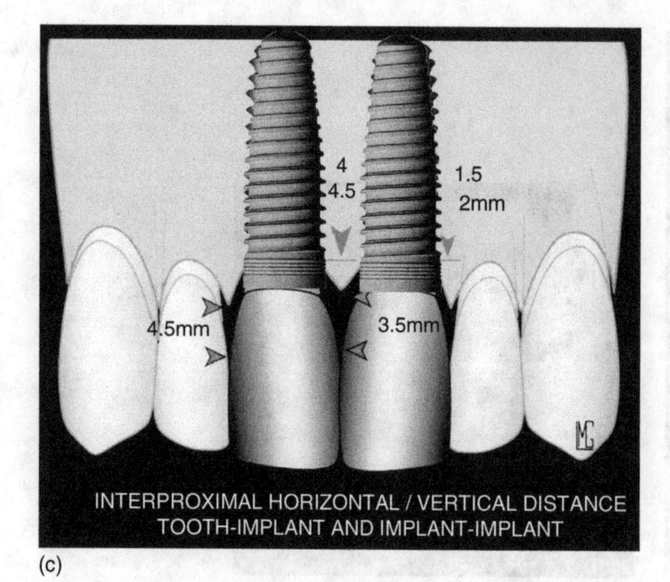

(c)

Figure 4.25 (c) Vertical biological criteria for single or multiple implant restorations.

- bone crest/implant–implant contact point restoration, 2.3–3.4 mm
- bone crest/implant–pontic contact point restoration, 5.5–6.0 mm
- bone crest/tooth–pontic contact point restoration, 6.0–6.5 mm
- bone crest/pontic–pontic contact point restoration, 6.0–6.5 mm.

The ability to restore and maintain the health, function, and esthetics of soft tissues (gingival margin level and interproximal papilla height) around a single implant restoration depends mainly on the integrity of the attachment apparatus of the adjacent teeth (Figs 4.26a–d).

The configuration of the interdental papilla relies mainly on the crestal bone and the overlying soft tissue volume, rather than on solid supracrestal

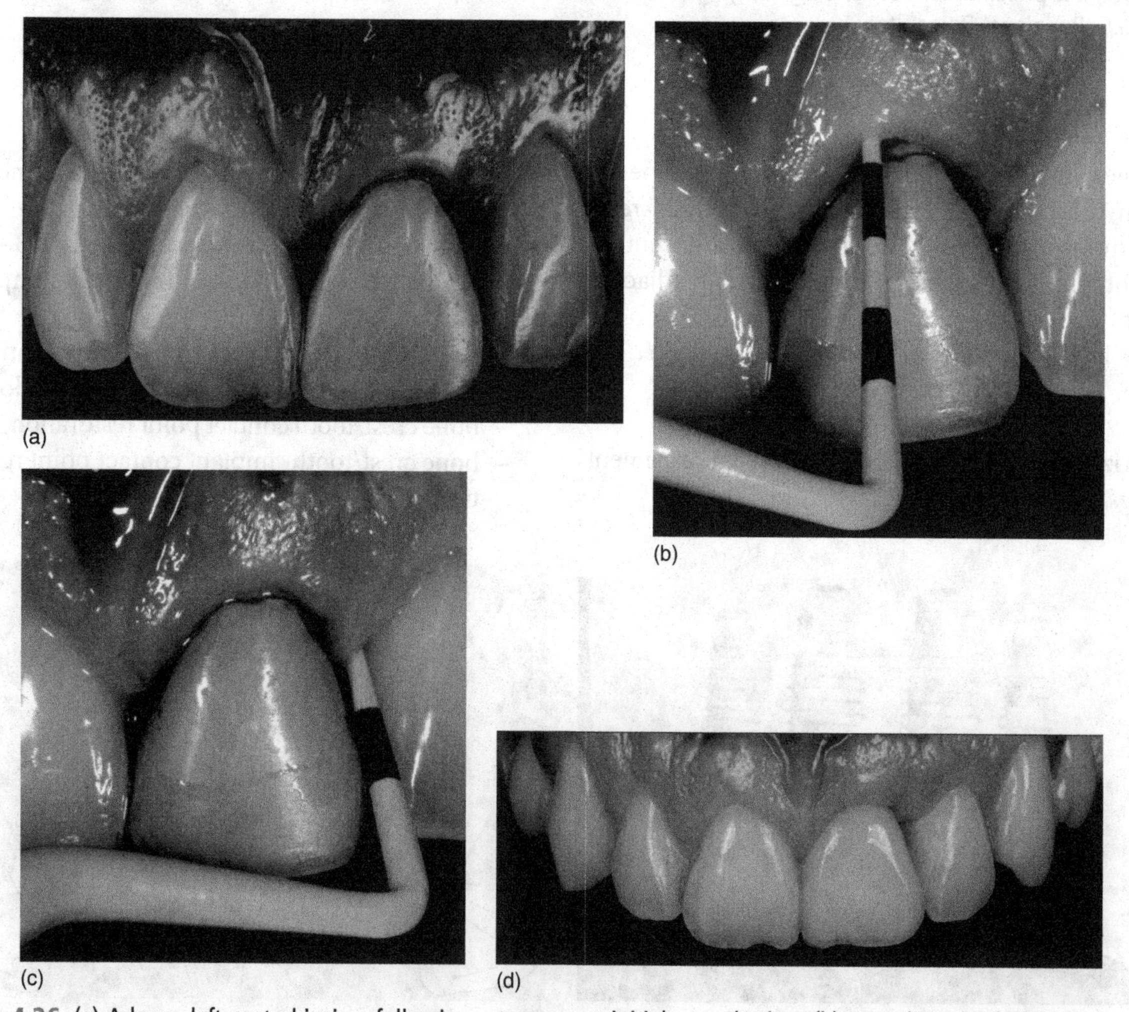

Figure 4.26 (a) A loose left central incisor following a trauma, at initial consultation. (b) Sounding the facial bone crest on the mesial interproximal bone peak at a normal distance. (c) Sounding the distal bone peak at an increased distance. (d) The final esthetic left incisor implant restoration, with a lack of distal papillae. (Courtesy of Dr. M. Groisman, Rio de Janeiro, Brazil.)

functional connective tissue fiber attachments (Landsberg, 2005).

The apico-coronal proximal biological width position and dimensions appear to determine the location of the papilla tip between adjacent implants. In a study by Kourkouta *et al.* (2009), there was a significant association between the provisionalization protocol and missing papilla height, which was also influenced by the horizontal distance between implants. Patient esthetic satisfaction was high, despite a less than optimal papilla fill.

Chow *et al.* (2010) reported that the appearance of the gingival papilla was associated significantly with subject age, tooth form and shape, proximal contact length, crestal bone height, and interproximal gingival thickness.

In a recent study (Kan *et al.* 2011), after a mean follow-up time of 4 years following immediate implant placement and provisionalization, the following were observed:

- The overall cumulative implant success rate was 100%.
- The changes in the mean mesial and distal bone levels (−0.72 and −0.63 mm, respectively) were significantly greater than those observed at the 1-year follow-up examination (−0.26 and −0.22 mm, respectively).
- The changes in the mean mesial and distal papilla levels (−0.22 and −0.21 mm, respectively) were significantly less than those observed at the 1-year follow-up examination (−0.52 and −0.39 mm, respectively), suggesting that in the presence of a proper interproximal embrasure form and underlying bony support, a certain degree of spontaneous papilla regeneration can occur over time following this procedure.
- The change in the mean overall facial gingival level (−1.13 mm) was significantly greater than that observed at the 1-year follow-up (−0.55 mm), suggesting that facial gingival tissue recession is a dynamic process and may continue beyond 12 months after implant surgery.
- Sites with a thick gingival biotype exhibited significantly less change in facial gingival level than sites with a thin gingival biotype at both 1 year after implant placement (−0.25 mm versus v−0.75 mm, respectively) and the most recent follow-up examination (−0.56 mm versus −1.50 mm, respectively).
- The effect of the gingival biotype on the peri-implant tissue response seems to be limited to facial gingival recession, and does not affect the interproximal papillae or the proximal marginal bone levels.

The pink/white esthetic score, or PES/WES

The PWES is defined by evaluation of the result of the gingiva, tooth, and implant restoration and is determined using the parameters in Table 4.9 (Fuerhauser *et al.*, 2005).

For the clinician, the problem is to adequately diagnose and determine the osseous and gingival state, as well as the treatment plan of choice that will lead not only to a good white esthetic score but, more importantly, a good pink esthetic score, wherein tissue defects will have been treated or compensated, thus rendering them invisible.

Table 4.9a The pink esthetic score (PES) (Figs 4.27a–c)

Score	The PES represents the final gingival contour defined by	Rate
1	Mesial papilla	0–2
2	Distal papilla	0–2
3	Level facial mucosa	0–2
4	Curvature facial mucosa	0–1
5	Root convexity	0–1
6	Soft tissue color	0–1
7	Soft tissue texture	0–1
Score (10 being the best)		0–10

Table 4.9b The white esthetic score (WES) (Figs 4.28a–c)

Score	The WES represents the final tooth restoration/appearance defined by	Rate
1	Tooth form	0–2
2	Tooth outline and volume	0–2
3	Color (hue and value)	0–2
4	Restoration surface texture	0–2
5	Translucency and characterization	0–2
Score (10 being the best)		0–10

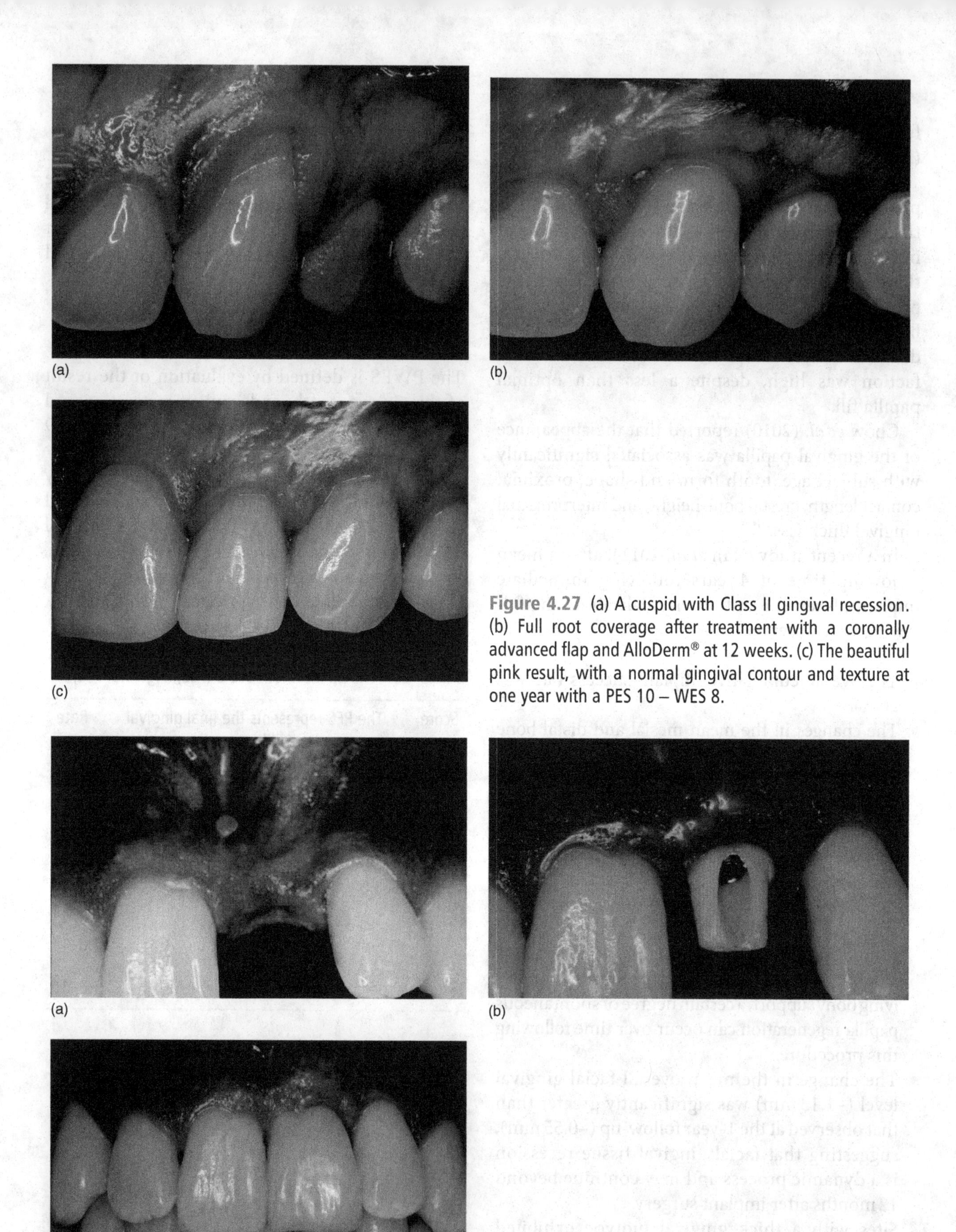

Figure 4.27 (a) A cuspid with Class II gingival recession. (b) Full root coverage after treatment with a coronally advanced flap and AlloDerm® at 12 weeks. (c) The beautiful pink result, with a normal gingival contour and texture at one year with a PES 10 – WES 8.

Figure 4.28 (a) A healed site, 6 months after the accidental loss of the central incisor. (b) A zirconium abutment with a thicker gingival margin. (c) Esthetic implant restoration with an optimal gingival contour and papilla height at one year with PES 10 – WES 10.

The biological space

Restorative dental care, in any capacity, depends on the clinician's understanding of the biological factors involved. The biological width was originally defined by Dr. D. Walter Cohen and described in Ingber *et al.* (1977), but the measurements were provided by Gargiulo *et al.* (1961) without the use of that term. It corresponds to the distance between the bone crest occupied by the connective tissue attachment to the coronal part of the junctional epithelium. This distance has an average value of 2 mm and includes the combined dimensions of the junctional epithelial attachment plus the connective tissue attachment. The gingival sulcus does not belong to the biological width. The biological width is, in fact, a biological seal which has fixed circumferential and volumetric dimensions for each specific tooth and is genetically predetermined. It could be transferred orthodontically by forced eruption or surgically by a crown lengthening procedure (Fig. 4.29a,b,c) (Ingber, 1974, 1976; Salama and Salama, 1993).

The presence of a dentogingival complex influences the biological response of the gingival tissues (junctional epithelium/connective tissue attachment) to intrasulcular margins created during esthetic dentistry (Ingber *et al.*, 1977). This dentogingival complex has been measured as 3 mm (biological space plus healthy sulcus) facially to nearly 4–5 mm interproximally, and affects the esthetic outcome of any restoration that is placed at the level of the free gingival margin (Kois, 2006).

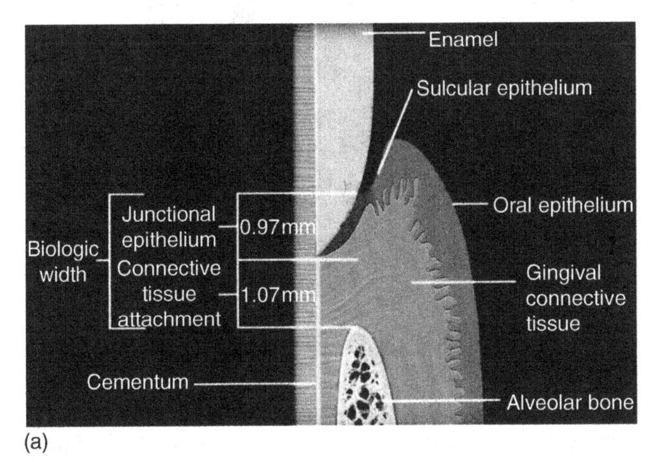

Figure 4.29 (a) A diagram of the natural tooth biological width.

If there is less than 2 mm of gingival tissue from the restoration margin to the alveolar bone, the gingival biological width will be altered, leading to gingival inflammation or recession, depending on the perio-biotype.

Clinically, any violation of the biological width, such as a tooth preparation or restoration that impinges on surrounding tissues, can lead to periodontal inflammation, altering the form and contour of the gingival tissues (a hyperplastic tissue reaction on a thick biotype and tissue recession on a thin biotype).

The dentogingival complex consists of connective tissue attachment, epithelial attachment or junctional epithelium, and the gingival sulcus:

- The most critical relationship for biological health when the clinician is placing a restoration below or at the free gingival margin is the location of the margin relative to the crest of the bone. The maximum distance from the free gingival margin to the osseous crest on the facial aspect is 2.5–3.0 mm, and 4.0–4.5 mm interproximally (Kois, 1994).
- There is approximately 2 mm at the osseous crest for root proximity.
- The clinician must first decide where the restorative margin will be placed. For all-ceramic restorations that do not need to block out undesirable dentin colors or core materials, it may be desirable to place the restorative margin at the juxta-free gingival crest (juxta-gingival) or slightly supragingival (Materdomini and Friedman, 1993).
- If an intracrevicular margin is required for esthetic reasons, however, it should be placed no further than 0.5 mm into the gingival sulcus (subgingival), to avoid adverse biological responses due to encroachment upon the biological attachment apparatus.
- Variations in biological width that compare the distance from the alveolar crest to the free gingival margin have been described and divided into three categories (Coslet *et al.* 1977; Kois, 1994):
  1. Normal bone crest – normal crest patients (about 70%) have an approximately 2 mm combined epithelial and connective tissue attachment and a 1 mm sulcus depth (a total dentogingival complex of 3 mm). If the sulcus depth is greater than 1 mm, the free gingival

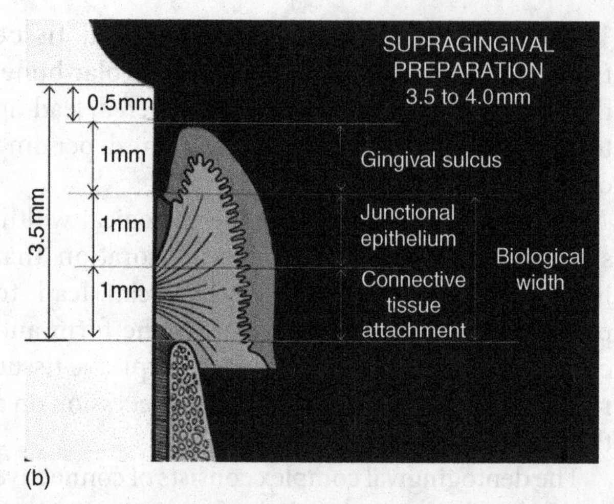

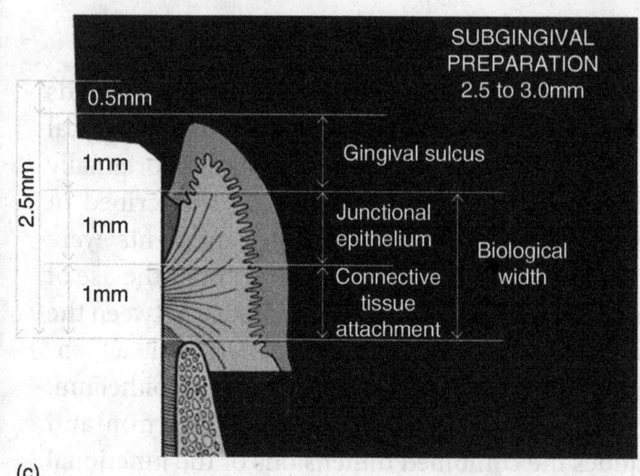

Figure 4.29 (b) A diagram of a supragingival preparation that respects the biological width. (c) A diagram of a subgingival preparation that is not jeopardizing the biological width.

excess can be safely resected and, upon healing, will result in a dentogingival complex measuring 3 mm on the facial aspect.

2. High bone crest – patients with a high crest often have a shallower sulcus depth and a combined dentogingival complex measurement of less than 3 mm. These patients have relatively stable free gingival margin positions and are not prone to recession upon manipulation of the tissues.
3. Low bone crest – patients with a low crest often have a normal sulcus depth (1–3 mm) and a combined epithelial and connective dentogingival complex measurement that is greater than 3 mm. These patients are more vulnerable to gingival recession.

Therefore, the most important factor in postrestorative gingival health and stability is the position of the restorative margin relative to the bony crest, not the preoperative health and/or position of the gingival tissues.

Adequate keratinized tissue may be more important around implants than around natural teeth for several reasons. On implant surfaces, supra/subcrestal collagen fibers are oriented in a parallel rather than in a perpendicular configuration, providing less resistance to local trauma and microbial penetration (Figs 4.29d, e). Peri-implant mucosa may have a reduced capacity to regenerate itself due to a compromised number of cells and poor vascular supply (Abrahamsson *et al.*, 1997).

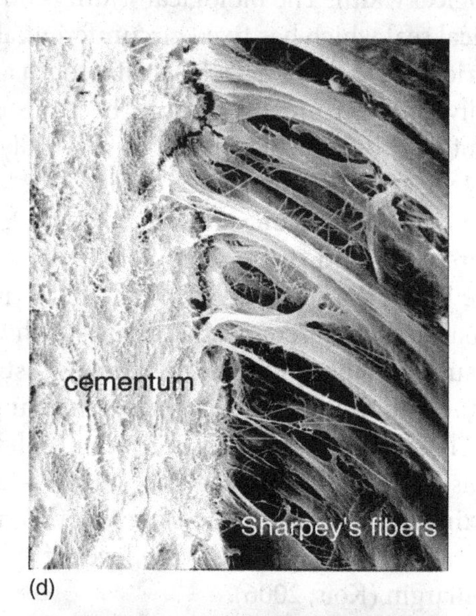

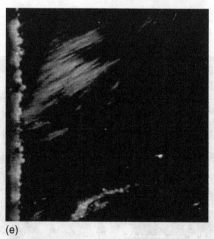

Figure 4.29 (d) Sharpey's fibers inserted on natural root cementum. (e) Functionally oriented connective fibers inserted on a TiUnite™ implant surface. (Courtesy of Dr. P. Schupbach, Zürich, Switzerland.)

Table 4.10 The biological width and bone remodeling around one- or two-stage implants and teeth

Biological components	Machined surface (mm)		Rough surface (mm)		Natural teeth (mm)
	Range	Average	Range	Average	
Gingival margin to junctional epithelium	3.00–4.30	3.65	1.77–2.14	1.95	1.76
Sulcus depth	1.00–1.50	1.25	0.77–0.96	0.86	0.79
Junctional epithelium	2.00–2.80	2.40	1.00–1.18	1.09	0.97
Connective tissue attachment	1.30–1.70	1.50	0.97–1.66	1.31	1.04
Biological width	3.50–4.30	3.90	1.97–2.84	2.40	2.11
Total soft tissue height	4.30–6.00	5.15	2.74–3.80	3.26	2.90
Bone remodeling around implant collar	1.00–1.60	1.30	0.70–1.20	0.95	N.A.

The oxidized and acid-etched TiUnite™ implant revealed less epithelial downgrowth, a smaller connective tissue seal, and less bone remodeling than machined implants (Adell *et al.*, 1990; Cochran *et al.*, 1997; Hermann *et al.*, 2000; Glauser *et al.*, 2003). The biological width of rough implant surfaces is becoming smaller in size and closer to that of natural teeth (Table 4.10).

Final remarks

The smile is dynamic and cannot be measured precisely. Furthermore, patients who have an esthetic deficiency often modify their smiles in order to hide the esthetic problem. The smile line should be evaluated in comparison with the quantity of uncovered gingiva and the number of teeth. Above all, it is necessary to consider the age and the sex of the patient.

Today, the promotion of various images of beauty by the media reinforce the notion that physical perfection can be achieved. Even people who are fundamentally satisfied with their appearance feel driven to maintain or enhance it.

However, the surgeon should be aware that the patient's demands and expectations may go beyond his or her abilities and the current dental possibilities. Therefore, it is important that surgeons present a clear explanation of the process, so that the patient's expectations will be realistic and the result satisfying.

The psychodynamics of esthetic surgery amounts to a kind of psychosurgery that allows a patient to bring out his or her hidden self in such a manner that a profound energy is released, which allows open communication with others. This new positive attitude encourages a complete change in personality and confidence. The majority of people enjoy their new appearance and, most of the time, better professional and familial integration are noticed (Saadoun, 2005).

In order to enhance the smile, esthetic teeth and gingival deficiencies could be treated in the following ways:

- Bleaching: in the office or at home.
- Orthodontics: buccal–lingual, mini-, or regular implants.
- Resin composites.
- Ceramic laminate veneers.
- Ceramic/zirconium crowns.
- Periodontal plastic surgery:
  - gingivo-osseous surgery for crown lengthening procedures;
  - mucogingival surgery for gingival recession coverage, to increase the thickness and harmonize the contour, or
  - peri-implant soft tissue management.
- Implant restorations.

In Chapters 5 and 6, we will limit the discussion to esthetic periodontal and implant treatment.

5

Esthetic periodontal treatment

A harmonious smile does not just depend on beautiful lips. It cannot be conceived without a perfectly healthy gingival frame and well-aligned natural teeth. Since the smile is a vital part of a beautiful face and there is a high patient demand for beauty, demands for smile enhancement with periodontal surgery, cosmetic restorations, or implant restorations continue to increase as patients live for longer.

The fundamental criteria of dentogingival esthetics are perfectly established and must be a part of the esthetic culture of every clinician. Each practitioner must adopt a scientific approach when analyzing dentogingival esthetic criteria, to establish the main alterations that are needed to their patients' smiles before proposing orthodontic, surgical, and/or restorative solutions.

The biological rationale

If the goal of a clinician is to reduce the depth of periodontal pockets, surgery remains the treatment of choice for moderate to deep pockets (4–6 mm and >6 mm). But if the goal is to gain a clinical attachment, root planing without raising a flap will yield better results than root planing with flap raising for pockets with little to average depth (1–3 mm and 4–6 mm). On the other hand, for deep pockets (> 6 mm) and esthetic gingival concerns, it is the surgical approach that will allow the pocket depth to be reduced and esthetic problems to be resolved (Heitz-Mayfield, 2000).

According to Claffey *et al.* (2004), surgical and nonsurgical therapies achieve similar results in terms of overall improvement of clinical conditions, and allow clinical attachment levels to stabilize within the context of regular follow-up therapy and with good personal plaque control.

The logic of active periodontal treatment today is therefore based on the association of four phases (Range, 2008) (Figs 5.1a–d):

- Initial therapy: to reduce inflammation by means of mechanical debridement and chemical irrigation.
- Reevaluation: to measure the patient's response and weigh the risks and benefits of possible surgical treatments.
- A possible corrective phase: to reduce the pockets if they pose a risk of progression of the disease. Resective procedures will reestablish a positive periodontal structure compatible with a high level of plaque control, and/or regenerate infrabony lesions, cover gingival recessions, and finally correct ridge deformities.
- Maintenance therapy: to reinform the patients about the disease, reinforce the patient's oral hygiene, eliminate etiologic factors, regain dental health, and prevent recurrence of disease.

It is important to understand the essential role of dental hygiene, because the absence of, or a deficiency in, dental hygiene induces more bacteremia than the surgery itself. The prescription of antibiotics

Esthetic Soft Tissue Management of Teeth and Implants, First Edition. André P. Saadoun.

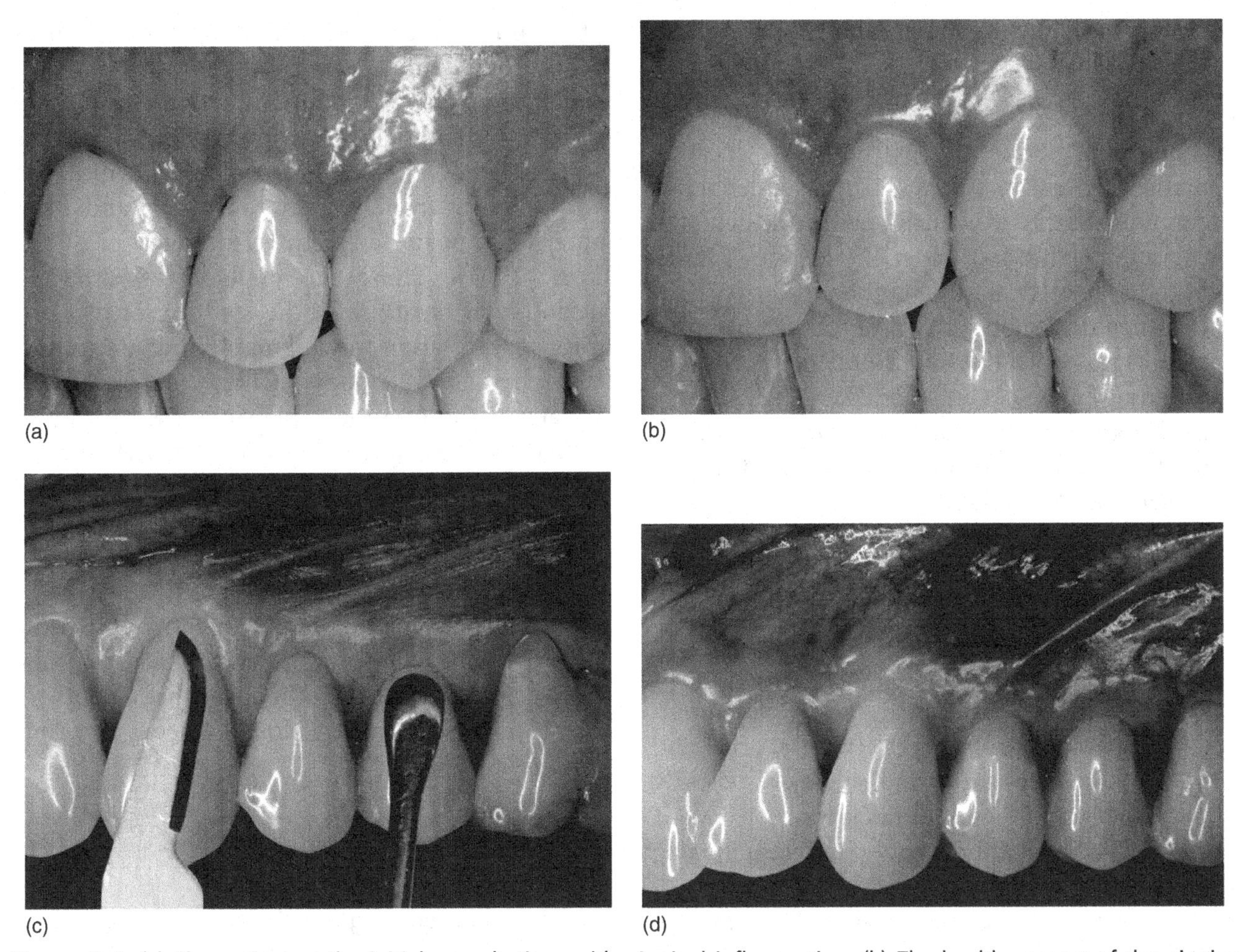

Figure 5.1 (a) The patient at the initial consultation, with gingival inflammation. (b) The healthy aspect of the gingiva 6 weeks after initial preparation. (c) Multiple gingival recessions on the left maxillary arch showing the instrument used for the incision and then raising the flap. (d) The healthy aspect of the gingival margin and interproximal papillae 3 months later.

cannot compensate for a lack of dental hygiene (Lesclous, 2011).

The composition of an esthetic and functional dentoalveolar gingival unit (DAGU) or periodontal restorative interface (PRI) must take into account the periodontal health of the gingiva, the bone, the interdental papillae, and the biological space. Periodontal therapy is concerned, first and foremost, with maintaining the health of periodontal structures and correcting any gingival disharmony to achieve a balanced gingival contour for each smile.

Disharmony in the gingival contour can be easily managed with periodontal plastic surgery through resective (gingival smile), additive, orthodontic, or biological procedures (gingival recession), but this treatment is much more challenging in implant surgery because of the differences between the tooth and implant surfaces. Eventual periodontal corrections cannot be envisioned without evaluating the position of the mucogingival line, the height and thickness of the keratinized gingiva (KG), the sulcular depth, the position of the interdental papillae, and the level of the alveolar crest (Levine and McGuire, 1979). Therefore, visual precision – without any guesswork or estimation based on emotional considerations – is vital for successful, predictable, and cost-efficient treatment.

More recently, instrumentation such as Chu's Aesthetic Gauges (Hu-Friedy Inc., Chicago, IL) has been created to diagnose and predictably treat esthetic tooth discrepancies and deformities. These new probes could also evaluate clinical and anatomical teeth dimensions, and could now secure the treatment through the application of quantitative standards (Chu, 2007):

- The metallic gauge helps to provide quick and simple analysis of the osseous crest location midfacially and interdentally. It has a deliberate curvature of the tip, which is coincident with the curvature of the tooth and root. This allows easier negotiation of the osseous crest location, particularly in the thin biotype. This increased dimension allows greater stability and confidence during the sounding process. Chu's metallic gauges can be used repeatedly to determine the amount of midfacial osseous tissue to be removed during surgery (see Figs 4.12b, c).
- The T-bar gauge is used to measure a noncrowded anterior dentition and the In-line gauge is used for a crowded dentition (see Fig. 4.19h).
- The measurements are mathematically aligned, with a preset individual tooth proportion ratio of 78%. The practitioner can accurately and simultaneously evaluate the length (vertical arm) and width (horizontal arm) and, therefore, visually assess the correct tooth size and proportion, before, during, and after the surgical crown lengthening procedure.
- The Crown Lengthening Gauge, or In-line gauge tip, is designed to measure the midfacial length of the anticipated restored clinical crown and the length of the biological crown (i.e., from the bone crest to the incisal edge). The short arm of the In-line tip is of the same length and cross-section as the long arm of the T-bar tip (see Fig. 4.19i).
- The color-coded marks on the shorter arm represent the clinical crown length, and the corresponding color markings on the longer arm represent the biological crown length at the bone level.

During the osseous resection procedure, the visualization of these two parameters compels the clinician to focus on the end-goal of the treatment, since the blueprint for bone removal is clearly delineated.

Crown lengthening procedures

Nowadays, crown lengthening procedures have come to be accepted as an esthetics-driven form of periodontal surgery. In crown lengthening procedures, the clinician must address the biological width and consider the different biotypes in order to avoid potential postoperative complications (Ingber *et al.*, 1977). The biological width can vary slightly from patient to patient and from anterior to posterior teeth (Gargiulo *et al.*, 1961; Kois, 1994). Thus, the biological width, the periodontal health, and the stability of the gingival margin after crown lengthening are important when one is trying to achieve ideal esthetics. Whatever the treatment plan option, the key to esthetic success depends on the preservation of the buccal cortical plate and interproximal bone of the alveolar sockets, and on the symmetry of the gingival contour which frames the natural teeth.

It is important that the same quantity of bone be removed or retained in order to create normal biological parameters. Authentic esthetic dentistry is only possible if the periodontal space is in perfect condition (Lowe, 2009).

The biological objectives

Indications

Crown lengthening procedures are indicated to provide adequate tooth structure in cases of subgingival tooth fracture (Hu *et al.*, 2008), subgingival caries (Hempton and Esrason, 2000), root resorption (Reddy, 2003), uneven gingival levels, unesthetic short crowns due to tooth wear, inadequate axial height for retention of restorations, altered passive eruption of a single or multiple teeth, and, finally, in cases of a gingival smile – called a "gummy smile" – with short natural crowns.

The objective of crown lengthening in restorative cases is to increase the axial length of the crown, and to strengthen the anchoring of the restored teeth, by surgically moving the alveolar crest bone to a more apical position, thereby providing adequate tooth structure to safely prepare the restoration. It also helps to reestablish the new physiological biological width.

The alveolar bone resection will depend on the type of the apical level of the restoration:

- If the restoration has a suprasulcular limit, the amount of bone resection should leave a minimum

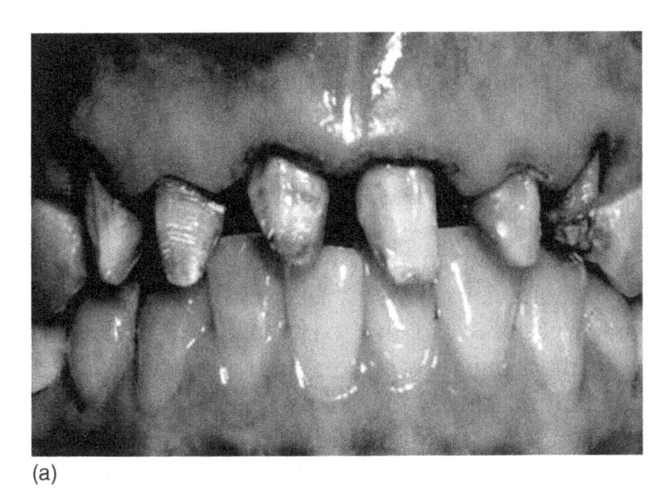

(a)

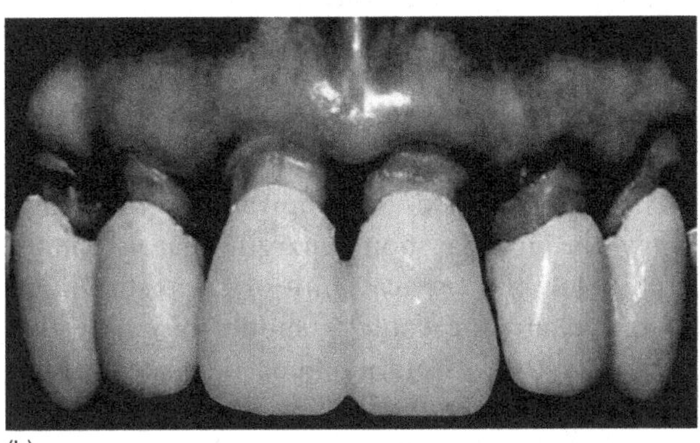

(b)

(c)

Figure 5.2 (a) Old anterior teeth preparation, violating the biological width, with irregular gingival contour. (b) The clinical aspect, with supragingival temporary crowns, 3 months after the bone has been surgically removed and the flap sutured more apically. (c) The final ceramometal anterior restorations after new subgingival preparation that respects the biological width 15 years later.

of 3.0–3.5 mm of sound tooth structure from the restoration margin (see Fig. 4.29b).

- If the restoration has an intrasulcular limit, the amount of bone resection should leave a minimum of 2.5–3.0 mm of sound tooth structure from the restoration margin (see Fig. 4.29c).

Subgingival preparation for esthetic restoration should not be initiated before a healthy sulcus is present (Figs 5.2a–c). This will take varying amounts of time, depending on the biotype (Rosenberg *et al.*, 1980).

In nonrestorative cases, crown lengthening is an independent procedure and is mainly performed to enhance esthetics. Excessively short teeth, lack of tooth display, and excessive gingival display require clinical crown lengthening, which can present a clinical dilemma for the esthetic-oriented periodontist.

The overall treatment of the gingival smile is multidisciplinary, leading to teamwork focused on the various elements that make up the smile, and most particularly on the position of the upper lip line (Miskinyar, 1983).

There is a specific treatment corresponding to each etiology, with which – in most cases – will be associated complex therapy, peripheral complementary treatments, or gingivoplasty, with or without restorative treatment (Toca *et al.*, 2008).

According to Goubron *et al.* (2011) the objective of the treatment should be to:

- Reestablish an ideal and symmetrical gingival margin.
- Obtain correct dimensions for the tooth crown.
- Harmonize the smile from the first and second premolars on the right side to the first and second premolars on the left side.

- Maintain a long-term result with the optimal biological width, and that has a distance of 3 mm from the new gingival margin to the reshaped (osteoectomy–osteoplasty) crestal bone.

The architecture of the gingival margin should follow the alveolar bone margin that is found 3 mm below the cervical limit of the restoration. The alveolar bone contour should resemble the margin of the restoration, but displaced 3 mm apically to respect, and allow for the reformation of, the normal biological width and sulcus (Lowe, 2004).

Any esthetic modification should take into consideration perfect knowledge of the position of the teeth and of the desired symmetry of the gingival profiles.

The rationale

The need to establish the correct tooth size and the proportions of the individual teeth drives the periodontal component of esthetic restorative dentistry (Chu, 2007).

Midfacial surgical crown lengthening has traditionally been performed to establish a healthy biological dimension of the dentogingival complex as an adjunct to esthetic restorative procedures. This procedure involves a multifaceted decision-making process, with the endpoint being whether or not hard and/or soft tissues can be excised and/or should be repositioned. Therefore, it is important to determine the position of the underlying bone in relation to the gingival tissue.

In order to obtain desirable final results in the esthetic region, preservation of the interproximal papillae is essential (Nemcovsky *et al*., 2001). Several authors have suggested that 3 mm of supracrestal tooth structure be established during surgical crown lengthening (Kois, 2006).

It is important to establish a consistent measurement that is representative of the dentogingival complex dimension, which is critical for health and for restorative success when performing surgical crown lengthening. Patients who exhibit asymmetrical gingival levels, and those with greater than 3–5 mm of maxillary gingival display, or both, may be candidates for surgical gingival and/or alveolar bone repositioning to improve their esthetics. Typically, these patient types have adequate amounts of attached gingiva to prevent the mucogingival junction from being encroached upon after the resective procedure. If an adequate amount of free gingiva exists, minor asymmetries can be corrected by means of internal gingivectomy or gingivoplasty alone. A minimum sulcus depth of 1 mm must always remain after any tissue resection, unless alveolar bone crest is repositioned in the apical direction as well.

Current crown lengthening procedures

The treatment modality for esthetic crown lengthening should be based on detailed diagnosis in each case, because the type of therapy selected by the clinician will have direct implications for the esthetics (Kao *et al*., 2008). Like the gingival margin and the bone level, the periodontal biotype can vary after crown lengthening surgery, depending on the patient's osseous biotype (Pontoriero and Carnevale, 2001).

Depending on the clinical situation regarding the amount of keratinized gingiva in the gingival margins, with or without disharmony in relation to the alveolar crest to the cemento-enamel junction (CEJ), there are two main clinical protocols for the treatment of these gingival anomalies:

1. Gingival resection and harmonization, with or without osseous resection, in natural passive eruption:
   - This is used without flap elevation and with a marginal incision to create, at a new level, a harmonious gingival margin contour without osseous resection, when there is an excess of gingival tissue (> 3–5 mm, Type I-A) with a correct marginal bone crest relation with the cemento-enamel junction (> 1.5–2.0 mm) (Figs 5.3a–v).
   - It is used with flap elevation, with a sulcular incision and osseous resection, when there is inadequate gingival tissue (≤ 3 mm, Type II-A) with a correct marginal bone crest

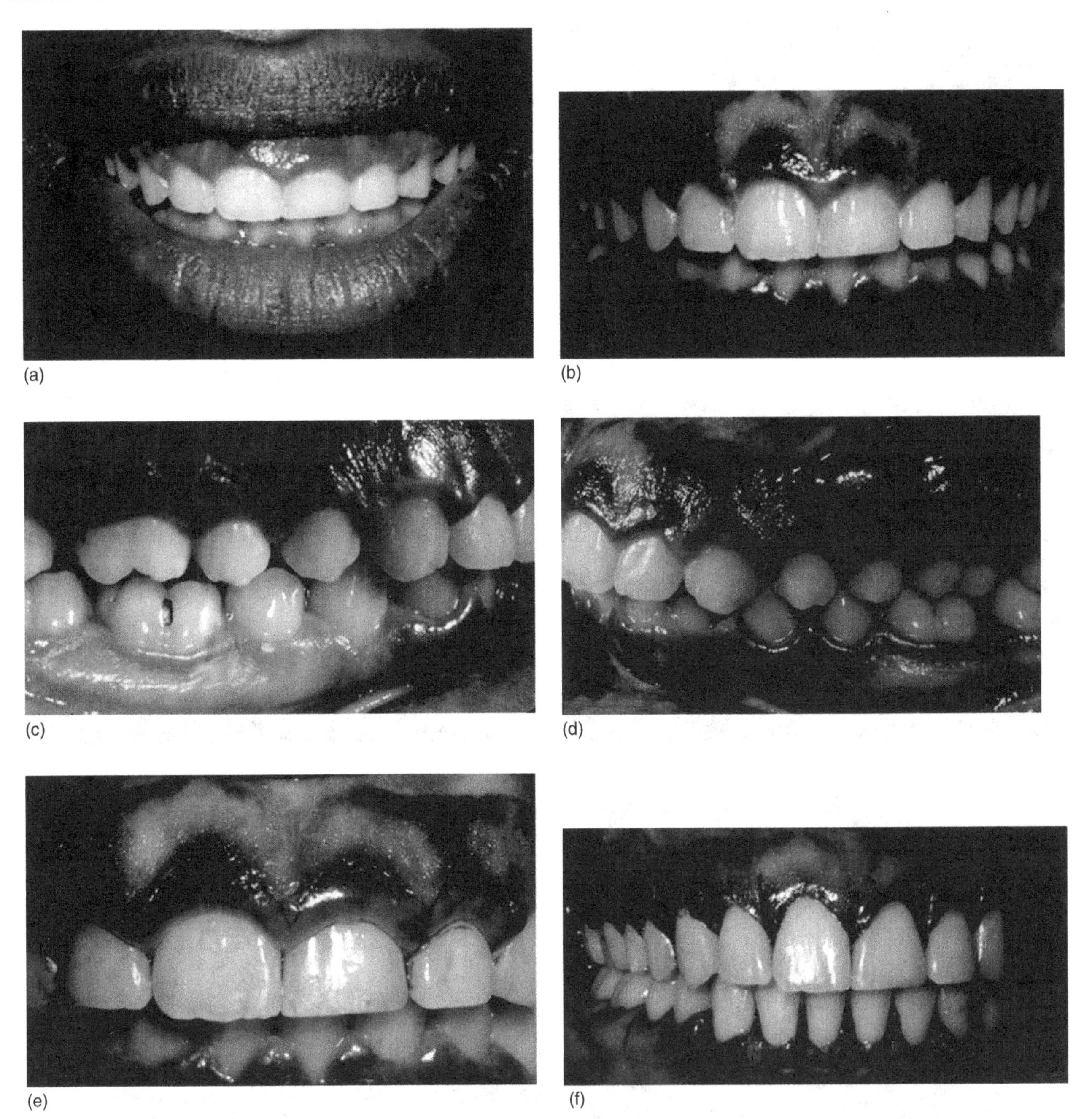

Figure 5.3 (a) A top model's gingival smile, with short crowns and an absence of make-up, to avoid drawing attention to herself. (b) A frontal view of the gingival smile, with pigmented attached gingiva. (c) The intrabuccal right profile, showing excessive amounts of KG. (d) The left profile, also showing a large band of KG (Type I-A). (e) An internal beveled supracrestal incision involving the tip of the papillae on the anterior teeth combined with a sulcular incision; the gingival margin is then removed. (f) Continuous silk sutures after surgery on the maxillary and mandibular teeth, leaving 3 mm of gingival tissue from the bone crest.

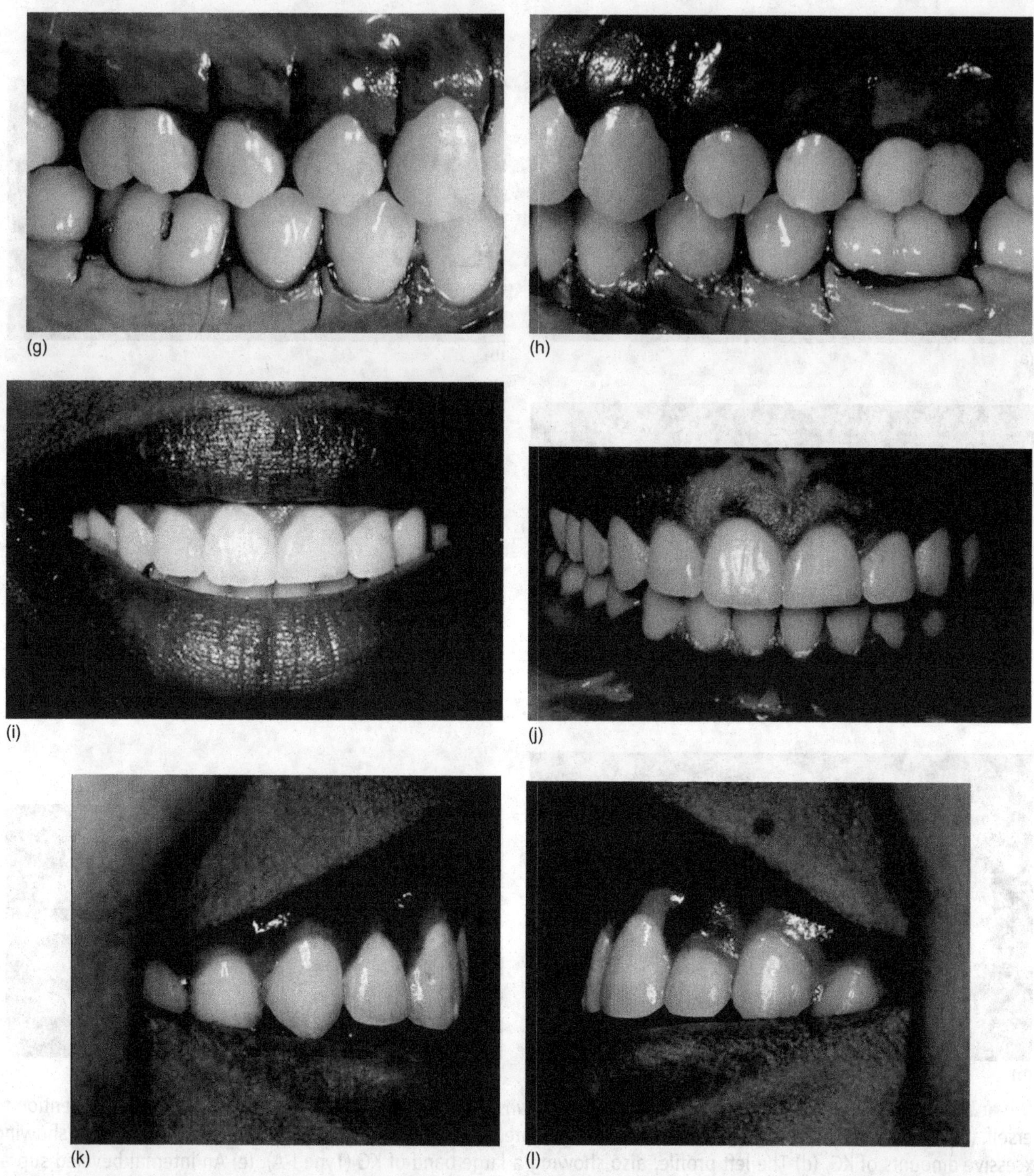

Figure 5.3 (g) After a scalloped internal bevel incision has been extended around all of the right maxillary and mandibulary teeth, the gingival margin is removed and continuous silk sutures are put into place. (h) After a scalloped internal bevel incision has been extended around all of the left maxillary and mandibulary teeth, with double contour incisions on molars, continuous silk sutures are put into place. (i) Her new confident and enthusiastic smile, now enhanced by make-up. (j) The frontal view of the patient's new smile, showing longer teeth. (k) The right profile aspect of an excessive gingival display (Type I-A). (l) The left profile with excessive gingiva, more pronounced than on the right lateral.

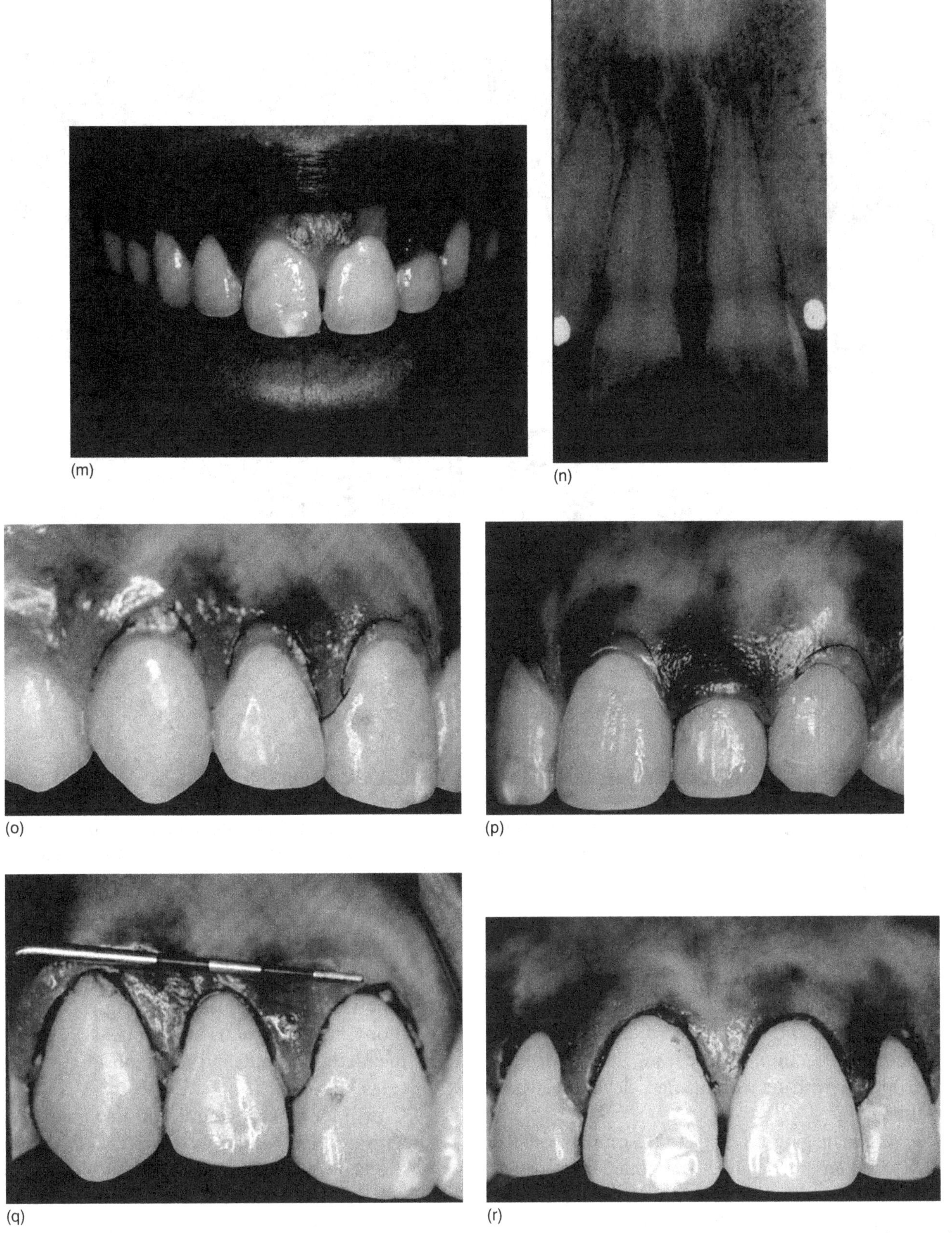

(m) (n) (o) (p) (q) (r)

Figure 5.3 (m) The frontal view, showing the excess of gingiva with gingival disharmony. (n) A semilunar marginal internal incision not involving the tip of the papilla. (p) The same type of incision as on the right side, with a higher incision on the lateral. (o) An X-ray of the central incisors, revealing the absence of a contact point and a correct interproximal bone level. (q) Checking the level of the gingival margin on the right anterior teeth. (r) The clinical aspect at the end of the surgical session.

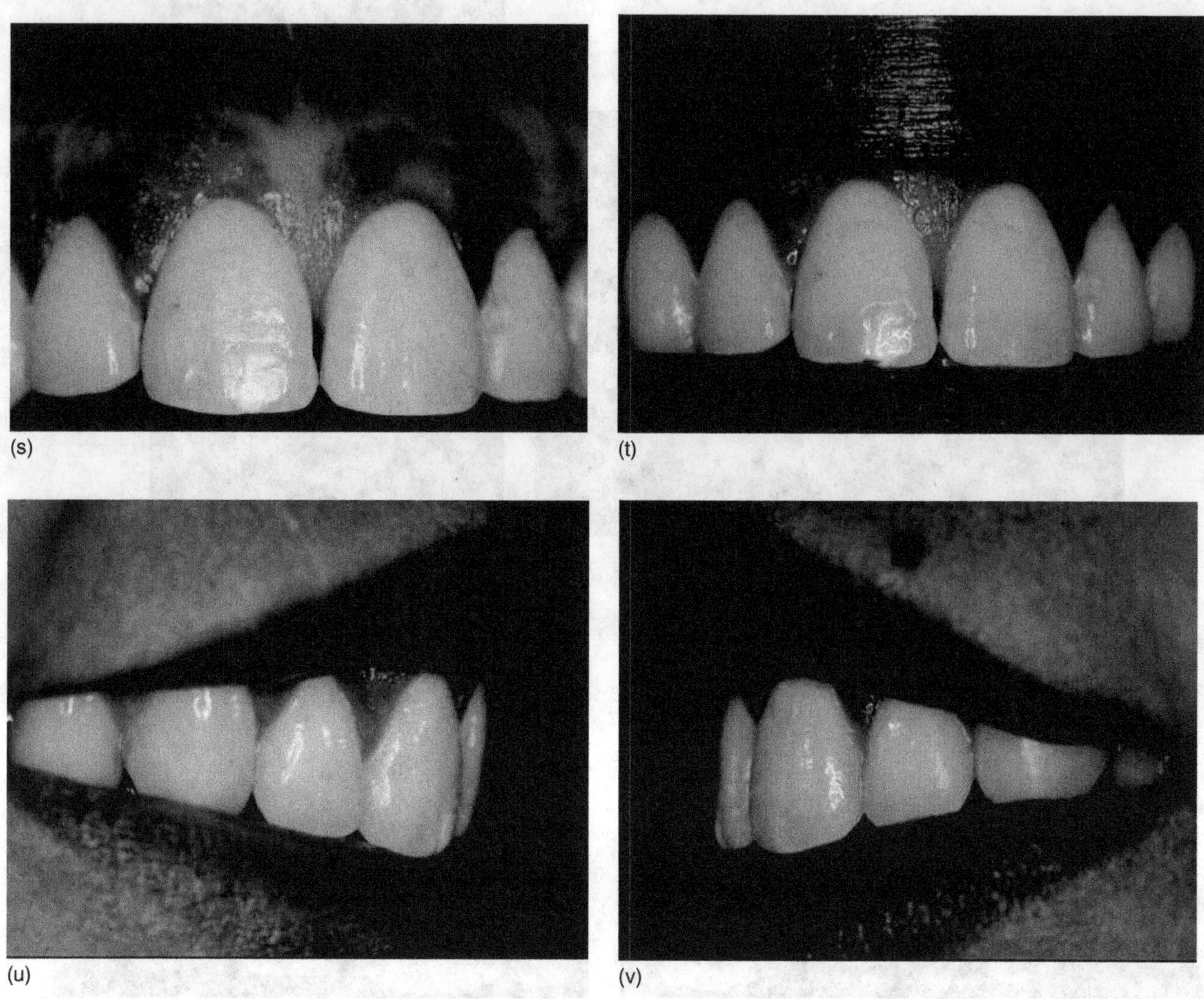

Figure 5.3 (s) The clinical aspect 2 weeks after surgery. (t) The 6-month postoperative result on the right profile of the smile. (u) The patient now feels good about herself and uses make-up. (v) A gingival display of < 1 mm on the left profile, in harmony with the lip contour.

relation with the cemento-enamel junction (>1.5–2.0 mm) (Figs 5.4a–f).

2. Gingival resection and harmonization, with osseous resection, is used in altered passive eruption, with or without flap elevation, when there is:
   - Adequate gingival tissue (>3–5 mm, Type I-B), with an inadequate marginal bone crest relation with the cemento-enamel junction (<1 mm). A marginal incision is recommended, with an apically repositioned flap (Figs 5.5a–f).
   - Inadequate gingival tissue (≤ 3 mm, Type II-B), with an inadequate marginal bone crest relation with the cemento-enamel junction (< 1 mm) and/or gingival disharmony. A sulcular incision is recommended, with an apically repositioned flap (Figs 5.5g–k).
   - Crown lengthening could be also combined with implant therapy, carried out during the same surgical session, to achieve a better planned and more esthetic result (Figs 5.5l–q).
   - Forced eruption is the most common procedure for restoring an isolated tooth in order to prevent gingival disharmony with the adjacent teeth after the procedure

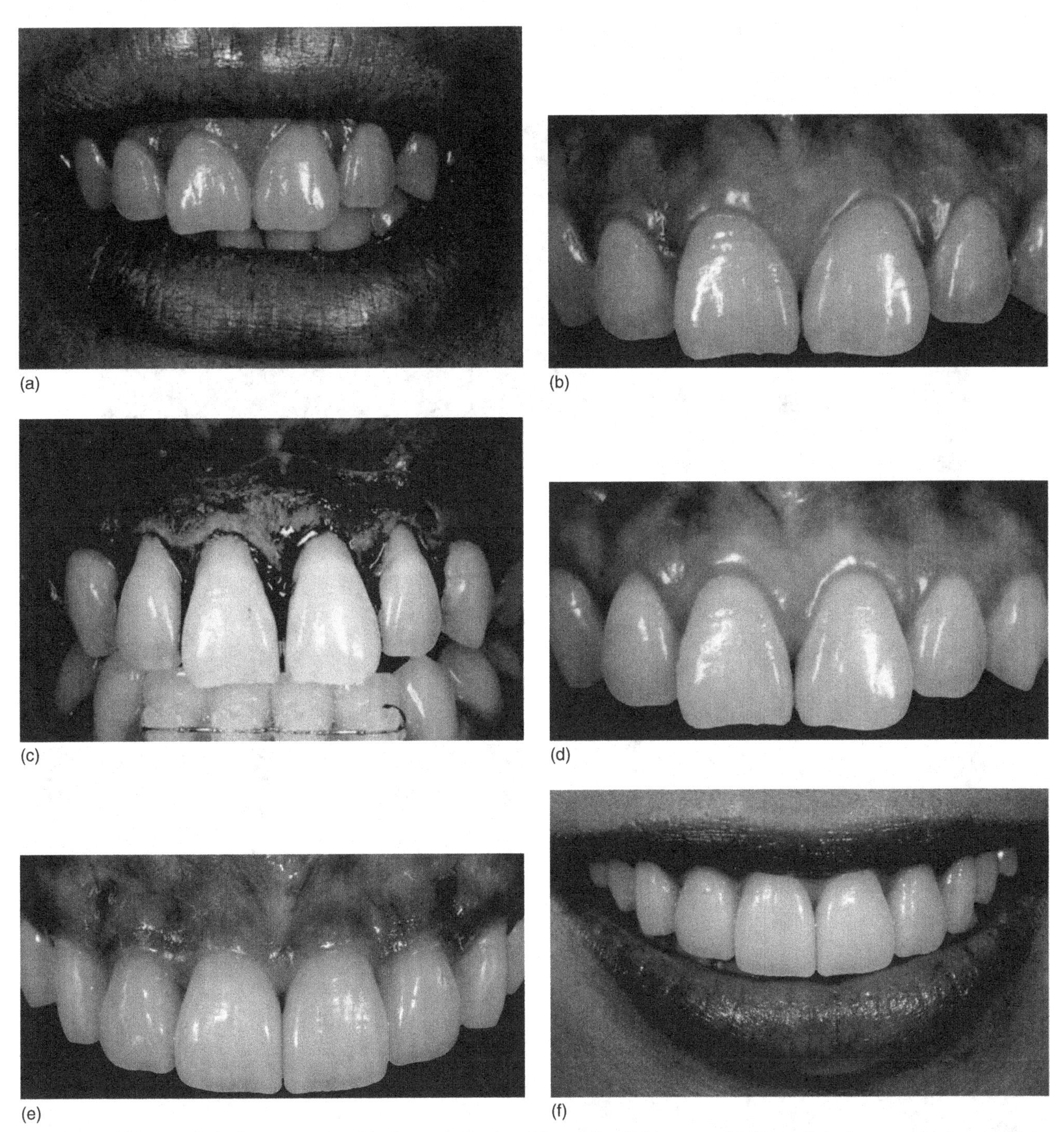

Figure 5.4 (a) A smile before surgery, with dentogingival and lower lip disharmony. (b) Short clinical crowns and an irregular gingival margin level on the right side (Type II-A). (c) Full thickness flap elevation, with harmonious apical bone resection. (d) Three months postoperative healing after an apically repositioned flap. (e) Laminate ceramic veneers from cuspid to cuspid with gingival harmony. (f) A beautiful smile, with the three components – the lips, teeth and gingiva – in harmony. (Courtesy of Dr. M. Okawa, Tokyo, Japan.)

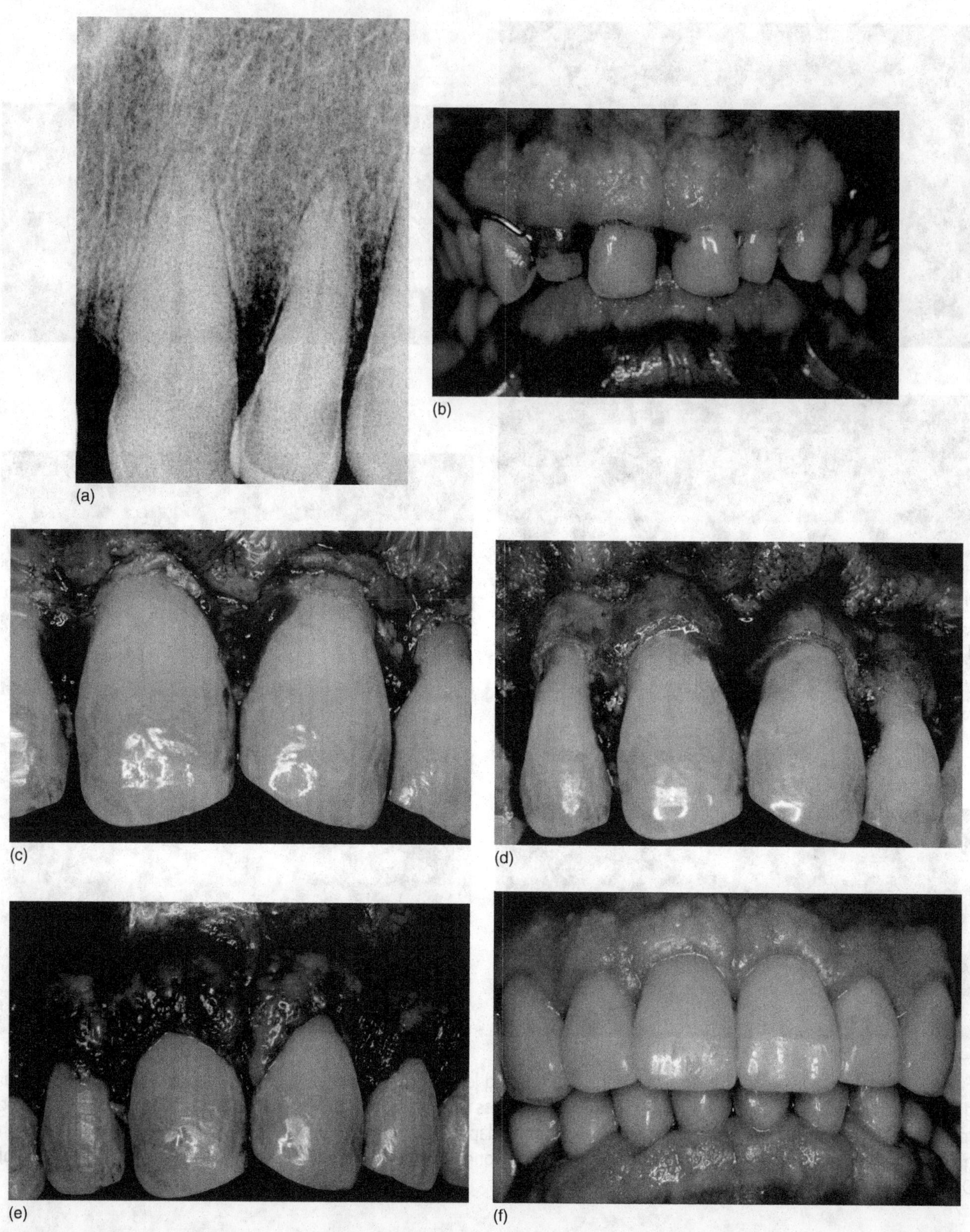

Figure 5.5 (a) X-rays of the right anterior teeth, with the interproximal bone level at the CEJ. (b) The patient's occlusal deep bite, with an excessive amount of KG (Type I-B). (c) After orthodontic treatment was completed, full-mouth flap elevation was performed after marginal incision, with the bone crest at the CEJ level. (d) Buccal osseous resection to restore the biological space between the CEJ and the BC. (e) An apically repositioned flap, showing longer teeth. (f) The full-mouth ceramic restoration, with a normal occlusal relation (Restoration Dr. Raygot C, Paris, France).

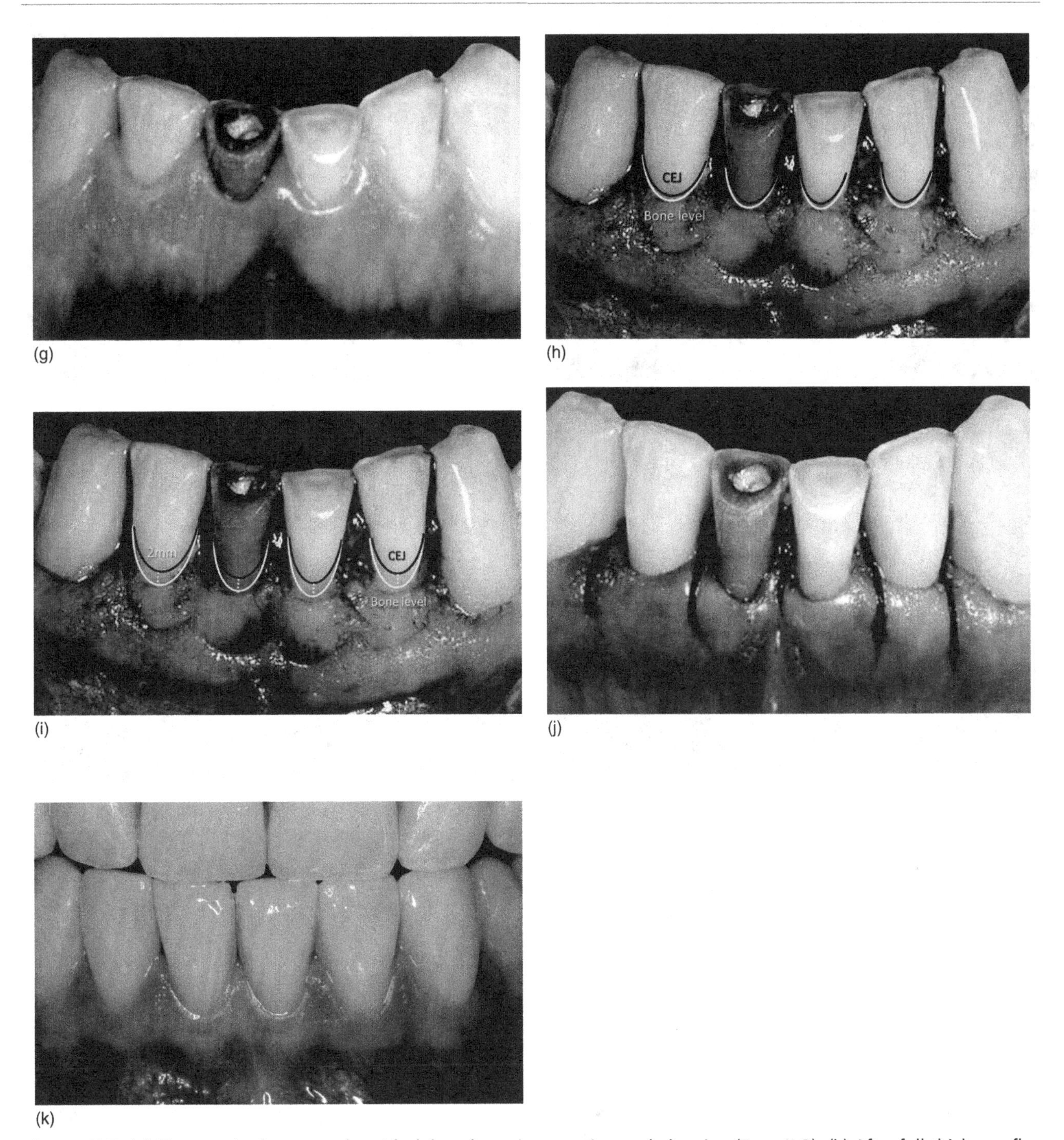

Figure 5.5 (g) The anterior lower teeth, with delayed passive eruption and abrasion (Type II-B). (h) After full-thickness flap elevation, the bone almost reaches the CEJ level. (i) The bone is resected apically and harmoniously 2 mm below the CEJ. (j) The sutures will be removed 1 week after the surgery. (k) Laminate veneer restorations on the eight lower anterior teeth (restorations by Dr. S. Koubi, Marseille, France).

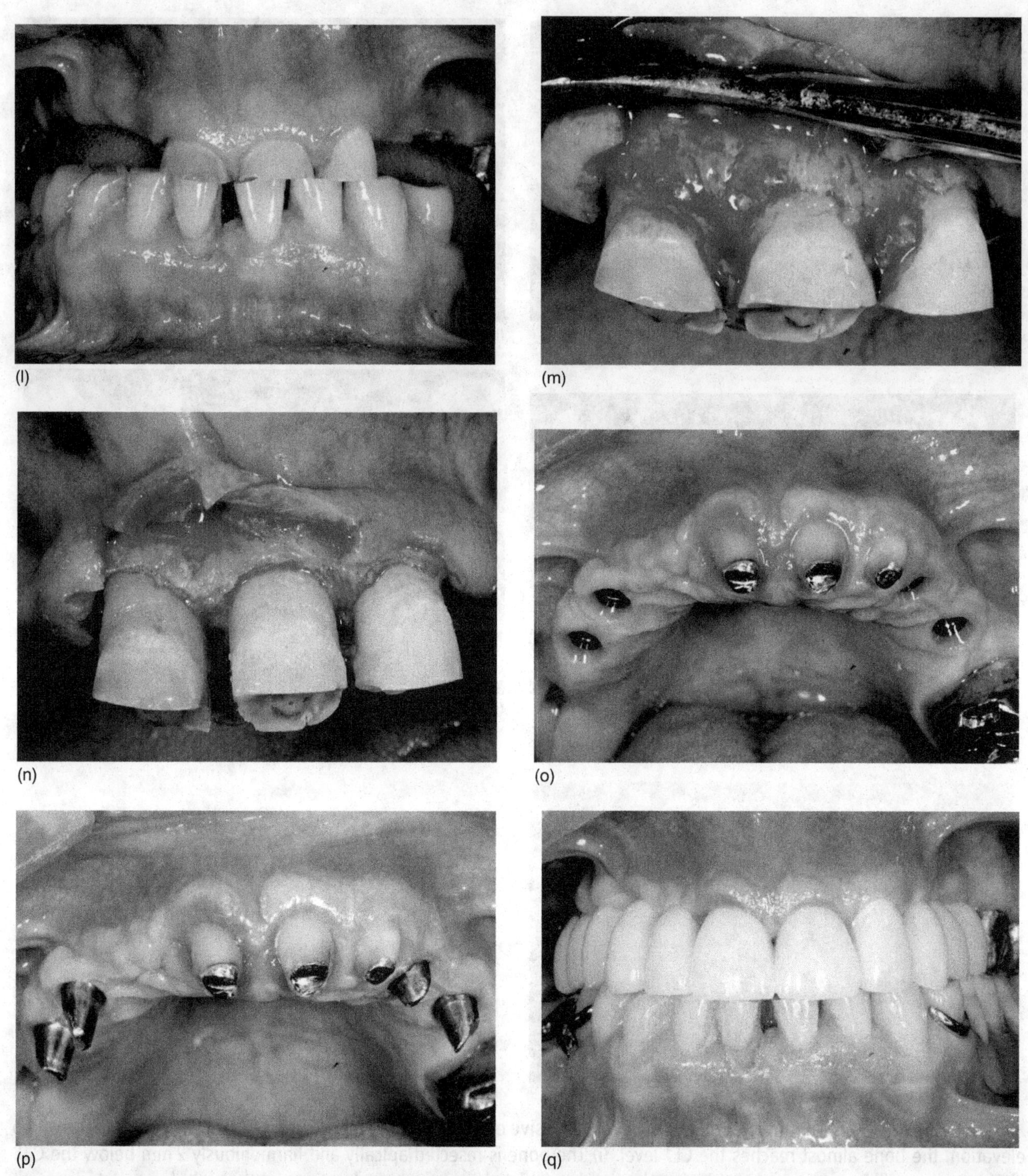

Figure 5.5 (l) Abrasion of the anterior teeth, with collapse of the posterior bite. (m) The bone crest level close to the CEJ. (n) Crestal bone resection to establish a minimum of 3–4 mm from the CEJ level and improve the structure of the teeth for preparation of the restoration. (o) The occlusal aspect of the ridge after implant osseointegration and soft tissue maturation. (p) The same occlusal aspect with the implant abutments. (q) The full mouth fixed and with rigid dento-implant restoration. (Courtesy of Dr. A. Peivandi, Lyon, France.)

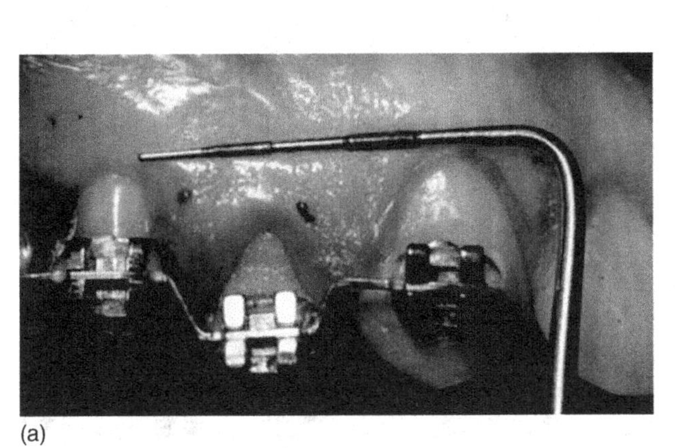
(a)

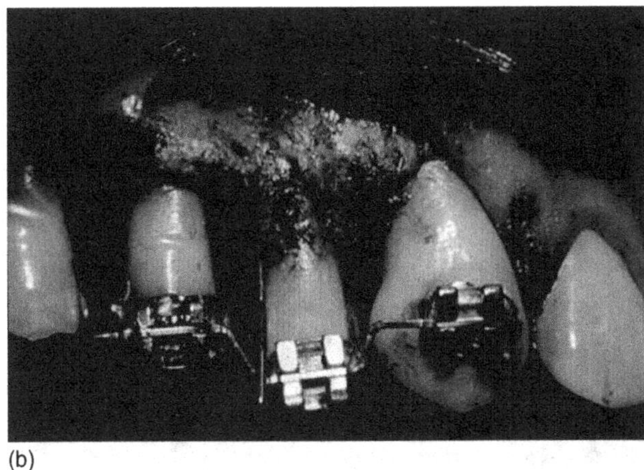
(b)

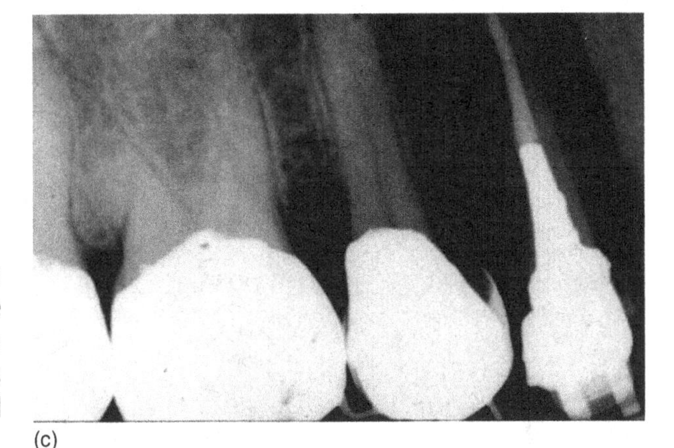
(c)

Figure 5.6 (a) Forced eruption performed before crown lengthening. (b) During the process of forced eruption, the KG increased in height in comparison to the adjacent teeth and the bone moved down. (c) The excess of bone was resected only on the premolar, keeping the correct bone level on the adjacent teeth.

(Figs 5.6a–c). If the bone is located below the mucogingival line, the amount of keratinized gingiva and bone will increase without changing the level of the mucogingival junction. On the other hand, if the mucogingival junction is below the bone crest, the amount of keratinized gingiva will remain constant, followed by a coronal movement of the mucogingival junction, but the bone will still move coronally (Chu and Hochman, 2011).

The two surgical approaches, more or less invasive, involving gingival resection with osseous resection are the closed flap technique and the open flap technique, as follows.

The closed flap technique on Type I-A

This technique can be used in lieu of a flap elevation procedure to make the correction and complete the restorative process without the healing time required for open flap crown lengthening surgery (Figs 5.7a–j). Patients with medium biotypes (i.e., moderate to thick keratinized gingiva with medium bone thickness) are good candidates for this procedure. For patients with a thick biotype (thick keratinized gingiva and thick bone), only a flap elevation procedure is recommended.

A marginal internal bevel incision located at the ideal gingival marginal position, preserving the papillae in order to retain the integrity of the papilla tissue, is performed according to the desired new smile of the patient.

The removal of the soft tissue margin, resected apically, creates the new esthetic coronal position and a scalloped free gingival margin and interproximal papillae. The osseous crest is sounded using a periodontal probe to determine the distance from the new free gingival margin to the alveolar crest. A small, round diamond bur is used to remove bone, holding the tip of the bur adjacent to the root and "walking" the tip across the buccal marginal bone area, using a "circular" (i.e., back and forth) movement to establish the corrected crestal level

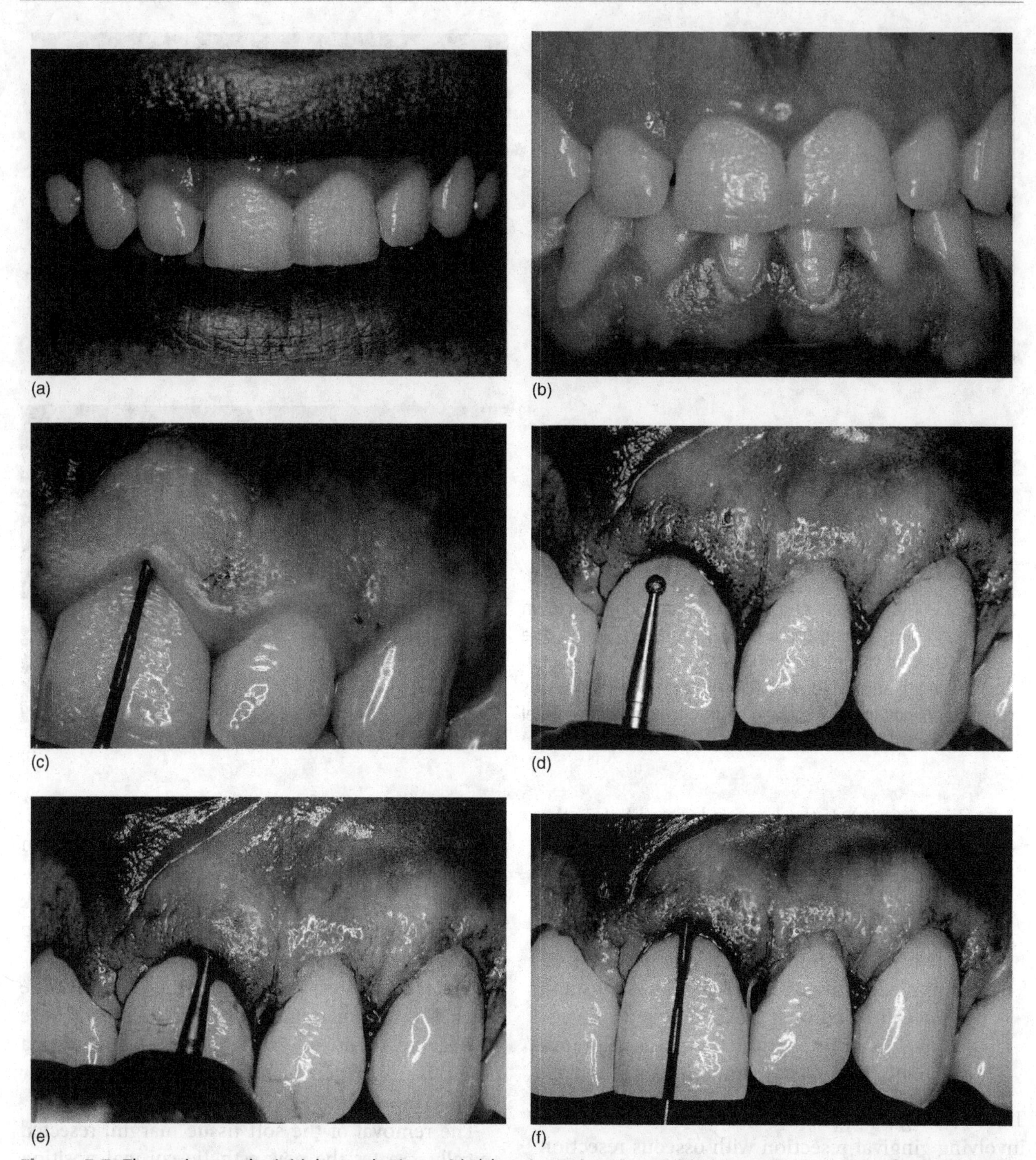

Figure 5.7 The patient at the initial consultation, with (a) a gingival smile and (b) short natural clinical crowns, an excess of gingiva, and gingival disharmony. (c) After papilla anaesthesia, bone sounding at 2.8 mm using a periodontal probe. (d) A marginal internal bevel incision is done at the ideal gingival level, without flap elevation. After suturing because of bleeding, a small, round diamond bur will (e) penetrate below the new gingival margin to resect just the buccal bone. A small diamond finishing bur will complete the bone recontouring. (f) Checking the proportions of the new clinical crown.

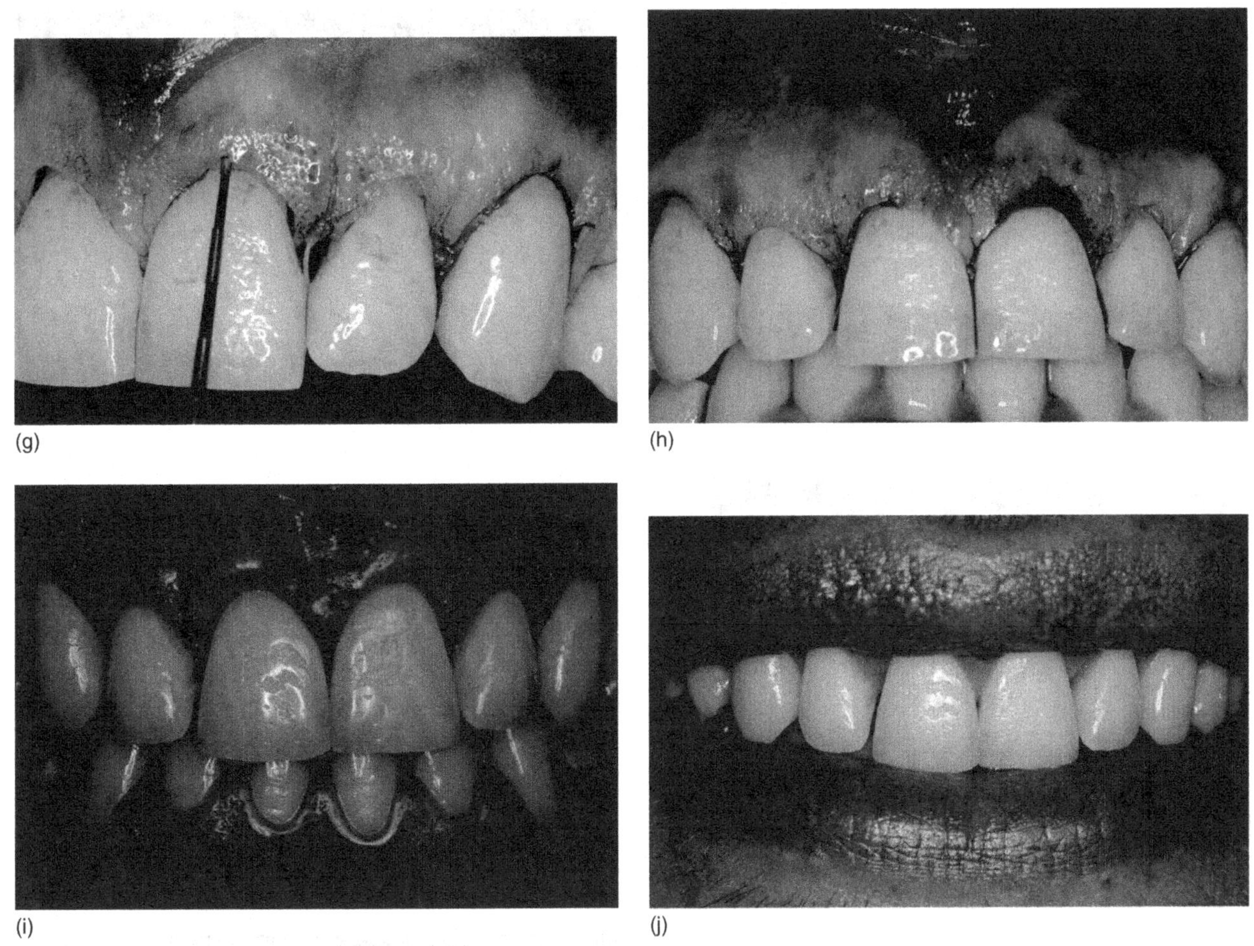

(g) (h) (i) (j)

Figure 5.7 (g) Checking the length of the crown by sounding the new cervical bone to the new gingival margin level (2.8 mm). (h) The end of the surgical session, with some bleeding due to aspirin intake. (i) The clinical aspect at 6 months after surgery. (j) The patient's new esthetic smile.

and to reach a 3 mm depth from the top of new gingival margin design, in order to reestablish the normal biological dentoalveolar gingival unit. A periodontal probe, or Chu's gauge, is then used to verify the depth by sounding to 3 mm. The interproximal bone, and the peak in particular, is not involved in this bone recontouring.

If a restoration is planned, these factors determine the restorative timing. Therefore, any definitive restoration can be seated 2–3 weeks after the closed crown lengthening procedure if the restoration is located supragingivally, and after a minimum of 12 weeks to allow for the reformation of the sulcus if it is located subgingivally.

The criteria for the clinical health of the dentogingival restorative interface complex are as follows:

- a pink color (i.e., the absence of inflammation), adequate texture, and a thin gingival margin
- the reestablishment of a shallow gingival sulcus a few months later, and
- the absence of bleeding upon probing.

The open flap technique on Type I-A or Type IB/Type IIB

To give the appearance of spatially moving teeth in the cervical direction and to alleviate excessive gingival display or asymmetry, oftentimes osseous correction must be performed in conjunction with soft tissue resection. Osseous resection is essential to the placement of apically positioned gingival margin; therefore, the usual periodontal flap surgery, giving access to the underlying bone for osseous resection, should be chosen (Figs 5.8a–m).

Following the objectives of the surgery and the guidelines for esthetic tissue levels, the perceived final gingival level is traced, creating heights of contour at the distolabial line angles. Furthermore,

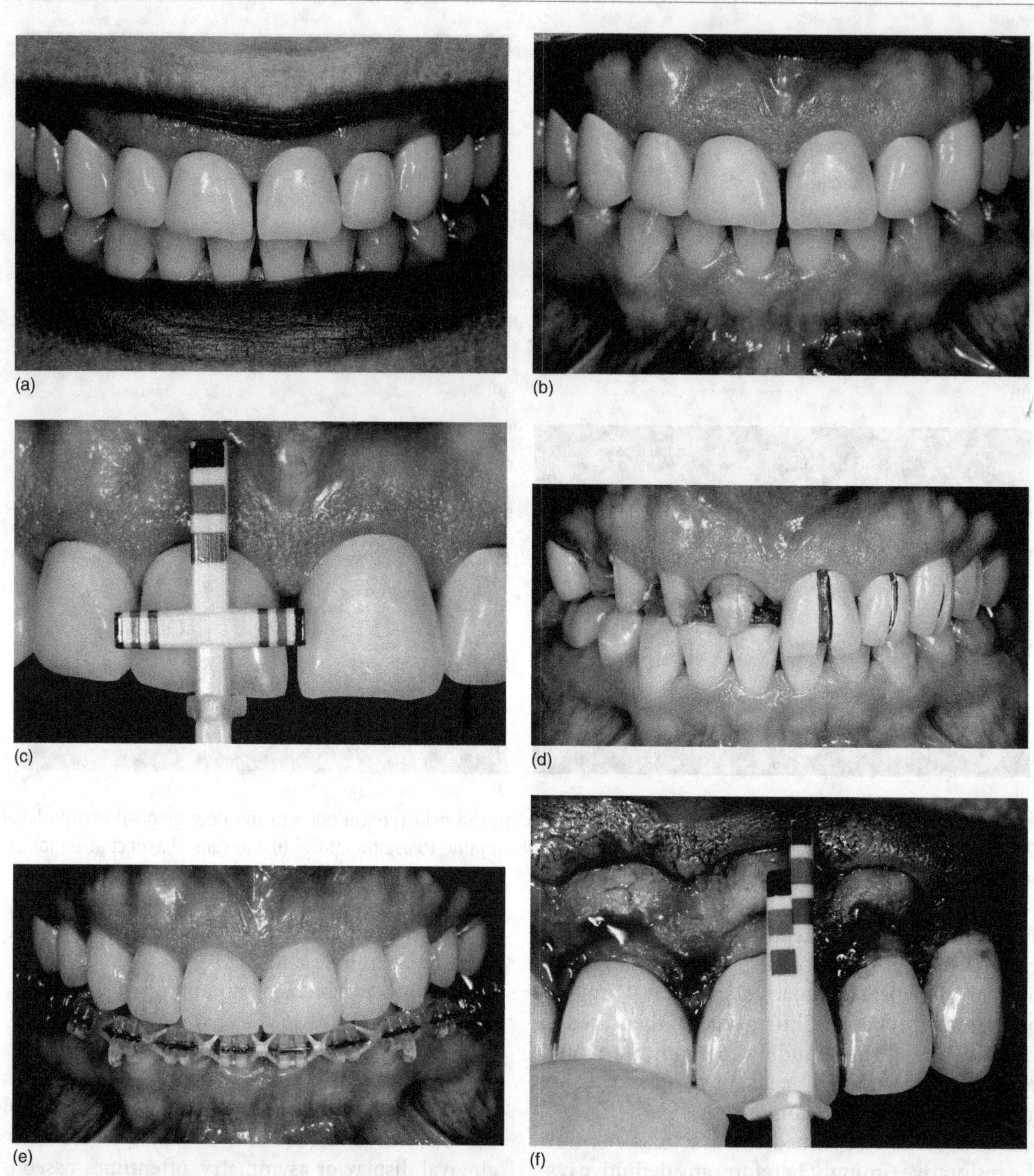

Figure 5.8 (a) The patient's smile, displaying an asymmetrical excess of gingiva and the metallic finishing line of the restorations. (b) Gingival disharmony, iatrogenic ceramometal crowns, and inflamed gingival margins. (c) A disproportion between the width and length of the crowns, measured using the T-bar gauge. (d) After removal of the crowns on the right side, the crowns on the left side are removed. (e) Presurgical temporary crowns are placed and orthodontic therapy is performed on the lower teeth. (f) The bone crest is resected buccally to restore the normal dimension between the bone crest and the apical part of the restoration, using the Probe or Chu's In-line gauge tip.

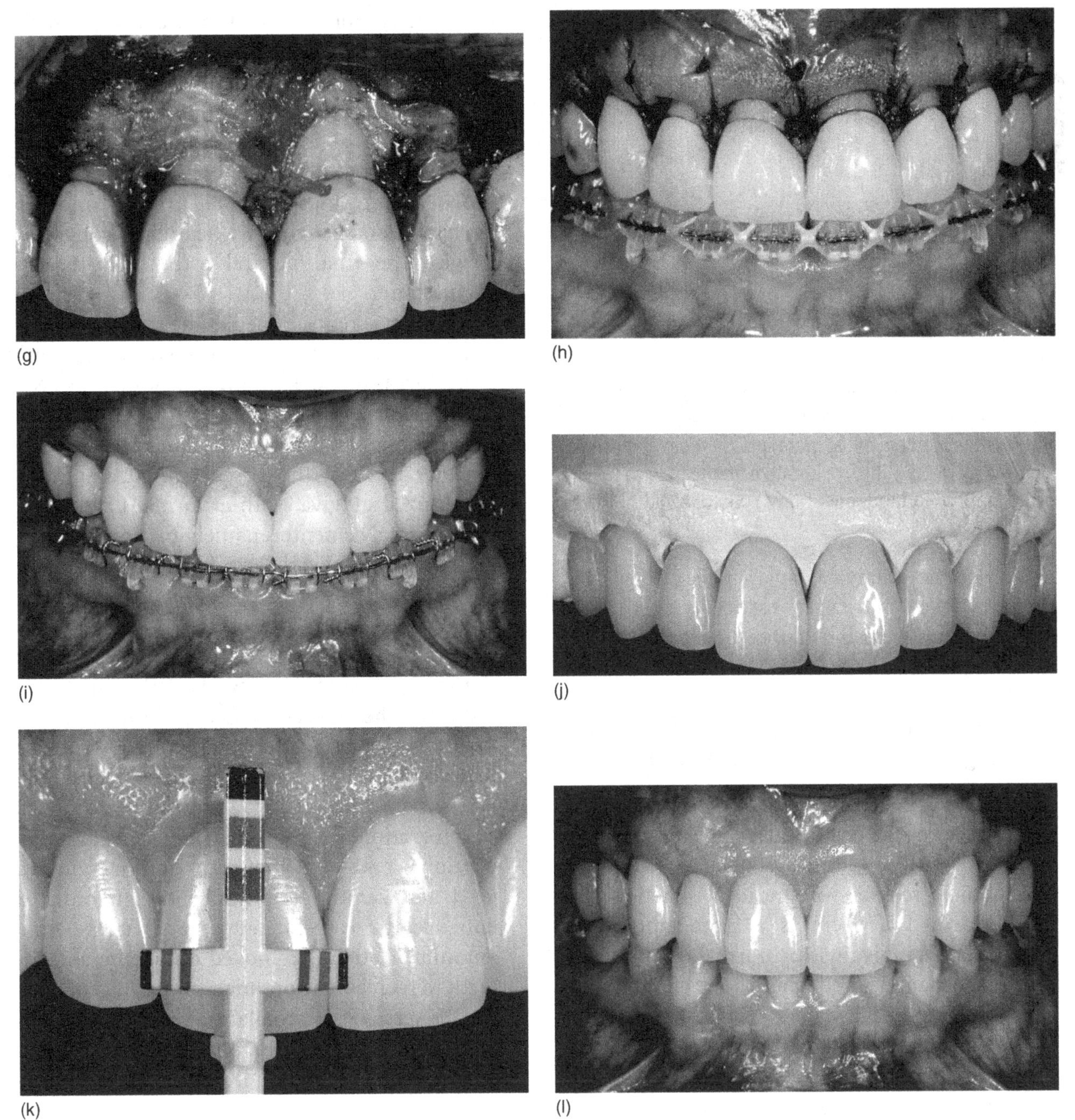

(g) (h) (i) (j) (k) (l)

Figure 5.8 (g) End of the surgical session, with a normal relation between the apical part of the temporary restorations, the preparations, and the scalloped contour of the alveolar bone crest. (h) The apically repositioned flap, with interrupted sling sutures away from the apical part of the restorations to allow normal healing of the gingiva. (i) Healing at 3 months, with a regular and symmetrical gingival margin contour. (j) At 5 months, final teeth preparation was done and final impressions were taken. The eight ceramic restorations are presented on the cast. (k) The adequate tooth proportion of the new restoration, measured using the T-bar gauge. (l) The final crown restorations, cemented 8 months after the crown lengthening procedure.

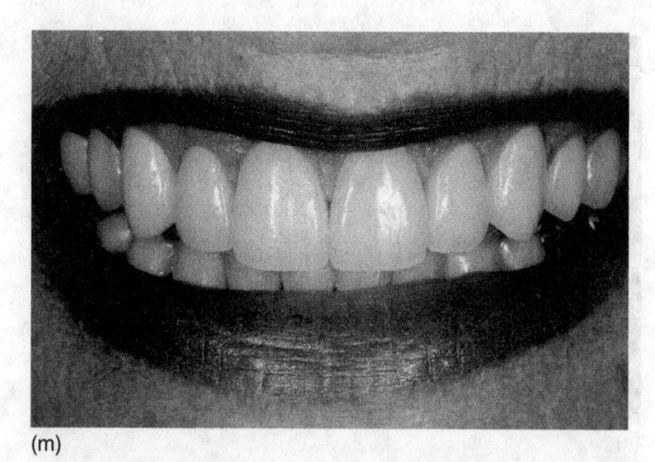

(m)

Figure 5.8 (m) The patient's new smile, with a harmonious relation between the teeth and the gingival contour, surrounded by a more pleasant lip line smile. (Courtesy of Dr. S. Chu, restorative dentist, and Dr. M. Hochman, perio-orthodontist, New York, USA.)

for an esthetic gingival display, it is critical that symmetry (right and left) – especially on the two central incisors – exists as far as the cervico-incisal tooth height and gingival zenith positions are concerned.

There are two possible approaches to incision, depending on the amount of keratinized gingiva:

- A marginal internal bevel incision, preserving the papillae, located at the ideal gingival marginal position with the dentogingival zenith, in a harmonious relation with the ideal esthetic smile, is performed if there is a large amount of keratinized gingiva with a normal or abnormal cemento-enamel junction and bone crest relation (Type II-A/Type I-B):
  - A full-thickness flap, including the new gingival margin and the papillae, is elevated. It is advisable to elevate a full-thickness buccal flap with the full papilla only and leave the interproximal bone and the palatal tissue intact. The initial buccal gingival margins remaining on the teeth are removed through a sulcular incision, and the buccal bone is resected with a positive architecture in order to create optimal tooth dimensions and proportions. The alveolar bone architecture should also mimic the restorative margin 3 mm apically, allowing the biological width and sulcus reformation to attain a normal crest position. In facial esthetic correction cases, the interproximal bone is not touched except in the instance of altered passive eruption.
  - The optimum tooth length and the future location of the free gingival margin are now established prior to and during crown lengthening surgery using the T-bar tip. This will ensure that the final tooth proportion that is established post-healing is congruent with the final natural esthetic restorative outcome.
  - The flap is repositioned at the initial predetermined level and then sutured continuously using 5-0 VICRYL™ (Ethicon, Somerville, NJ).
- An internal bevel sulcular incision is performed, over the direct facial and proximal surface of the anterior teeth, if there is a limited amount of keratinized gingiva, with a normal (Type II-A) or abnormal cemento-enamel junction and bone crest relation (Type II-B). A full-thickness mucoperiosteal flap is elevated to expose the underlying crest and the facial alveolar bone topography. Direct clinical assessment utilizing the In-line tip of the Crown Lengthening Gauge indicates the proper vertical position and the amount of osseous resection required to reestablish a biological width of 3 mm. The buccal bone is resected with a positive architecture, according to integration of the tooth dimensions and proportions, and to achieve an optimal gingival level and zenith. It is important, in order to enhance the esthetic outcome, that the same amount of bone is removed on all the anterior teeth to recreate the optimal soft tissue biological parameters. The alveolar crest correction is made using a round diamond bur and/or bone chisel.

An apical partial flap dissection will allow the apical repositioning of the initial flap using vertical interrupted periosteal sutures using 5-0 VICRYL™ material, to hold the gingival margins in the predetermined positions.

There should be a time interval of 3–6 months after surgery, depending on the biotype before any final restoration. This is to allow the buccal dentogingival junction to mature and support the regeneration of the original, healthy, pre-operative sulcular levels, and to let the interproximal papillae rebound to a height greater than 4 mm before the preparation and impression of the final teeth restorations (Rosenberg *et al.*, 1999).

Discussion

Using the previous biological parameters of the dento-restorative gingival interface, it is now possible to perform closed or open periodontal flap procedures both facially and interdentally, and to predict where the level of the tissues will heal, on the basis of the position of the restorative margin or the correct tooth proportion. It is important for the clinician to use a periodontal probe and sound from the free gingival margin to the alveolar crest to determine the patient's biological parameters prior to preparing teeth for restorative purposes. This makes it possible to take the final impressions on the day of preparation and surgery. The clinician will then deliver the definitive restorations several weeks later, and can be confident that the gingival tissues will heal to the appropriate esthetic levels. The clinician must, however, still adhere to proven healing and surgical principles (Lowe, 2006).

Whether a closed or an open approach is adopted, the following concepts must be addressed in any crown lengthening procedure:

- A closed intrasulcular approach to remove bone and reestablish biological width can be performed only in patients with a medium biotype, where the thickness of the osseous crest is approximately 1–2 mm. The procedure may be limited to 1–2 mm of osseous removal as the bone width increases apically.
- However, the thick osseous ledge cannot be shaped or thinned in an intrasulcular way. In a patient with a thick biotype, a full-thickness flap is necessary to gain access to the alveolar bone and perform significant osteoectomy–osteoplasty.
- In the thin, highly scalloped biotype, the laser or the round diamond bur can remove the thin bone of 1 mm or less thickness when performed in a closed approach, but could result in excessive recession thereafter. Therefore, crown lengthening is not really recommended in the thin biotype.
- In the first year after a crown lengthening procedure, the marginal soft tissues tend to grow in a coronal direction.

Gingival recession coverage

Gingival recession occurs when the location of the gingival margin is apical to the cemento-enamel junction. Clinically, it results in an exposed root surface, loss of marginal tissue, and loss of attachment, with or without associated root and/or enamel abrasion (Horning *et al.*, 2008). This phenomenon will induce hypersensitivity, and has functional and esthetic repercussions.

Biological objectives

An *inadequate band of attached keratinized tissue* has been associated with chronic inflammation and progressive recession in the presence of poor oral hygiene. However, recession is a common clinical finding in populations with high standards of oral hygiene or after orthodontic treatment.

While factors such as tobacco use, incorrect or excessive hygiene, and various aspects of successful periodontal surgery can contribute to the general health and habits of the patient, it is mainly the presence of defective soft tissue morphology, the degree of root and/or enamel abrasion, the amount of keratinized gingiva apical to the recession, the details of the surgical technique, and the dexterity of the clinician that make the difference between success and failure.

The amount of root coverage after surgery will depend on the Miller classification. The root coverage should be complete and highly predictable in Classes I and II, partial in Class III, and nonexistent in Class IV (Miller, 1985).

To be more precise, the line of root coverage (the level at which the soft tissue margin will be positioned after the healing process of the root coverage surgical technique) is predetermined by calculating the ideal vertical dimension of the interdental papillae of the teeth adjacent to the marginal recession (Zuchelli *et al.*, 2006).

Tested individually by a group of periodontists, the root coverage esthetic score (RES) after treatment of gingival recession seems to be a reliable method (Fig 5.14k) for assessing the esthetic outcomes of root coverage procedures (Cairo *et al.*, 2010).

Operative restorative treatment should be considered with hybrid composite resin, a ceramic onlay and chip, or a laminate veneer when the lesion (enamel abrasion) is coronal to the cemento-enamel

Table 5.1 Several modalities for increasing the amount of keratinized gingiva and root coverage

Pedicle flaps	Grafts	Bioengineering materials
CAF Lateral pedicle Rotation pedicle Double papillae	ECG • one-stage • two-stage Submerged CTG	GRT with R/NRM EMD (Emdogain®) ADM (AlloDerm®, Dermis®) PRF gel/membrane Collagen matrix (Mucograft®)

CAF, coronally advanced flap; EMD, enamel matrix derivative; ECG, epithelial-connective graft; ADM, acellular dermal matrix; CTG, connective tissue graft; R/NRM, resorbable/nonresorbable membrane; GRT, guided tissue regeneration.

junction, and should be performed after healing of the soft tissue (Terry *et al.*, 2006).

Several modalities for increasing the amount of keratinized gingiva and root coverage are described in Table 5.1. The evaluation of root coverage after plastic mucogingival surgery with different types of procedures – pedicle flap or coronally advanced flap, free gingival graft or connective tissue graft – has shown that the coverage reaches 72% on average. The increase in the height of keratinized gingiva is more important with the free gingival graft in comparison to the coronally advanced flap or pedicle flap and the connective tissue graft. Less esthetic results are obtained with the free gingival graft. The height of the keratinized gingiva is negatively correlated with the overall esthetic (Dersot, 2011). The probability of the connective tissue graft attaining full coverage is increased to 78% if the graft is harvested from the tuberosity in comparison to the palatal. On maxillary teeth, smokers have a 64% chance of not obtaining full coverage, in comparison to 49% of nonsmokers.

The submerged connective graft was initially developed to increase the volume of the edentulous deformed crest. It was rapidly adopted to correct a lack of keratinized tissue, attain root coverage in cases of gingival recession, and resolve patients' esthetic demands (Langer and Langer, 1985; Wennström, 1996). There are many ways to harvest the palatal connective tissue graft, using different lines of incision. The least traumatic way is one horizontal line of incision (Figs 5.9a, b) that will allow full coverage of the donor site and better primary healing.

With regard to complete coverage, the connective tissue graft is superior to the other methods. To increase the amount of keratinized gingiva (Figs 5.10a–f), however, the free gingival graft is the most effective approach (Kerner *et al.*, 2009).

Today, the use of nonresorbable, regenerable membrane has a limited indication, because of the

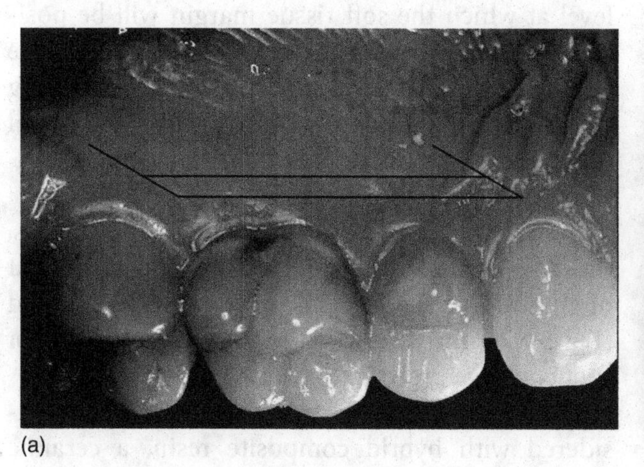

(a)

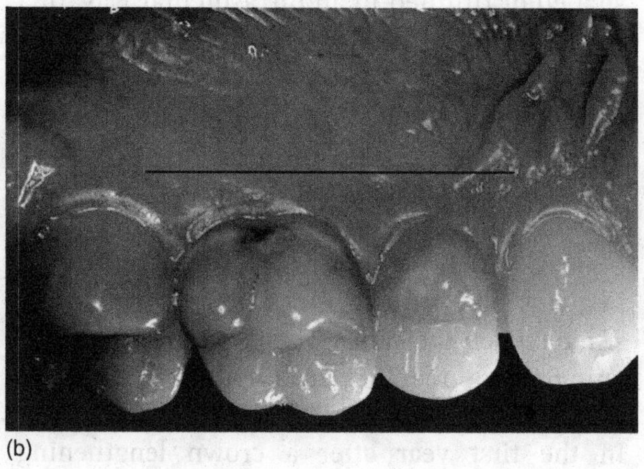

(b)

Figure 5.9 (a) A four-line palatal incision to harvest CTG (very traumatic). (b) A one-line horizontal palatal incision to harvest CTG (least traumatic).

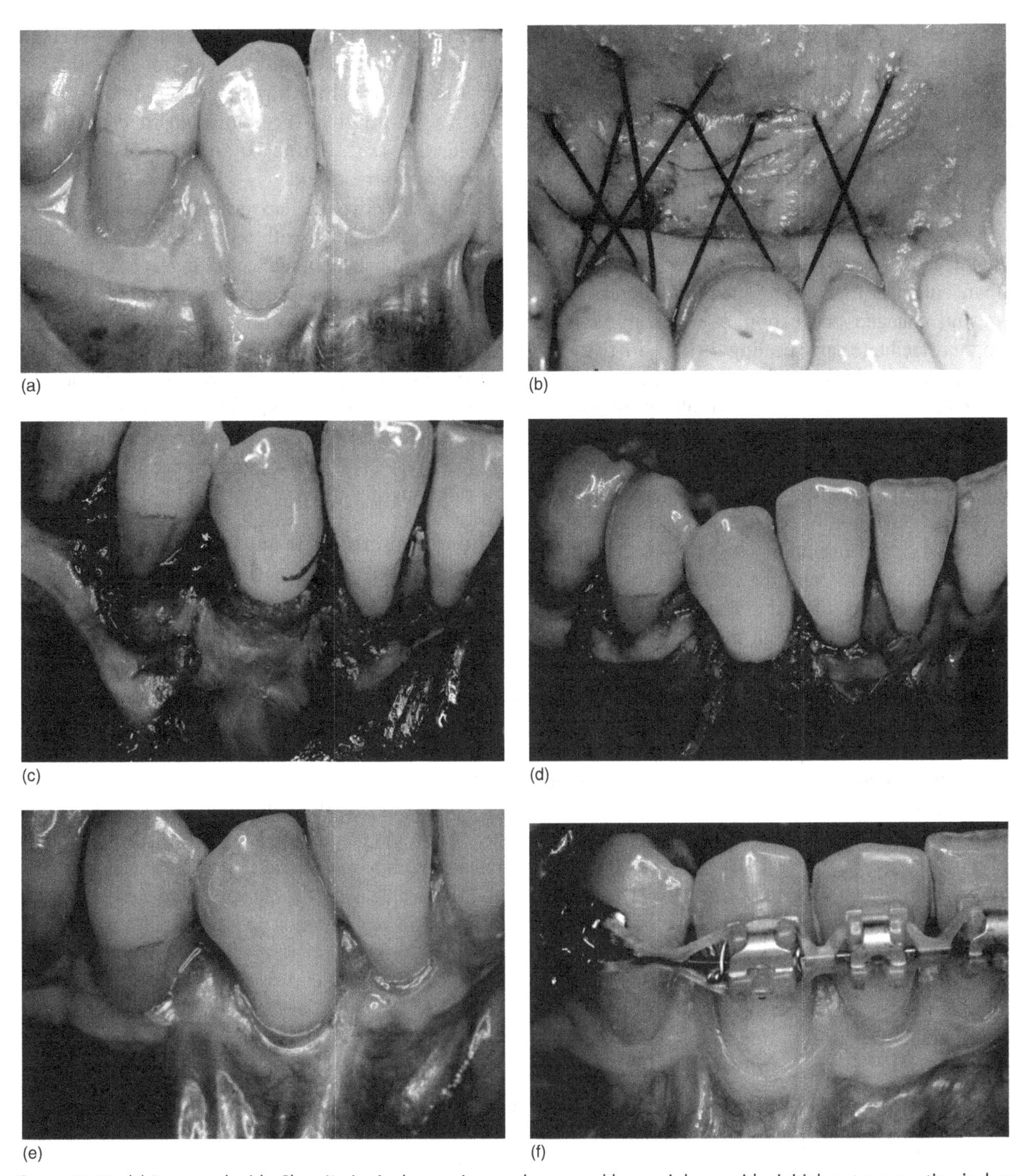

Figure 5.10 (a) Deep and wide Class II gingival recession on the rotated lower right cuspid – initial root preparation is done before and after raising the flap. (b) A one-line incision will permit harvesting of the CTG with immediate suspensory sutures around the teeth. (c) A thick and large palatal connective tissue graft is well stabilized around the root surface with resorbable suture. (d) A coronally advanced flap using suspensory silk sling suture is achieved. (e) Full coverage of the gingival recession on the cuspid at 3 months. (f) After 1 year of orthodontic therapy, the tissue remains at the same level with an aligned lower right cuspid.

two stages of surgery and the frequent risk of complications (Tinti *et al.*, 1992).

The enamel matrix derivative (EMD) has been shown to possess the potential to stimulate and promote the formation of new connective tissue, new bone, new periodontal ligament, and new cementum (Harris, 1997). It has been reported that enamel matrix derivative applied to instrumented root surfaces may remain active up to 10 days. It may influence the enhancement of PDL cell proliferation, increase protein and collagen production, promote mineralization, and facilitate early healing of the soft tissue in the dentogingival region (Sculean *et al.*, 1999).

Acellular dermal matrix (ADM) also presents several advantages: no need for palatal autograft harvesting or other secondary surgical sites, an unlimited supply of material, the ability to treat larger areas of multiple recession in one surgical session, a decrease in surgical chair-time, an increase in patient motivation and acceptance, and the achievement of excellent esthetic results (Shepherd *et al.*, 2009).

The principal intent of all these procedures is to cover single or multiple gingival recessions, create a tissue barrier that is more resistant to further recession due to trauma, simultaneously treat mucogingival root and/or ridge defects, and meet the increasing esthetic demands of the patients (Langer and Langer, 1985).

Current connective tissue graft procedures

Several techniques for the connective tissue graft procedure have now been described, but the currently most used ones are discussed below. Prior to any surgical procedure, all patients receive scaling, root planing, and prophylaxis. Full-mouth periapical and bitewing radiographs are taken to evaluate the interproximal alveolar bone level and to determine the gingival recession classification of the teeth exhibiting recession defects. Only teeth with gingival recession defects classified as Miller Classes I, II, and III are selected for plastic-periodontal treatment.

The usual envelope flap raising the buccal tissue and the proximal papilla with a coronally advanced flap, but without palatal tissue harvesting, is indicated only where there is a thick gingival margin or where there is a minimum of 3 mm of keratinized gingiva (Zuchelli and De Sanctis, 2000). In all other clinical situations, a combined palatal connective tissue graft or allograft membrane, submerged under the coronally advanced flap or using the tunneling pouch procedure, will be used for gingival recession coverage or ridge augmentation.

The connective tissue graft, the tunneling pouch technique, and recession coverage

This complex mucogingival procedure is selected to simultaneously treat multiple roots under Class I/Class II gingival recession (Figs 5.11a–m).

The procedure presents some definite advantages, as well as some drawbacks and disadvantages (Table 5.2) (Blanes and Allen, 1999; Zabalegui *et al.*, 1999; Saadoun, 2006).

The design of the sulcular incision is developed using a round blade or a #15c blade. An envelope full-thickness mucoperiosteal flap reflection is extended to 3 mm apical to the alveolar bone crest using a microperiosteal elevator, followed at the mucogingival junction by a partial-thickness flap dissection. A split-thickness flap dissection, using a #15 blade or the microperiosteal elevator kept in close contact with the contour of the periosteum, will prevent cutting of

Table 5.2 The advantages and disadvantages of the CTG mucogingival procedure

Advantages	Disadvantages
Excellent adaptation on the recipient site	Delicate harvesting of the graft
High visualization by the advanced flap	Traumatic surgery for the patient
Increased thickness of the KG	Requires two surgical sites
Decreased healing time	Difficult stabilization of the graft
High coverage success rate	Limited quantity and/or thickness of palatal tissue
Harmony in the gingival color/texture	Lengthy surgery and/or healing
Highly esthetic results	More technique-sensitive
	Postoperative discomfort for the patient

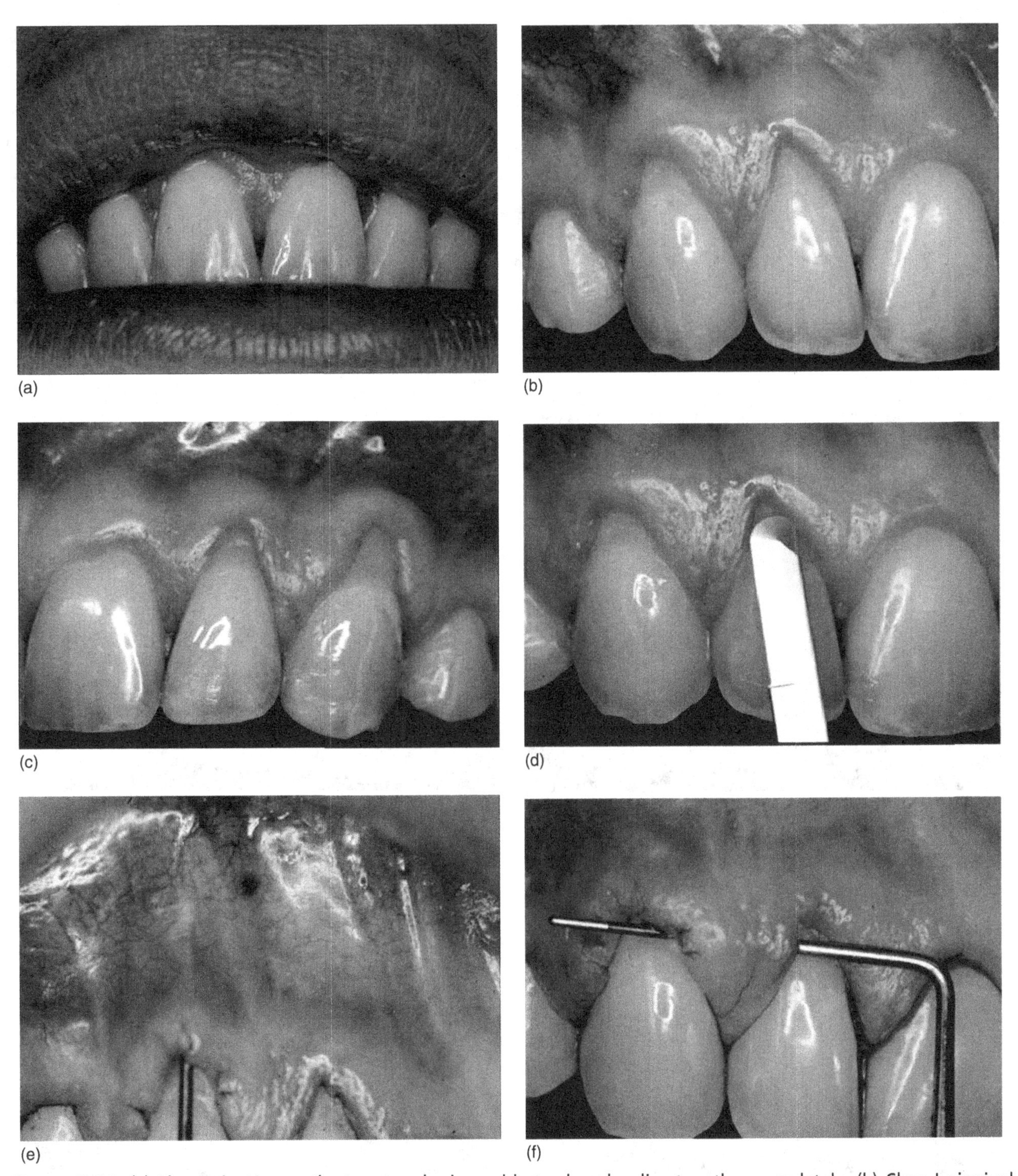

Figure 5.11 (a) The patient's mouth at rest – she is unable to close her lips together completely. (b) Class I gingival recession on the right maxillary canine and lateral incisor. (c) Class II gingival recession on the left maxillary canine and lateral incisor. (d) A rounded ophthalmic blade to initiate the circular incision. (e) Vertical sounding of the tunnel with a probe created beyond the MGJ. (f) Transversal sounding of the tunnel without detaching the peak of the papillae.

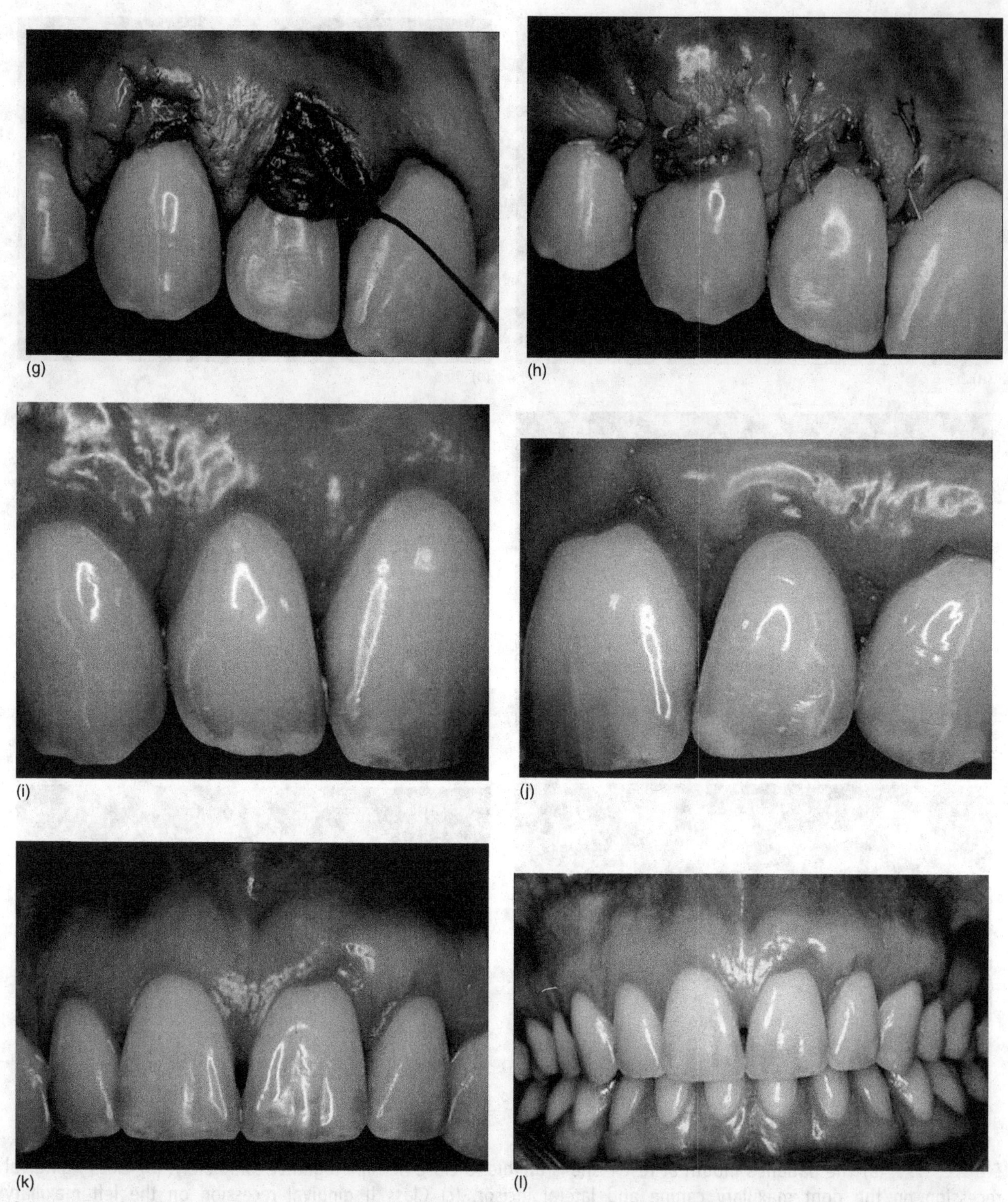

Figure 5.11 (g) After palatal harvesting, a large and thick CTG is inserted into the tunnel using a silk suture. (h) The flap is coronally advanced with sling sutures, stabilizing the CTG. (i) The postoperative right maxillary aspect at 6 months. (j) Improved gingival thickness and color harmony can be seen in this left maxillary view. (k) The postoperative frontal view at 6 months, with no more tooth sensitivity. (l) The full-mouth view 1 year post-op, showing total coverage of the gingival recession on both sides, with a thicker and stable gingival margin following the CEJ contour and enamel deformities on the left central incisor.

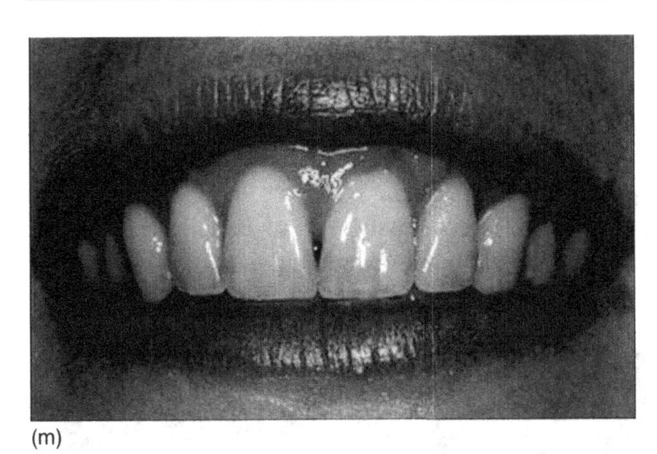

(m)

Figure 5.11 (m) The patient's new smile, showing gingiva, with no more gingival recession on the lateral incisors and canines.

the muscle fibers. This incision is extended mesially and distally without vertical releasing incisions, and apically to facilitate adequate mobility and coronal positioning of the flap without tension. This partial dissection is carefully performed in order to create a deep pouch beyond the mucogingival junction – care being taken not to perforate the alveolar mucosa, while keeping the tip of the interproximal papillae attached to the teeth below the proximal contact point.

The root surfaces are planed thoroughly, using curettes to remove contaminated cementum, and are then prepared using a fine diamond bur to flatten the prominent root surface as necessary. The root preparation is finished using a prophyjet.

The connective tissue graft is usually harvested from the palate on the same side as the gingival tunneling defect, with one line of incision instead of two horizontal and two vertical incisions, to minimize the bleeding and decrease postoperative discomfort. The graft should be as thick as possible, but when the primary palatal flap has a thickness of about 1.25 mm, the risk of palatal necrosis decreases (Horning *et al.*, 2008).

Using a 4-0 silk or Vicryl™ suture and a needle, the connective tissue graft is delicately inserted into the distal tunnel extremity below each papilla, and pushed apically and laterally inside the pouch. The CTG is then stabilized, with the flap advanced coronally using 5-0 Vicryl™ suspensory sling sutures with palatal knots. It is important that the flap totally cover the CTG to prevent partial exposition of its coronal part and lack of vascularization from the flap, which could induce complications.

However, in a study by Han *et al.* (2008), the intentional small exposure of connective tissue grafts resulted in successful root coverage and a greater increase in the width of the keratinized gingiva, but a greater amount of root coverage was observed when the connective tissue graft was completely covered by the flap. However, the difference in the outcomes was not statistically significant in the long term.

A prescription of ibuprofen, amoxicillin, and chlorhexidine gel is prescribed to the patient. Healing usually progresses uneventfully, with the possible exception of some postoperative edema in the days following the surgery. It is important to prevent as much swelling as possible, because clinical experience has shown that edema can disrupt graft stability and cause the sutures to pull through the papillae, resulting in apical flap displacement. The prescription of corticoids is therefore recommended before and after the procedure.

The patient is seen at weekly postoperative visits to evaluate healing and plaque control. The sutures are not removed until the 2-week postoperative visit. The patient is instructed to resume gentle mechanical tooth brushing on the treated sites, using a soft brush and roll technique, after 4 weeks. Professional plaque control, consisting of debridement and oral hygiene instruction, is performed weekly during the first 4 weeks, and scaling is performed at the 3-month and 6-month recalls.

After 6 weeks to 3 months of healing, the gingiva is usually observed to have a healthy appearance. The gingival margins appear thicker and more resistant to trauma. Sensitivity to air or cold has been eliminated and the sulcular probing depths are 2 mm or less. In approximately 6 months, the tissue will mature with a smooth contour. Gingivoplasty could be performed to remove the remaining irregularities.

The extent and predictability of root coverage procedures for the treatment of recession defects are dependent on the quality of the vascularity that is maintained at the surgical site. The tunnel/envelope technique optimizes vascularity by eliminating the need for vertical releasing incisions. Furthermore, when adjacent recession defects are present and connected by an esthetically critical papilla, the tunnel technique is an excellent approach to protect the positional height of the papilla. This flap design, combined with partial-thickness dissection, creates the most optimal and vascular subgingival environment for the placement of subepithelial or acellular collagen matrix types of grafts (Salama *et al.*, 2008).

The connective tissue graft, the tunneling pouch technique, and ridge augmentation

The purpose of this surgery is to resolve gingival recession, whether or not it is associated with deformed vertical and/or horizontal ridges adjacent to the teeth, by combining the tunneling pouch procedure and soft tissue ridge augmentation, using several stages of submerged connective tissue grafts (Figs 5.12a–g).

The first step consists of an incision below the mucogingival junction, and a sulcular incision around

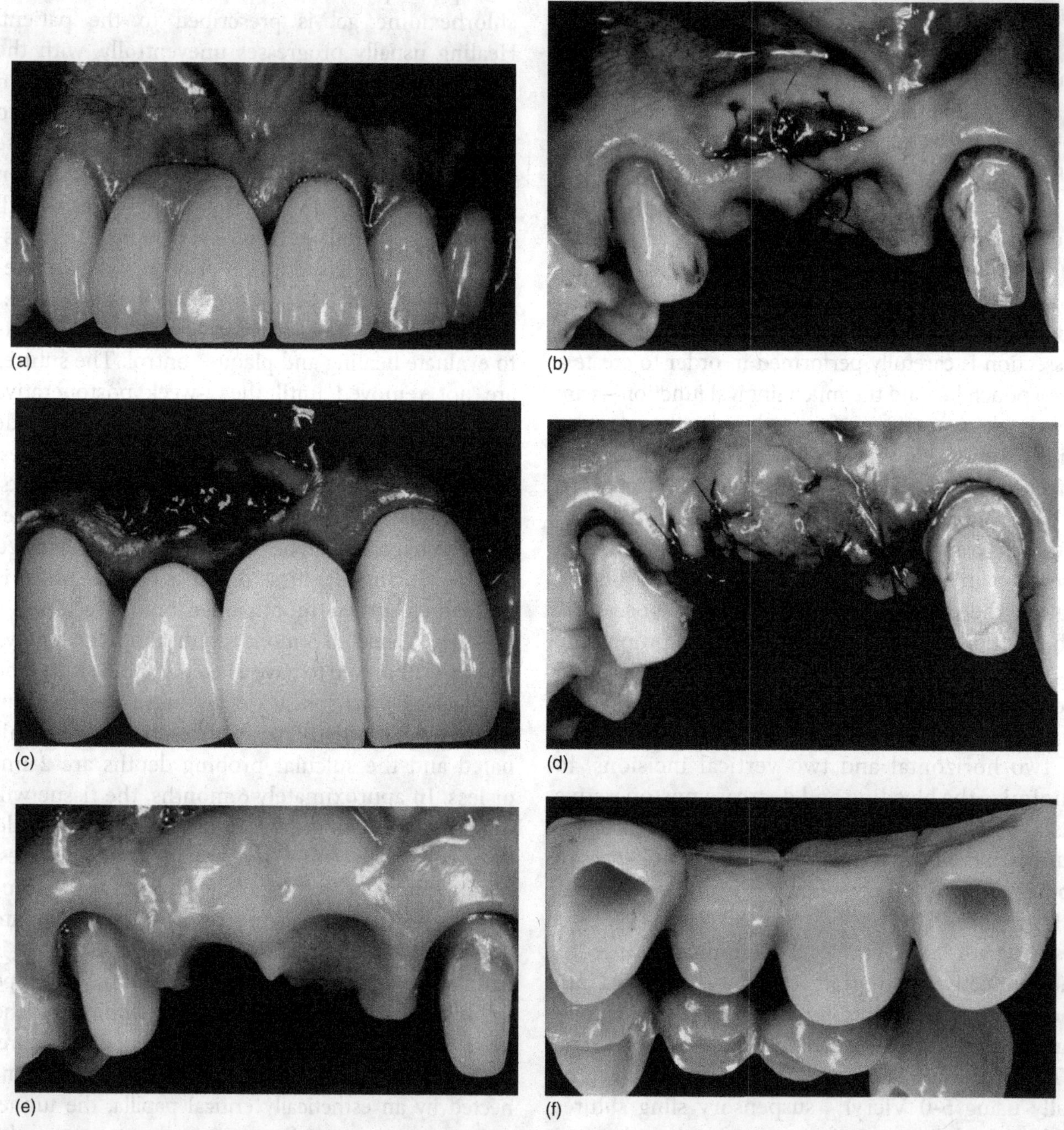

Figure 5.12 (a) A bridge from the right cuspid to the left central incisor, with pink ceramic above the pontics. (b) Apical connective tissue graft tunneling with a coronally advanced soft tissue ridge. (c) The new modified temporary bridge at the end of the initial surgical session. (d) The submerged connective tissue graft on the ridge. (e) Development of the pontic site, and the creation of new papillae, with minimal surgery and a temporary bridge. (f) The apical aspect of the final ceramic bridge.

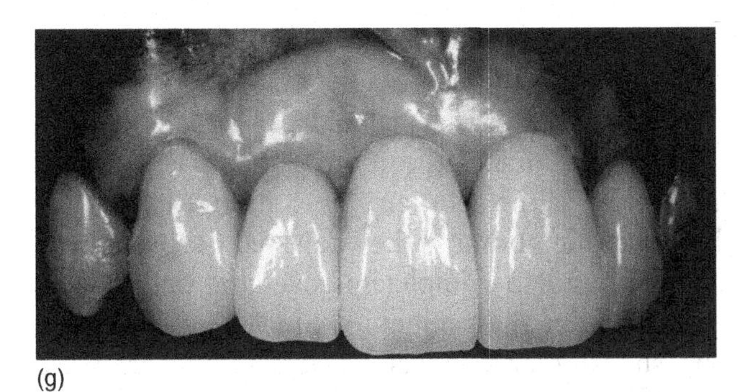

(g)

Figure 5.12 (g) The new four-unit ceramic bridge restoration with two convex pontics, showing an excellent PES/WES. (Courtesy of Drs. M. Okawa and M. Suzuki, Tokyo, Japan.)

the adjacent teeth bordering the edentulous crest, to undermine all of the soft facial tissue. The creation of the buccal pouch permits the coronal displacement of all of the labial tissue and the ridge tissue.

A palatal connective tissue graft is harvested and inserted apico-coronally into the pouch, and all the tissues are then coronally repositioned, covering the adjacent gingival recession and moving the ridge more coronally. Following 8 weeks of healing, another connective tissue graft is placed between the buccal and palatal flap of the ridge, in order to increase its length and width, resolving the initial ridge deformity. After 2 months, the healed ridge is recontoured with a round diamond bur, and the placement of a temporary bridge with convex pontics assures elegant gingival scalloping and the creation of new interproximal papillae. The final ceramic restoration, using a convex pontic, is cemented 6–8 weeks later.

Discussion

The connective tissue graft procedure remains very complex for many clinicians, due to its indications and the technically demanding aspects.

More recent modifications of this technique tend to simplify both parts of the procedure. For example, the graft harvesting may involve only one incision line; it is no longer necessary to retain an epithelial strip or place releasing incisions. The graft can also be thinner than originally suggested (1–2 mm) in order to improve the acceptance of the graft at the recipient site, to create a more natural and esthetic result, and to avoid palatal necrosis (Mattout and Mattout, 2008).

The residual height of the attached keratinized gingiva does not seem to influence the root coverage. However, the partial flap dissection should allow more flexibility for the coronally advanced flap to be sutured over the graft without any tension, decreasing postoperative discomfort and improving the esthetic result. The phenomenon of "creeping attachment" after a soft tissue graft corresponds, on average, to a gingival margin migration of about 1 mm coronally within 1 year, or up to 2.5 mm in 18 months (Pollack, 1984).

Current bioengineering materials

Nowadays, the goal of periodontal plastic mucogingival procedures is to perform surgery as atraumatically as possible at the recipient and donor sites.

Recently, as an alternative to autogenous gingival grafts in root coverage procedures, Emdogain®, or enamel matrix derivative (Emdogain®, Straumann, Andover, MA), and AlloDerm®, or acellular dermal matrix allograft (AlloDerm®, Bio Horizons, Dermis® Zimmer), alone or combined (Shin *et al.*, 2007; Saadoun, 2008), have been utilized to correct these gingival defects, negating the requirement for a second palatal surgical procedure (Mellonig, 1999; Cueva *et al.*, 2004; Harris, 2004; Sallum, 2004). Enamel matrix derivative alone or combined with acellular dermal matrix offers an excellent alternative to the use of a connective tissue graft for patients who do not desire a second surgical site, or have limited tissue available to harvest and transplant to cover multiple gingival recessions.

A new resorbable collagen matrix, the Mucograft® (Geistlich Pharma AHG Company, Wolhusen, Switzerland), is now available and is used to fulfill the same objectives.

In a study by Miller (1985), prior to the surgical procedures, all patients received scaling, root planing, and prophylaxis. Full-mouth periapical and bitewing radiographs were taken to evaluate the interproximal alveolar bone level, to assist in the gingival recession classification of teeth exhibiting recession defects. Only teeth with recession defects classified as Miller Classes I, II, and III were selected for treatment.

Two types of procedure presented in this chapter have been used to treat these patients: the flap elevation technique and the pouch tunneling technique, using enamel matrix derivative and acellular dermal matrix alone or combined.

The flap elevation technique

After periapical and intrapapillary anesthesia on the buccal site – but not on the palatal one – bleeding points equivalent to the length of the buccal recession are marked with a probe at the base of the adjacent interproximal papillae, to determine the location of the tip of the new interdental (from the tip to the base) papillae. Scalloped sulcular incisions are made from the bleeding reference points on the existing papillae to create new papilla tips and the flap design.

The design of the sulcular incision, using a round ophthalmic blade, or a #15c blade, enables limited-envelope, full-thickness mucoperiosteal flap reflection. The incision is extended to the nearest mesiodistal line angle of the adjacent non-defective tooth. The flap is reflected to 3 mm apical to the alveolar bone crest using a macroperiosteal elevator, followed by a partial-thickness flap reflection. The split-thickness flap dissection close to the periosteum is extended using a #15 blade mesially, distally, and apically, to facilitate adequate mobility and coronal positioning of the flap without tension. The flap should be free of any tension before suturing and should be made passive through the utilization of an apical partial thickness flap. The remaining interdental papillae are then de-epithelialized to ensure good vascularization of the connective tissue bed. The root surfaces are planed thoroughly, using curettes to remove contaminated cementum, and prepared as necessary using a fine diamond bur to flatten the prominent buccal root surface.

The exposed root surfaces are conditioned with 24% EDTA (PrefGel™, Straumann, Andover, MA) for 2 minutes in an attempt to remove the smear layer. After acid application, the area is rinsed with saline solution or tap water and then dried.

The flap is then advanced coronally onto the de-epithelialized gingival margins without any resistance, and sutured using a double-sling suture technique with palatal notches (Saadoun, 2008). The enamel matrix derivative gel is applied with a syringe on the root surface before or after the suturing of the coronally advanced flap (Figs 5.13a–f).

If acellular dermal matrix is used, the flap dissection remains the same as previously described. The dried acellular dermal matrix graft is sized with a #15 blade out of the mouth and is rehydrated in a water saline solution for 15 minutes. The soft hydrated membrane is then adjusted precisely to fit the area and to completely cover the defect. It is positioned at the cemento-enamel junction, while the superior and lateral borders of the graft are extended at least 0.7–1.0 mm apically beyond the alveolar defect margins. The acellular dermal matrix graft is placed with the basal membrane side (with smaller concavities) against the bone and roots, while the connective tissue or dermal side (with larger concavities) faces the overlying flap (Figs 5.14a–k).

The stretching adaptation to the underlying periosteal surface may also aid in the development of a new blood supply for the graft by opening microspaces in the graft to allow the ingrowth of blood vessels from the adjacent tissue (Imberman, 2007).

Correct suturing of the acellular dermal matrix with sling sutures with palatal knots is critical for the success of this procedure, as it must immobilize the graft and stabilize for the underlying blood supply.

Postoperative medication and postsurgical instructions are given to the patient as described in the next section. If some gingival marginal deformity remains after a few months of healing, a light gingivoplasty is performed to harmonize the tissue.

The tunneling pouch technique

This procedure is carried out following the same guidelines as described previously for the connective tissue graft until the root surfaces are planed, but it will contribute to the combined use of acellular dermal matrix and enamel matrix derivative. Then, the exposed root surfaces are conditioned with PrefGel™ for 2 minutes in an attempt to remove the smear layer. After acid application, the area is rinsed with saline solution and the root surfaces are dried. The rehydrated acellular dermal matrix material should be oriented with the epithelial basal membrane side against the bone and teeth, while the dermal connective tissue site should face the overlying flap.

Using a 4-0 suture, floss, and a needle, the acellular dermal matrix is delicately inserted into the distal tunnel extremity below each papilla, and pushed apically and laterally inside the pouch

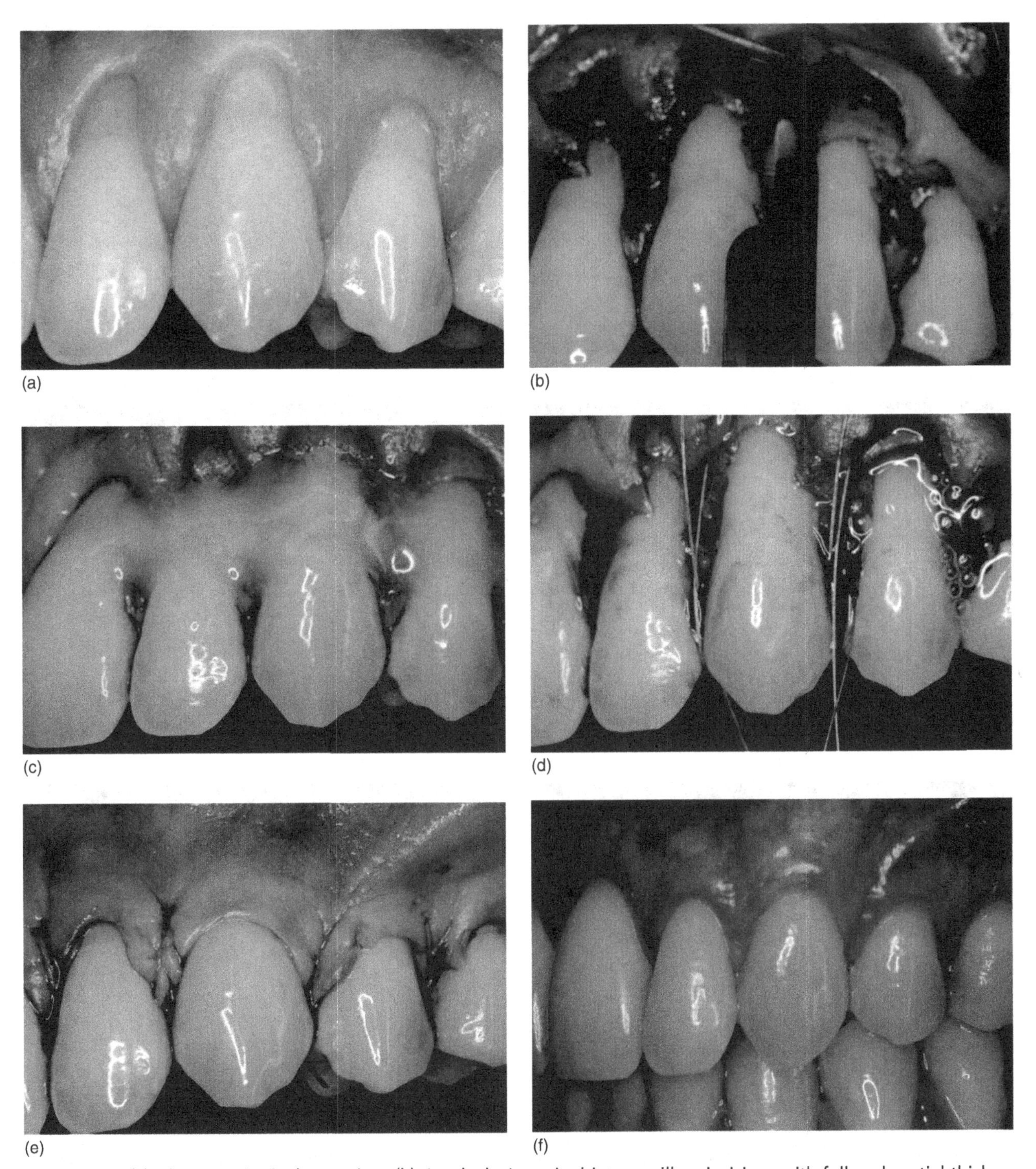

Figure 5.13 (a) Class I/II gingival recession. (b) A sulcular/marginal intrapapillary incision, with full and partial thickness flap elevation. (c) The application of PrefGel™ after root planing and epithelial removal on papillae. (d) The application of Emdogain® gel on the root surface after the root has been washed and dried. (e) The coronally advanced flap (CAF), with sling sutures. (f) Full gingival recession coverage 1 year post-op.

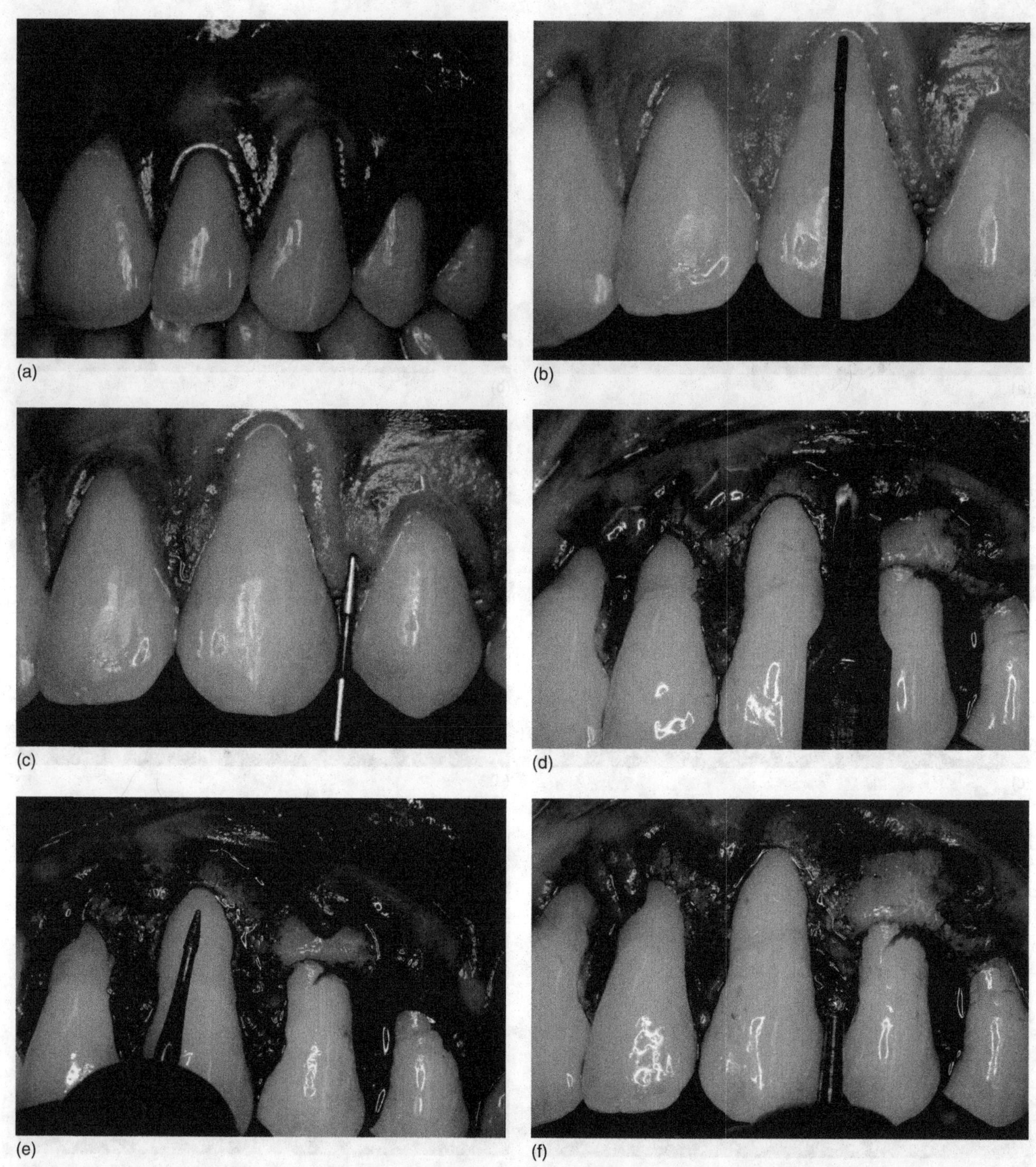

Figure 5.14 (a) Class I/II gingival recession to be treated with Emdogain® and AlloDerm®. The depth of the buccal recession (b) is noted on the adjacent papillae (c) from the tip to the base. (d) Full and partial thickness dissection to increase the flexibility of the flap. (e) Root planing and flattening, using a thin diamond bur without any pressure. (f) The epithelium of the papilla is removed with a round diamond bur.

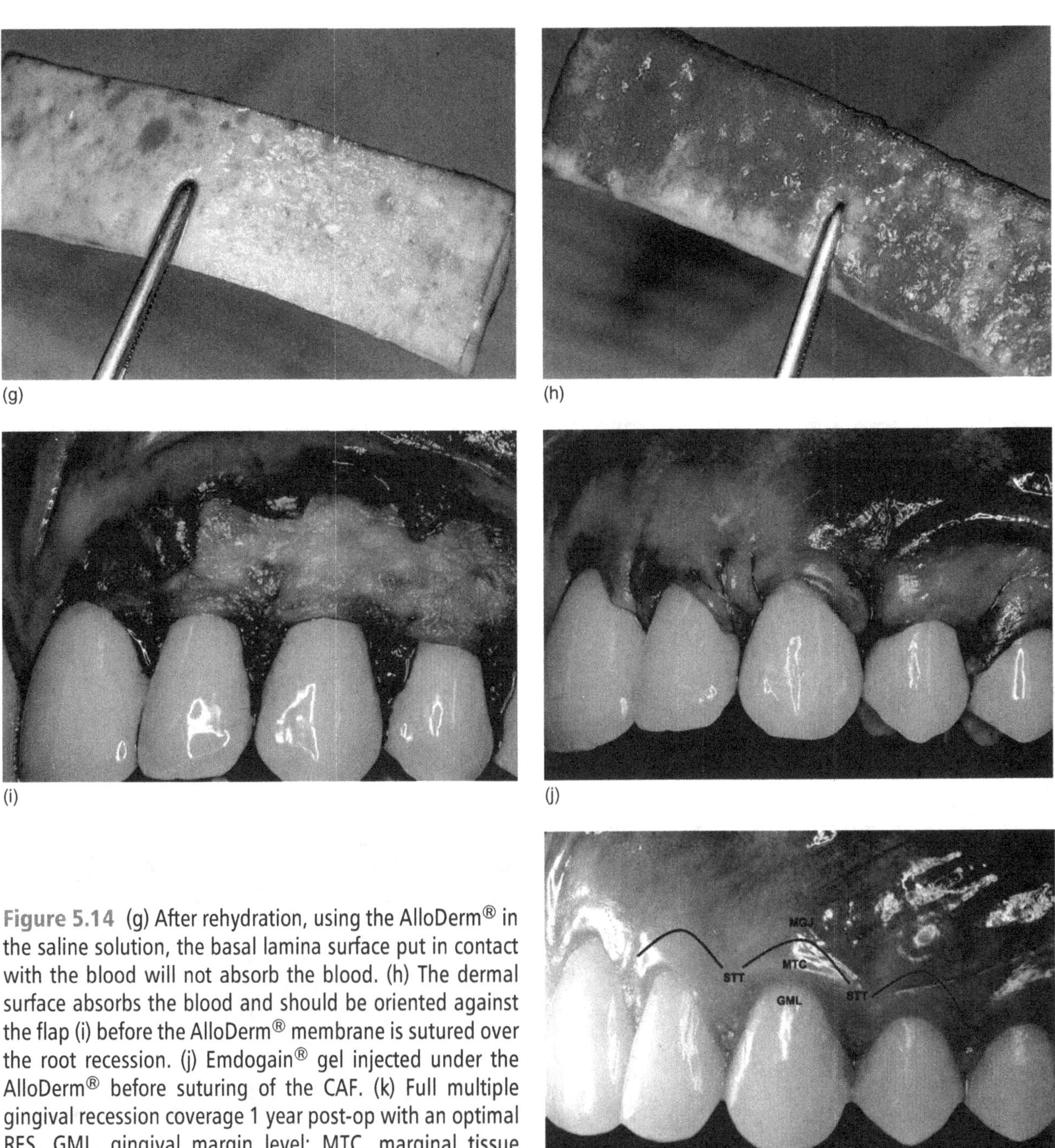

Figure 5.14 (g) After rehydration, using the AlloDerm® in the saline solution, the basal lamina surface put in contact with the blood will not absorb the blood. (h) The dermal surface absorbs the blood and should be oriented against the flap (i) before the AlloDerm® membrane is sutured over the root recession. (j) Emdogain® gel injected under the AlloDerm® before suturing of the CAF. (k) Full multiple gingival recession coverage 1 year post-op with an optimal RES. GML, gingival margin level; MTC, marginal tissue contour; STT, soft tissue texture; MGJ, muco-gingival junction (according to Cairo et al 2010).

(Figs 5.15a–i). Then the acellular dermal matrix is stabilized with the coronally advanced flap, using the same 5-0 Vicryl™ polyglactin 910 sling suspensory sutures. It is important that the flap totally cover the membrane to prevent partial exposition of its coronal part and bacterial colonization that could induce complications. Enamel matrix derivative gel is then injected under the flap below the acellular dermal matrix, over the prepared root surfaces (Saadoun, 2008). The excess gel remains on the outer surface of the flap protected by a post operative guaze with chlorhexidine.

Immediately following surgery, an ice pack is applied intermittently, at 15-minute intervals for the first 2 hours, at the surgical site. All patients are advised to discontinue mechanical oral hygiene measures for 4 weeks following surgery, to mini-

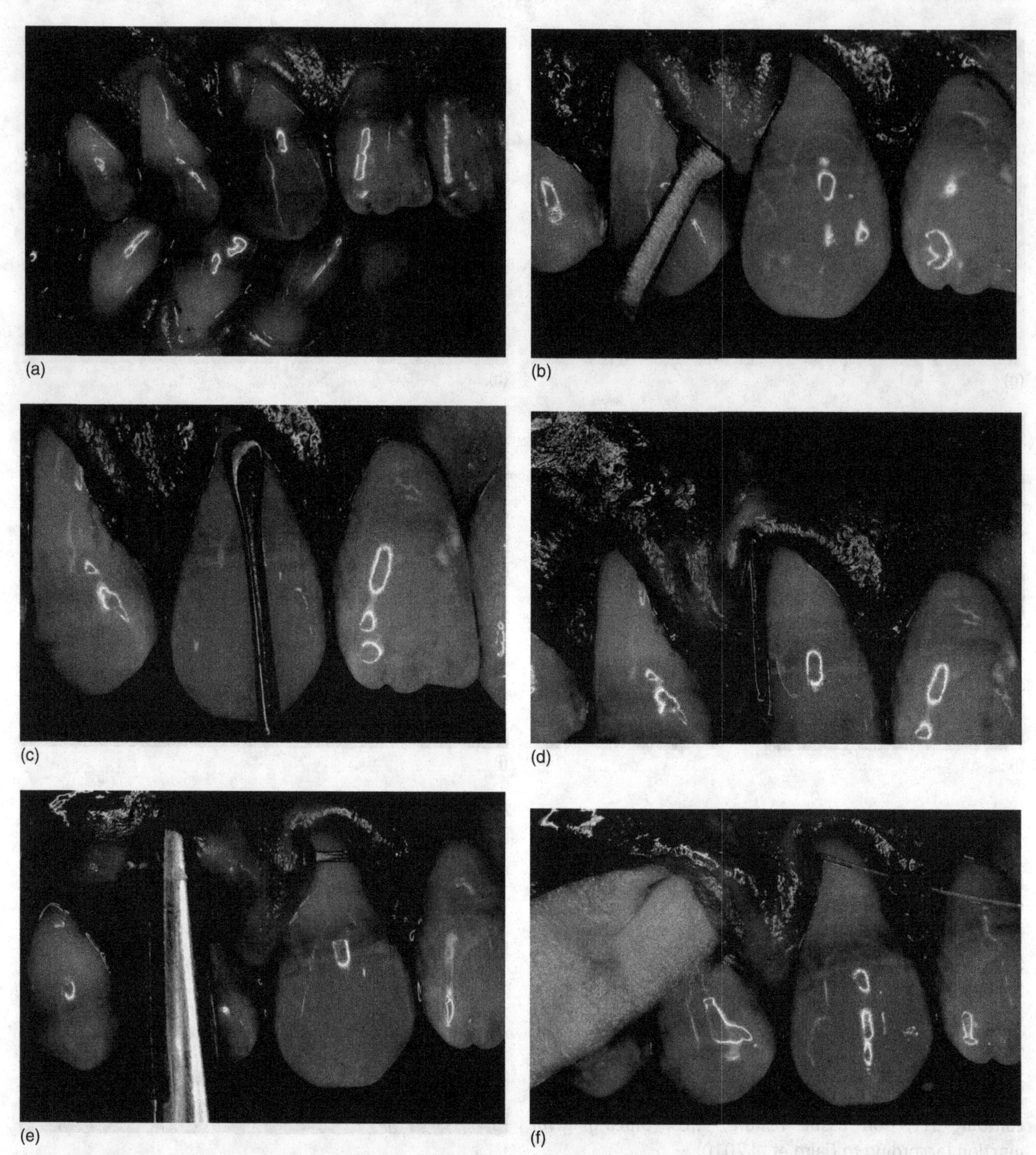

Figure 5.15 (a) Full-mouth gingival recession on a patient with stained teeth. (b) The macropapilla elevator, raising the base but not the tip. The instrument in place (c) prior to the creation of (d) a deep partial buccal pouch. (e) The needle is prepared, attached to the membrane, to go under the papillae. (f) Then, the needle pulls the AlloDerm® under the papillae.

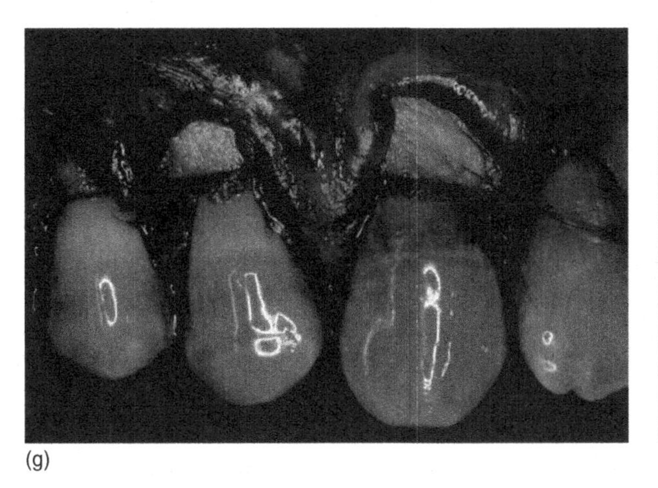
(g)

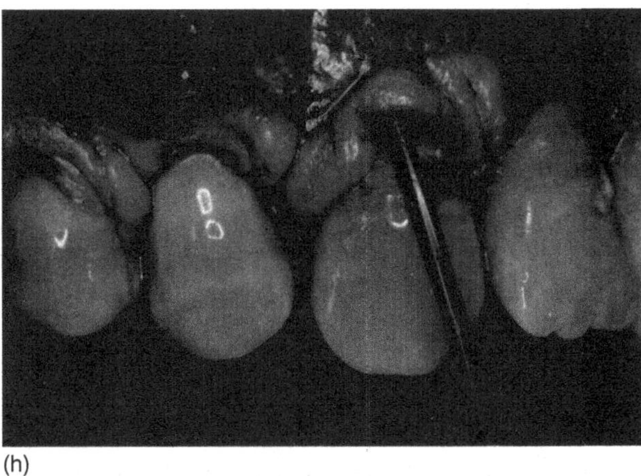
(h)

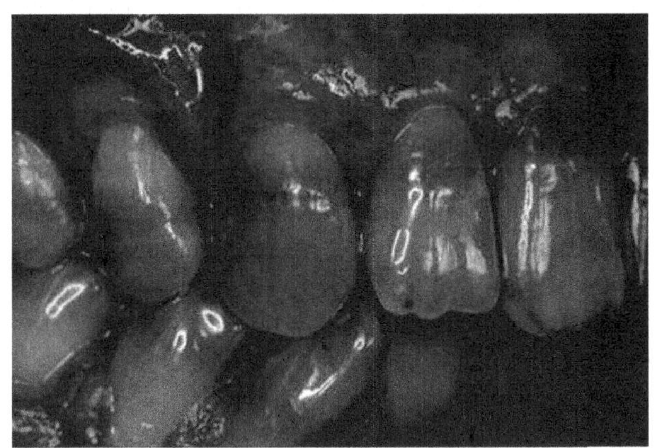
(i)

Figure 5.15 (g) The AlloDerm® is adjusted under the pouch and sutured. (h) The flap is advanced coronally with sling sutures, and the gel is injected underneath. (i) Full-mouth gingival recession coverage 1 year post-op.

mize trauma to the surgical sites. A cold liquid diet is suggested for the first 24 hours.

Several medications are recommended and prescribed to the patient: chlorhexidine gluconate gel (0.2%), to be applied six times a day for 4 weeks; amoxicillin (500 mg) three times a day for 7 days; ibuprofen (400 mg) three times a day; and methyl prednisolone (20 mg) per 40 kg for 3 days.

Healing usually progresses uneventfully, with the exception of some habitual postoperative edema in the days following the surgery. It is important to prevent as much swelling as possible using an atraumatic procedure and medication, because clinical experience has shown that edema can disrupt graft stability and cause the sutures to pull through the papillae, resulting in apical flap displacement.

The patient is seen at weekly postoperative visits to evaluate healing and plaque control. The sutures are not removed until the 1-month postoperative visit.

In a study by Scarano *et al.* (2009), after 6 weeks to 3 months of healing, the gingiva was observed to have a healthy appearance and the acellular dermal matrix was completely substituted and re-epithelialized in 10 weeks, according to the histological and ultrastructural results. The gingival margins appeared thicker and more resistant to trauma. In this way, sensitivity to both air and cold is eliminated and the sulcular probing depths are 2 mm or less. In approximately 6 months, the tissue will mature with a smooth contour. If not, a gingivoplasty can be initiated to remove the gingival irregularities and to blend the soft tissue with harmonious tissue. Scarano *et al.* achieved complete root coverage in both surgical techniques, in addition to increasing the thickness of the marginal tissue.

Discussion

One of the limitations of the use of autogenous grafts is the limited supply of donor connective tissue. Multiple recession sites often require several surgical procedures, which is not well accepted by patients. Biology-based approaches, with bioactive substances, are now being used to mimic nature's formation of functional periodontal soft and hard tissues.

Emdogain® fulfills all of the requirements for an established product in regenerative periodontal treatment. The coronally advanced flap alone, with a minimum keratinized gingiva of 3 mm or with enamel matrix derivative, is an effective procedure to cover localized gingival recessions. The addition of enamel matrix derivative significantly improves the amount of root coverage and tissue thickness (Castellanos *et al.*, 2006).

Enamel matrix derivative stimulates connective tissue growth factor (CTGF) expression, and the interaction is modulated via TGF-beta in osteoblastic cells. Connective tissue growth factor affects EMD-induced osteoblastic mineralization, but not cell proliferation. These results provide new insight into EMD–CTGF interactions, which have therapeutic relevance for tissue engineering and regeneration (Heng *et al.*, 2007).

In a comparative study by Mahajan *et al.* (2007), between the coronally advanced flap (CAF) and the acellular dermal matrix, the mean recession was 4.0 ± 1.0 mm and 3.7 ± 0.7 mm for the acellular dermal matrix and coronally advanced flap groups, respectively. For the acellular dermal matrix group, defect coverage was 3.85 ± 0.89 mm, or 97.14%, compared to the coronally advanced flap group, in which the defect coverage was 2.85 ± 0.89 mm, or 77.42%. A coronally advanced flap plus acellular dermal matrix produced a defect coverage of 95%, whereas the tunnel procedure plus acellular dermal matrix produced only 78% coverage. Also, the predictability of achieving $\geq 90\%$ defect coverage was 50% for the tunnel group.

Enamel matrix derivative is used alone if there is more than 3 mm of keratinized gingiva. Enamel matrix derivative is combined with acellular dermal matrix if there is less than 3 mm of keratinized gingiva, but acellular dermal matrix could be used in any situation, whatever the thickness or width of the keratinized gingiva. These products offer an excellent alternative to connective tissue grafts for the treatment of gingival recession in patients who do not want a second surgical site, or have limited tissue available to harvest and transplant (Hirsch *et al.*, 2005).

These bioengineering materials have become more and more popular as substitutes for donor connective tissue in single and multiple gingival recession and augmentation procedures, because they eliminate the aforementioned disadvantages of the autogenous graft materials.

The unlimited supply of enamel matrix derivative and acellular dermal matrix allows for extended elevated flaps or pouch preparations to achieve multiple site root coverage, which proves to be practical and predictable (De Queroz *et al.*, 2004).

In the presence of gingival recession with abrasion on the root and/or enamel surface, mucogingival surgery should be performed before resolution of the enamel abrasion. Operative restorative treatment should be considered using a hybrid composite resin or ceramic chip when the lesion is coronal to the cemento-enamel junction.

Control and prevention of the advancement of hard and/or soft tissue destruction is accomplished by using an occlusal guard (Terry *et al.*, 2006).

Final remarks

Esthetics is an inseparable part of today's oral therapy. In esthetic dentistry, development of the proper tooth size, form, and color or restoration (white esthetic, WE) is critical to clinical success. It is also mandatory to take the gingival frame (pink esthetic, PE) into account. The soft tissue component is the key factor, and must be addressed for a predictable esthetic outcome in any periodontal, implant, or restorative treatment. Among perio-plastic surgical procedures, the treatment of gingival excess and/or gingival disharmony and buccal gingival recessions are the most frequent indications (Roccuzzo and Romagnoli, 2006). To fulfill this objective, several procedures are proposed nowadays to preserve or enhance the patients' smiles. The current perio-plastic procedures have been developed to treat a variety of gingival deformities using resective or additive techniques.

An unattractive excessive gum display, which can be caused by multiple factors, can be treated successfully – after a detailed esthetic and etiologic diagnosis – by means of various crown lengthening approaches.

Multiple gingival recessions with or without ridge deformities can be treated in several ways. Despite the recent development of biologically based strategies (enamel matrix derivative, acellular dermal matrix, and platelet-rich fibrin) rather than mechanical strategies (connective tissue graft) for periodontal regeneration, techniques using connective tissue grafts are still used with success in some specific cases.

In truth, the connective tissue graft remains today one of the most fundamental options in periodontal plastic surgery, especially when the patient is unwilling to accept new bioengineering materials. Therefore, in order to meet patient demands, it is important to continue to perfect the technique.

6 Esthetic implant treatment

The demand for beauty and smile enhancement through cosmetic restoration or esthetic implant restoration continues to increase in our modern society. However, in the area of the smile, it is challenging and difficult to achieve highly esthetic results using implants. It is easy to understand that the patient's tooth is still the best implant. Therefore, in order to become the treatment of choice, implant restoration has to offer a more natural look, beyond the results of conventional prostheses.

A modern concept of implantology should be based on predictable osseointegration associated with the harmonious integration of soft tissues. Osseointegration is attained if the basic surgical implant principles are respected, but esthetic predictability in the anterior zone is a different issue, and is more challenging to achieve, for a variety of reasons:

- Anatomical and biological considerations, and the patient's immune potential.
- The patient's local and general parameters, and any aggravating risk factors.
- Choices between invasive or less invasive surgical approaches.
- The clinician's high degree of responsibility toward the demanding and well-informed patient!
- The patient's high expectations with regard to the clinician's dexterity and expertise!
- Scientific, clinical, and technological progress.

The objective of any esthetic implant treatment is to ensure that the restoration has a pleasant aspect and that the alignment of the soft tissue is correct.

Osseointegration, one of the most important revolutions in dentistry, represents a real answer to the patient's needs, by offering a solution for total, partial, or single edentation. Implant protocols for the replacement of missing anterior teeth or compromised ridges have evolved considerably and modern approaches are much less invasive. But a predictably beautiful result is difficult to obtain using implants and more challenging to achieve in the anterior zone.

Replacing a single tooth in the esthetic zone with an implant restoration is one of the most demanding tasks in implantology. Therefore, the anterior region represents the most critical area from an esthetic standpoint and the most complex one with regard to the osseous and gingival architecture.

The anterior sector always becomes even more esthetically challenging during the replacement of a central incisor, because of the presence of the contralateral tooth and the adjacent teeth; thus the gingival tissues will serve as references for the volume, position, color, texture, marginal contour and interdental papillae, and so on at the end of the treatment (Touati, 2011).

Replacing a maxillary anterior tooth with an implant becomes extremely challenging in patients with a high smile line or gingival recession (Figs 6.1a, b). Therefore, implant placement in the anterior esthetic zone can be esthetically risky.

Esthetic Soft Tissue Management of Teeth and Implants, First Edition. André P. Saadoun.

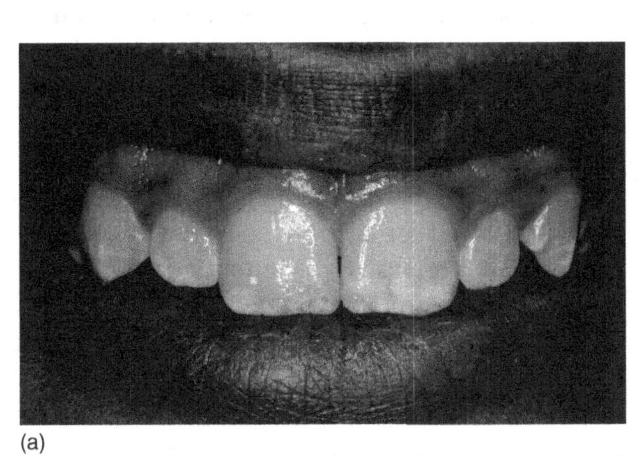

(a)

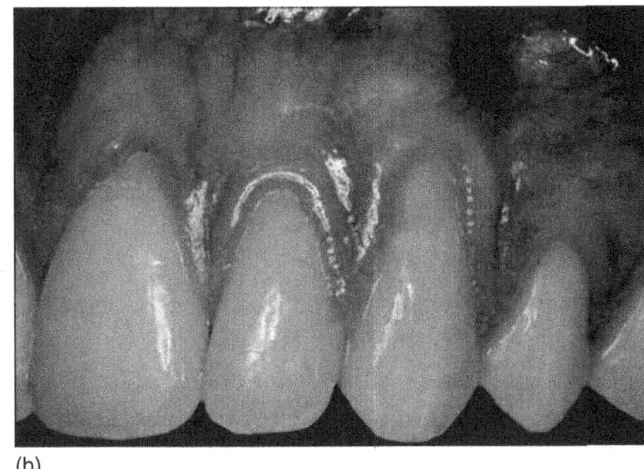

(b)

Figure 6.1 (a) A gingival smile, with an excess of gingiva on the lateral side. (b) Multiple Class I/II gingival recession.

In the area of the smile, immediate implantation after an extraction, or delayed implantation in a healed site with a thin biotype, generally also represents a great clinical challenge (Saadoun, 2010).

When a single central incisor is to be replaced by an implant crown without accompanying restoration of the adjacent teeth, the esthetic risk is even greater, as no compromises are acceptable with regard to the restoration and the surrounding gingiva (Goldstein *et al.*, 2010).

The esthetic difficulties involved in implant dentistry are managing the soft tissue, and mimicking the natural appearance of the patient's teeth and gingiva. Indeed, achieving the ultimate esthetic results in the anterior zone with implant restoration should be similar to achieving esthetic results with conventional restorative dentistry.

Radiography, cone beam, and CT scanning allow the clinician to evaluate the complexity of the case. It is imperative to assess the osseous and gingival states with precision before any treatment, since this information will guide the clinician in determining the best time for implant placement (immediate or delayed) as well as the type of temporization.

The presence of a thick cortical bone is one of the prerequisites for obtaining an adequate gingival profile. The use of biomaterial will give the best result, as long as it is combined with an immediate implant placement, allowing the clinician to correctly maintain the initial volume of the alveolar socket. When it comes to bone loss, there is no difference between immediate and delayed implant placement.

An esthetic gingival contour includes a harmoniously scalloped gingival line, the avoidance of abrupt vertical differences in clinical crown lengths between adjacent teeth, a convex buccal mucosa of sufficient thickness, and distinct papillae (Ahmad, 1998).

Esthetic success can really be predictable only through the development of a comprehensive treatment approach and a proper understanding of the biological parameters that can influence the esthetic outcome at the dental/implant restoration interface (Van Dooren, 2000).

For all of the surgical and/or prosthetic steps to culminate in a predictable esthetic result, there is an optimal treatment time, which is necessarily proportionate to the complexity of the case and the chosen treatment modality (Zuhr, 2011).

Peri-implant risk factors

With an increase in the average lifespan and a higher esthetic demand from older patients, a multidisciplinary approach enables the clinician to control facial and periodontal damage induced by tissue aging, combined with ongoing or aggressive periodontitis.

Our role is to diagnose what damage is caused by bacterial aggression on the periodontium and what is due to the normal aging of the dental and periodontal structures in these patients.

There is a consensus on the etiologic diagnosis of periodontal diseases. The infection cycle will only take place when four conditions are satisfied (Socransky and Haffajee, 1992):

- virulent bacteria are present
- saprophytic bacteria are absent
- the environment is favorable to the colonization of virulent bacteria (thin versus thick biotype), and
- the immune system does not react normally because of very bad habits (smoking or alcoholism) or an acquired deficiency (such as diabetes) or immune deficiency (such as AIDS).

The classic treatment of periodontal disease requires precise chronological therapy. The teaching of oral hygiene is an indispensable and essential step in the therapy prior to implant placement. Training patients to modify their bad dental habits, or their consumption of tobacco and alcohol, is part of a comprehensive approach to the treatment of the "patient" and not just the "disease". Nonsurgical therapy is the starting point of any periodontal treatment. The physicochemical disinfection of the teeth and the oral cavity is a prerequisite for the initial therapy.

Antiseptics such as chlorhexidine mouthwash must be prescribed before and after scaling and root planing. This initial treatment step alone solves the problem in the majority of cases.

In a recent study by Elter *et al.* (2008), the adhesion of bacterial plaque on implant supragingival areas was significantly higher than in subgingival areas. The accumulation of biofilm in supragingival areas increased significantly on rough surfaces, whereas this influence was not detected in subgingival areas. Consequently, there was a significant influence of surface localization (supra- and subgingival) as well as surface modification on biofilm.

Surgical treatment, in the form of flaps with or without osseous surgery, combined with bone grafts, is necessary if the periodontal pockets are deep. This is a prerequisite for all other tissue regeneration techniques and root coverage (Dersot, 2011).

The procedures for periodontal surgery on natural teeth are much less challenging than implant surgery because of the differences between the tooth and implant surfaces. The maintenance phase is indispensable in evaluating the risks for recurring loss of attachment, especially when the patient has a family history of severe periodontitis and is a heavy smoker.

A prospective study over 5–15 years (Kehl *et al.*, 2011), performed with sophisticated CT scanning on loaded implants placed on partially edentulous patients treated for chronic periodontitis (CP) or generalized aggressive periodontitis (GAP), has shown more significant buccal bone resorption on generalized aggressive periodontitis patients (2.3 mm) than on chronic periodontitis patients (1.75 mm). This study has also shown a significant thickness of keratinized gingiva in the mandible of the generalized aggressive periodontitis patient (1.12 mm) in comparison with the chronic periodontitis patient (0.85 mm). This decrease in gingival thickness is significantly correlated with the increase in bone resorption in the generalized aggressive periodontitis patient relative to the chronic periodontitis patient. The importance of the thickness of keratinized gingiva as the behavior of the bone resorption around the implant varies, according to the type of periodontal disease, is a new parameter that is becoming increasingly evident.

The logic of active periodontal treatment today, to be performed before any implant treatment, is to eliminate all etiologic, biological, and iatrogenic factors. An increasing number of scientific articles suggest that there is a tendency for smokers to have a higher number of pathogenic bacteria than nonsmokers, without an increase in the quantity of bacterial plaque (Figs 6.2a, b). This hypothesis confirms that tobacco has a harmful effect not on the subgingival environment, but primarily on the immune response (Nato, 2010).

The majority of publications agree that tobacco constitutes a major risk factor for periodontal disease. The link between smoking and calculus has not yet been clearly established. However, smoking is associated with higher susceptibility to periodontal disease and it induces a higher level of, and more rapid, bone destruction, with angular defects. Bone loss is increased by a factor of 2.3 among moderate smokers (ten cigarettes per day) and a factor of 5.3 among heavy smokers (17 cigarettes per day).

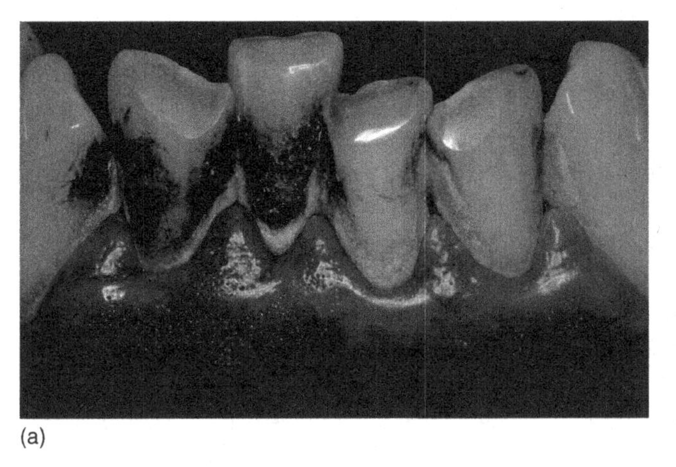
(a)

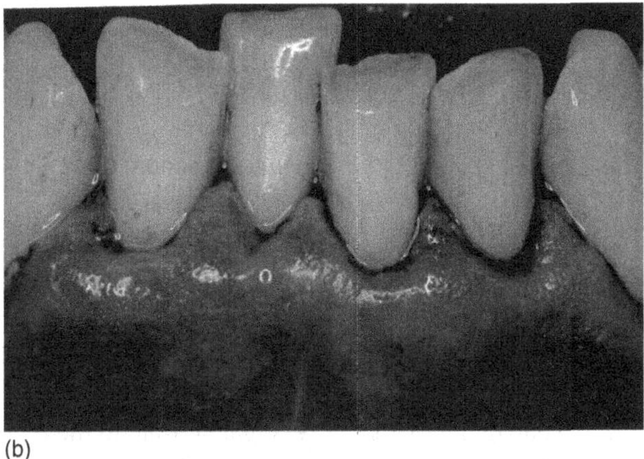
(b)

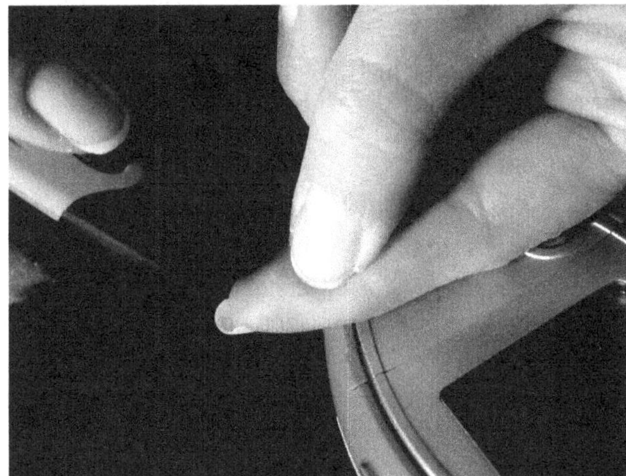
(c)

Figure 6.2 (a) The patient's teeth, full of calculus and heavy nicotine staining. (b) The same patient after periodontal dental prophylaxis. (c) A diabetic patient checking her blood sugar, using medication in tablet and injection form.

Tobacco significantly reduces the benefits of non-surgical and surgical periodontal therapy in terms of attachment gain, periodontal pocket reduction, bone gain, and root coverage. Augmenting the risk of failure in surgery, tobacco could become a major contraindication and obstacle to any surgical implant treatment. There is a consumption-related effect among these risk factors: the higher the consumption, the higher the risks (Nguyen, 2010).

It appears that the habit of tobacco smoking has a negative influence on periodontal healing. Even though its action mechanism is not totally understood, it has been shown that there is a link between smoking habits and factors such as systemic vasoconstriction, decrease in blood flow, polymorphonuclear leukocyte blood cell dysfunction, lymphocyte deficiency in the immune system, and inhibition in fibroblast proliferation and/or function. All these negative factors can be reversed if the patient stops smoking (Nato, 2010).

Are systemic factors affecting implant survival?

The various studies do not qualify the role of diabetes and smoking in implant failure, but together they support our continuing need to question the influence of systemic factors on implant survival in view of the possible complications and potential benefits that implant therapy may offer (Fig. 6.2c). Therefore, the benefit of implant therapy may be denied to some patients because of systemic conditions, which should be evaluated against the risk and our level of understanding of those risks. All of the systemic conditions should be under control before implant therapy is undertaken, to prevent any risk (Oates, 2011).

Selected personality traits may be used to predict patients' satisfaction with implant-supported prostheses prior to treatment, and may also provide valuable information for the prediction of a satisfactory outcome before implant treatment is started – which could save time and money if the prediction is

Table 6.1 Local implant risk factors

Parameters	Favorable factors	Unfavorable factors
The level of the FGM	Identical, or more coronal to the margin of the adjacent teeth	More apical than the GM of the adjacent teeth
The periodontal biotype	Thick and flat; rectangular-shaped teeth	Thin and scalloped; triangular-shaped teeth
Proximal bone sounding of the adjacent teeth of the implant	The presence of bone at a 3 mm distance from the buccal side, and a maximum of 4.5 mm from the proximal side	Bone architecture with more than 3 mm on the buccal side, and more than 4.5 mm on the proximal side
The location of the tooth/implant restoration contact point	Less than 4.5 mm to the bone peak, and less than 3.5 mm between two implants	More than 5 mm to the bone peak, and more than 3.5 mm between two implants
The mesiodistal length of the edentulous crest	Enough bone space (1.5–2.0 mm) between the implant and the natural teeth, and a minimum of 3 mm between two implants	Less than 1.5 mm space between the natural teeth and the adjacent implant, or less than 3 mm between two implants
The bucco-palatal width of the edentulous crest	More than 6 mm, leaving > 2 mm of buccal bone from the implant	Less than 6 mm, leaving < 1 mm of buccal bone from the implant
The timing of the procedure	Immediate implant placement within a short time following the extraction; < day 0 to 8 weeks	Delayed implant placement: > 8 weeks
The surgical technique	No flap or incision, hence preserving the papilla	An incision affecting the papilla
Temporization	More than 6 months: stability of the peri-implant HST	Less than 4 months: recession of the peri-implant HST

GM, gingival margin; FGM, free gingival margin; HST, hard and soft tissue.

unfavorable. Dentists could be more cautious when faced with the possibility of patients' rejection or dissatisfaction, before carefully deciding whether to opt for expensive and time-consuming treatment, or to modify the treatment plan in favor of a more reversible or less expensive one (Al-Omiri *et al.*, 2011).

All peri-implant procedures should respect the basic principles of periodontal surgery, taking into account the difference between the two entities – teeth and implants – and the role of local, general, and psychological risk factors, as described in Table 6.1.

The implant/mucosa interface differs in composition and measurement (Glauser *et al.*, 2005), depending on whether the interface is with the implant's machined surface (3.19 mm), the implant's rough surface (2.40 mm), or the natural teeth (2.11 mm) (see Figs 4.29d–f), and these differences are important in understanding the susceptibility of implants to infection (Listgarten *et al.*, 1991). The supracrestal collagen fibers are oriented in a parallel rather than a perpendicular configuration (Abrahamsson *et al.*, 1997; Schupbach and Glauser, 2007). This creates a much weaker mechanical attachment compared to natural teeth. In addition, the ability of the peri-implant mucosa to regenerate itself is limited by its compromised number of cells and poor vascularity (Lindhe and Berglundh, 2000). Therefore, peri-implant and periodontal tissues may differ in their resistance to bacterial infection (Lindhe *et al.*, 1992; Ericsson *et al.*, 2000).

Soft tissue management

An optimal gingival frame surrounding implant-supported restorations is important in completing the illusion of natural teeth in the esthetic zone (Fig. 6.3a). The soft tissue framework (PES) plays a critical role in the visual perception of any anterior implant restoration (WES) (Fig. 6.3b). Without a pleasing gingival framework, even the most skilled restorative

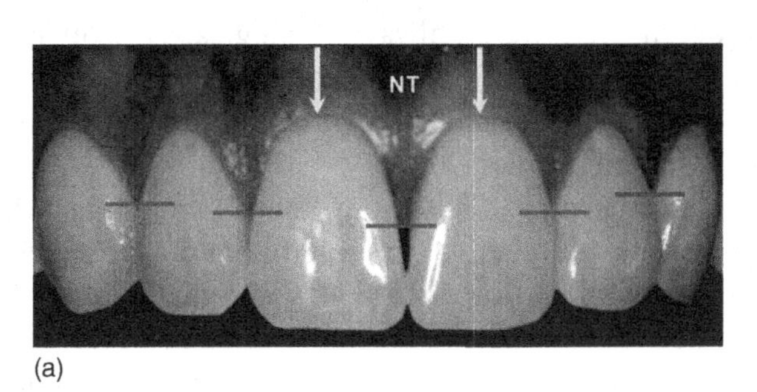

(a)

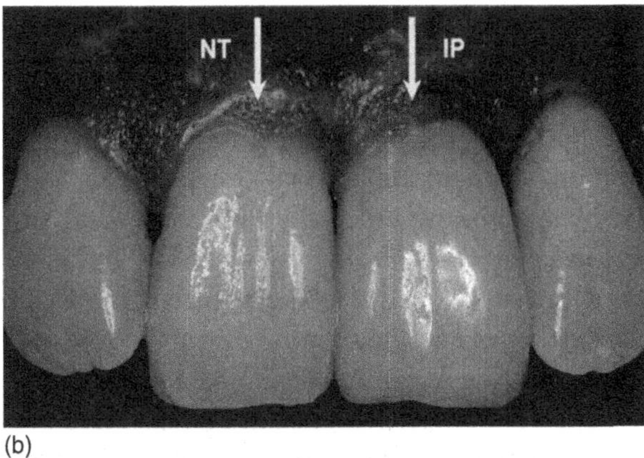

(b)

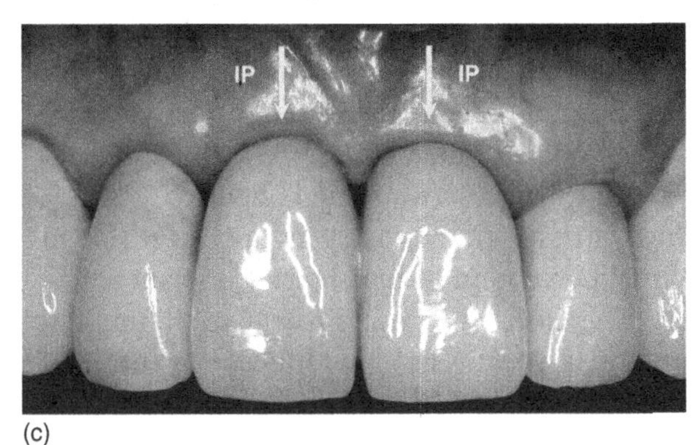

(c)

Figure 6.3 (a) Natural teeth with optimal proportions and a harmonious gingival contour. (b) The optimal esthetic result on the left central incisor implant restoration, with a harmonious gingival contour (with respect to the gingival zenith enamel deformity). (c) An unpleasant esthetic result on the two adjacent implant restorations (the zenith of the gingival margin is on the mesial instead of on the distal), with a disharmonious gingival contour on the central/lateral incisor restoration.

dentist and ceramist cannot predictably deliver an esthetically pleasing result (Leziy and Miller, 2008b); but without an implant restoration that respects and reproduces the optimal harmonious natural tooth gingival contour (Fig. 6.3c), it is also impossible to achieve an esthetic outcome (Saadoun, 2008).

Therefore, the functional and esthetic success of implant treatment in the anterior zone depends not only on the quality of the restoration, but on preserving or regenerating the favorable hard and soft tissue architecture, and mainly on the final and long-term aspects of the contour and stability of the marginal gingival and proximal papillae, in harmony with the adjacent teeth (Rompen *et al.*, 2003; Saadoun, 2010).

Around natural teeth, the techniques of plastic periodontal surgery allow a harmonization of the gingival contour and coverage of gingival recession while respecting the cosmetic quality of the tissue with regard to thickness, texture, and color. This is made possible through the use of lateral pedicle flaps or gingival grafts and, in particular, connective tissue grafts. The surgical protocol varies for partial or total coverage of the graft under an envelope, a tunnel, or a pedicle flap moved coronally or laterally.

In peri-implant cases, these plastic surgery procedures vary greatly according to the clinical situation: replacement of single or multiple implants, the morphology of the edentulous crest, the quality of the implant system, the biocompatibility of the material, and so on. Therefore, a robust general knowledge of plastic surgery is a prerequisite. Even though the *savoir-faire* with regard to teeth can also be applied to implants, it is not always sufficient for the recreation of an ideal gingival margin contour and interproximal papillae.

The facial tissue height and contour are important anatomical features for an esthetic restorative result, the other being bone levels at adjacent teeth, as already pointed out (Choquet *et al.*, 2001; Ryser *et al.*, 2005). The height and thickness of the facial bone wall determine the position of the midfacial mucosal margin and the contour of the alveolar ridge (Buser *et al.*, 2004; Grunder *et al.*, 2005).

Peri-implant soft tissues are more fragile and more delicate to manipulate, and even unpredictable during the healing phases, because they are inevitably traumatized due to the loss of the tooth and the several surgical sessions required to replace it with an implant that is integrated well into the hard and soft tissues. The more traumatized the implant site is, the more the potential for natural healing decreases. This limits the esthetic result, increases the frustration of the clinician, and leads to patient disappointment (Romagna, 2009).

It is a challenging task to achieve acceptable gingival esthetics around single anterior implants. Maintaining such an implant esthetic over time can be equally demanding, especially if the teeth that had to be extracted showed gingival recession initially and/or the absence of attached keratinized gingiva.

In the esthetic zone, the morphology of the soft tissues plays a central role in the achievement of satisfactory final results (Covani *et al.*, 2007). The apical zenith of the facial gingival outline is located slightly distal to the mid-axis of the maxillary incisor. Although an implant-supported central incisor crown may closely duplicate the adjacent teeth, if the free gingival margins do not match, visual disharmony will ensue and the illusion will be lost (Kinsel and Capoferri, 2008).

The soft tissue framework plays a critical role in the visual perception of any anterior implant restoration. Therefore, it is necessary that an implant restoration respects and reproduces the optimal harmonious natural tooth gingival contour, to achieve an esthetic outcome. It is then equally important to create harmony between the restoration and the remaining dentition and soft tissue framework (Saadoun, 2008; Tucker, 2009).

Thus, during treatment, a considerable amount of effort is focused on enhancing the balance of the pink and white esthetics, using a combination of surgical and restorative treatments (see Fig 6.3b). It is usually easy to create such a balance, as long as the various stages of treatment are appropriately timed (Leziy and Miller, 2009).

The optimal esthetics can be maintained when the various components of the tissue are in a physiological relation and work in harmony. Therefore, if this relation is not biologically correct, an esthetically pleasing result will not be achieved (Salama and Jundslalys, 2003).

The risk of marginal tissue recession is more predictable with thin marginal mucosa in implantology than in periodontics. The objective of connective tissue grafting is to obtain a thicker zone of keratinized soft tissue, regain attachment to the tooth, and cover the radicular surface to restore the esthetics and eliminate hypersensitivity. This soft tissue thickening in implantology augments the tissue biotype, preventing peri-implant soft tissue recession, and allows for a more stable and predictable tissue level after tooth extraction, at the time of abutment placement and the taking of impressions, and after the temporary and final restoration.

It must be considered that when something is lost or removed, there is always a biological consequence. This often means that a soft and hard tissue deficiency will develop following the loss of a tooth (Leziy and Miller, 2007).

Furthermore, following tooth extraction, the osseous and gingival tissues are often altered, with horizontal and/or vertical loss, and the implant site is often insufficient for ideal implant placement. Some forms of socket preservation or augmentation invariably become necessary to treat horizontal and/or vertical deformation (see Table 4.6).

In the majority of machine submerged implants (Fig. 6.4a), approximately 0.9–1.6 mm of crestal bone is lost in the first year of functioning after abutment connection and/or restoration, with the crestal bone being located at the first thread of the implant below the "microgap"; that is, the connection between the implant body and the prosthetic abutment. Moreover, the peri-implant soft tissue recession is 0.7–1.0 mm (Saadoun, 1997; Grunder, 2000; Small and Tarnow, 2000; Small *et al.*, 2001).

This ongoing gingival recession remains a reality today. It reveals the fragility of the peri-implant structure (bone and soft tissue), and it also creates an esthetic prejudice without jeopardizing the functional aspect of the restoration (Cardaropoli *et al.*, 2006; Kan *et al.*, 2007; Saadoun and Touati, 2007; Evans and Chen, 2008).

A wide range of factors are known to have a deleterious effect on crestal bone resorption (Figs 6.4b–d) and affect early crestal bone loss in the majority of endosseous dental implants (Koszegi Stoianov, 2010):

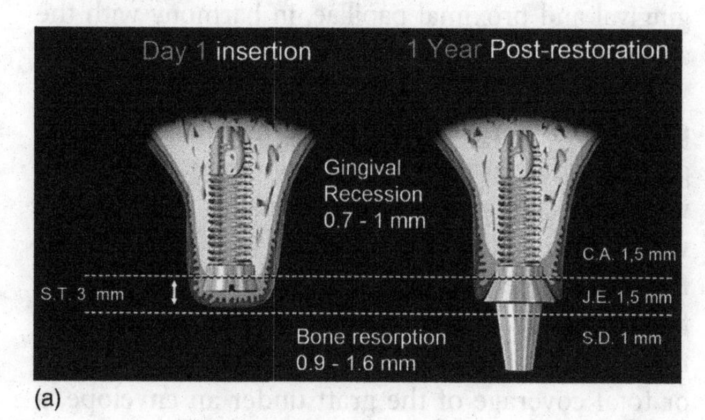

(a)

Figure 6.4 (a) The majority of submerged implants lose 0.9–1.6 mm of crestal bone after implant/abutment connection in the first year of functioning.

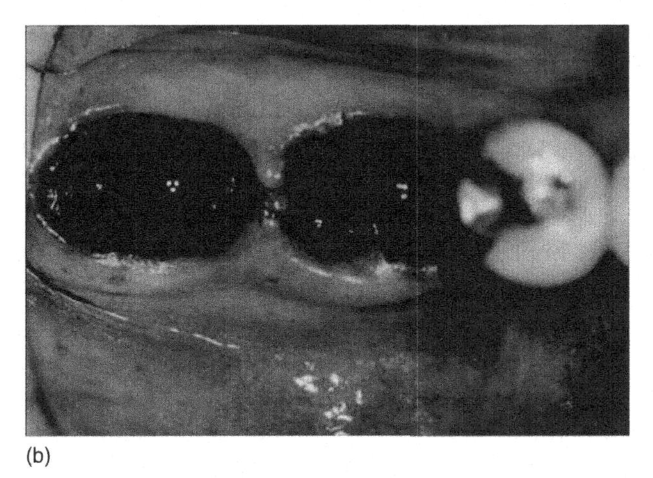

(b)

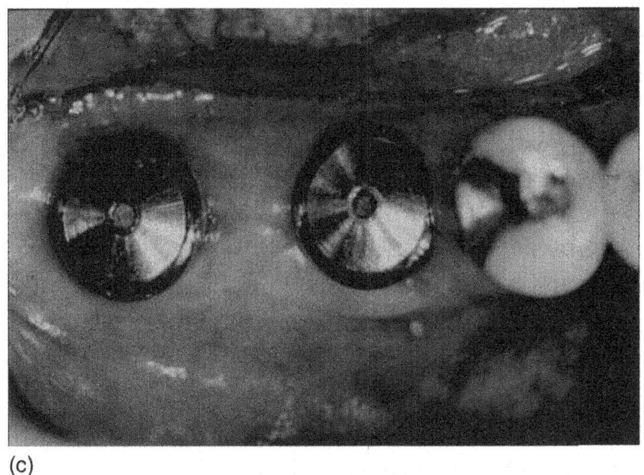

(c)

(d)

Figure 6.4 (b) The alveolar socket after premolar and molar extraction. (c) Immediate implants placement with healing abutments. (d) Switch platform prosthetic abutments were able to maintain the crestal bone at the top of the Mega-Gen implant platform. (Courtesy of Dr. K.B. Park, Seoul, S. Korea.)

- surgical and anatomical considerations
- the amount of keratinized gingiva
- the design of the mucoperiosteal flap
- bone quality and/or density
- an implant design with a divergent collar
- trauma during the surgical procedure
- the thickness of the buccal and lingual cortical plates of the bone remaining after osteotomy
- the healing process in the submerged or nonsubmerged implant protocol
- exposure of the implant during healing of the soft tissue
- the level of the microgap connection in relation to the bone crest
- the tooth–implant or inter-implant horizontal distance
- the establishment of the implant's "biological width"
- the lack of a soft tissue seal in the peri-implant mucosa
- the use of an abutment with a diameter equal to or less than that of the implant body
- the repeated removal and replacement of the abutment, with disruption of the soft tissue seal
- preloading and loading restorative phases with a functional occlusion
- excessive occlusal forces due to parafunctional occlusion, and
- the patient's oral hygiene, and local and systemic aggravating factors.

It is evident that full control of all the variables that play a role in bone loss around implants after implantation, especially around the implant crest module during the first year of implantation, is beyond any clinician's domain, given the biological (patient), human technical (clinician), and engineering (implant divergent collar design and connections) aspects that contribute to this complex problem (Marincola *et al.*, 2009).

Human implant histology over a 3-year period has shown that the apical migration of the implant junctional epithelium (JE) is halted by the attachment of the connective supracrestal fibers to the Laser-Lok® microchannel collar surface and hence resorption of cervical bone is prevented (Nevins *et al.*, 2008). The supracrestal position of the implant's Laser-Lok®

collar limits the apical migration of the junctional epithelium, allows the attachment of perpendicular connective fibers, and prevents crestal bone loss.

The analysis of 49 implants in a recent study by Shapoff *et al.* (2010) showed a mean crestal bone loss of 0.44 mm at 2 years postrestoration, and 0.46 mm at 3 years. All bone loss was contained within the height of the collar, and no bone loss was evident at the level of the implant threads.

Literature reviews on the topic of peri-implant recession over the past 5 years have proven that bone resorption has been limited to an average of 0.46 mm following the evolution of:

- precise diagnosis, with less invasive surgery
- improved implant design – with regard to the body, surface, collar and diameter, and micro-threads, and
- precise abutment/crown restoration connection (Zadeh, pers. comm., 2010).

When tooth extraction is planned, clinicians must decide when to extract, how to manage the extraction sockets to minimize ridge remodeling, and what method of tooth replacement will be used (immediate, delayed, or late). The residual or reconstructed ridge is generally the weak link in an esthetic oral rehabilitation, because the hard and soft tissues can never predictably be regenerated to the previous natural level, despite preservation and augmentation procedures.

Maintaining the buccal part of the root at the time of the tooth extraction may be another way of preventing crestal bone level change and soft tissue recession. However, further long-term studies are needed. At 4 months, new cementum develops at the apical part of the tooth and bone loss of 0.2 mm is observed on the buccal gingival margin (Hürzeler *et al.*, 2010).

After an extraction, preservation of the peri-implant soft tissue architecture and texture, combined with maintenance of the marginal bone levels, are absolute prerequisites for long-lasting esthetic success. Regardless of the implant approach (immediate implant placement with flapless surgery, immediate implant placement and loading, or delayed/late implant placement), several issues are of paramount importance to an ideal treatment outcome: atraumatic extraction techniques, ideal three-dimensional implant placement, supplemental ridge augmentation when necessary, and adjunctive soft tissue regeneration augmentation to enhance the soft tissue biotype and tissue volume. Under the right conditions, nature itself takes care of the major part of the healing process (Leziy and Miller, 2007).

An association exists between bone and soft tissue preservation around implants, and this has a direct influence on esthetics. As a support for the soft tissue, this stable marginal bone is a determinant of the long-term esthetic stability, and vice versa.

The preservation of crestal bone around dental implants cannot be attributed to a single factor. The final esthetic outcome is the result of a number of important parameters, especially in the challenging esthetic zone (Saadoun, 2010; Sonick *et al.*, 2012) (Fig. 6.5):

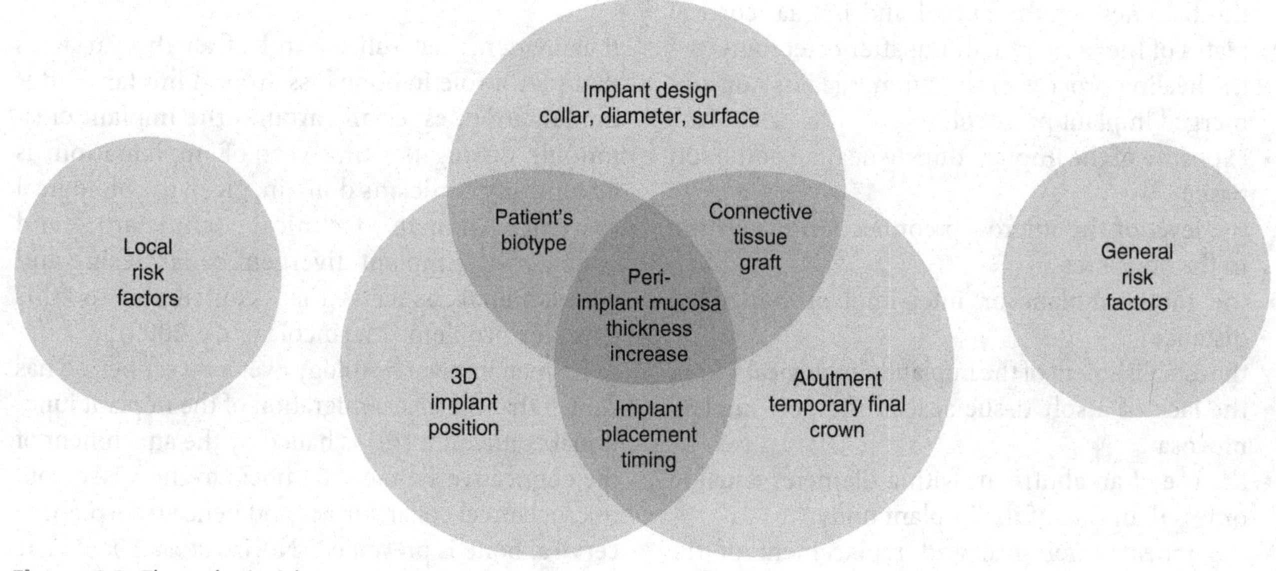

Figure 6.5 The esthetic risk management parameters.

- the implant design, collar, surface, and diameter
- the patient's biotype – thick or thin
- the biological width
- the timing of the extraction and of placement of the implant
- forced eruption before tooth extraction
- flap design – flapless versus pedicle roll or flap elevation
- the tridimensional position and orientation of the implant
- the timing of placement of the connective tissue graft
- the implant/abutment connection
- temporary or final restoration, and
- occlusal loading with or without functional occlusion.

All these various and multiple parameters are considered as posing risk to the esthetic zone, especially if they do not work together in synergy, to achieve the objective of a final increase the peri-implant mucosa.

Implant biomechanical considerations

There is a major management protocol for the parameters that aim to enhance the patient's soft tissue thickness biotype around an implant restoration (Fu *et al.*, 2011):

1. *Implant design* – a platform with a diameter less than that of the implant body, with a tapered wall, and with a convergent or sloping implant-shaped module of the platform shoulder, can be considered as the ideal implant design for homogenous occlusal force distribution, prevention of bone loss around the implant collar and crestal bone, and improvement of the gingival esthetics (Figs 6.6a–c):
   - From an engineering perspective, it is widely accepted that the bone loss around the implant's crest module is multicausal in nature. These factors are related to the design of the implant collar (the design of the crest module/implant connection).
   - From a mechanical standpoint, if same-diameter implants with the three different available crest module designs (divergent, parallel, and convergent) are to be placed in a given region, the convergent-shaped crest module implant will be less likely to lead to a loss of cervical bone, due to the higher level of bone around the crest module, which will help to dissipate the functional loads (Shi *et al.*, 2007).
2. *Implant position* – more palatal, more apical combined with a connective tissue graft (CTG):

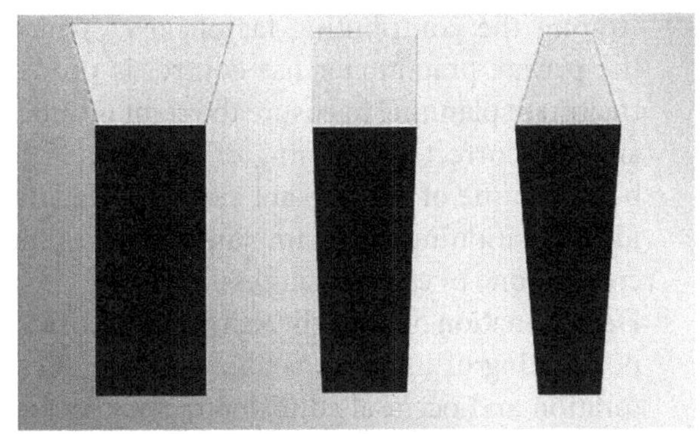

(a)

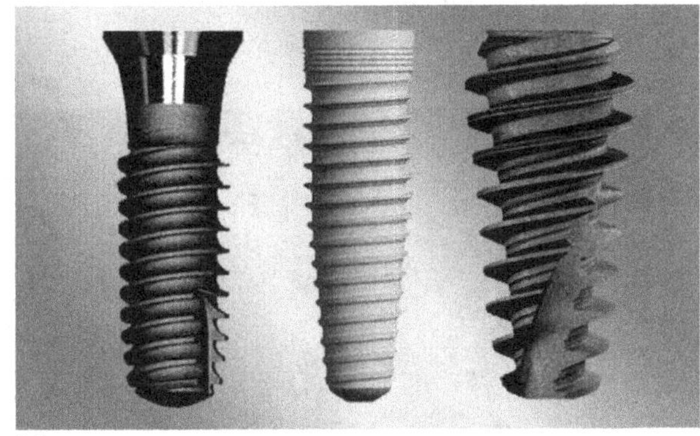

(b)

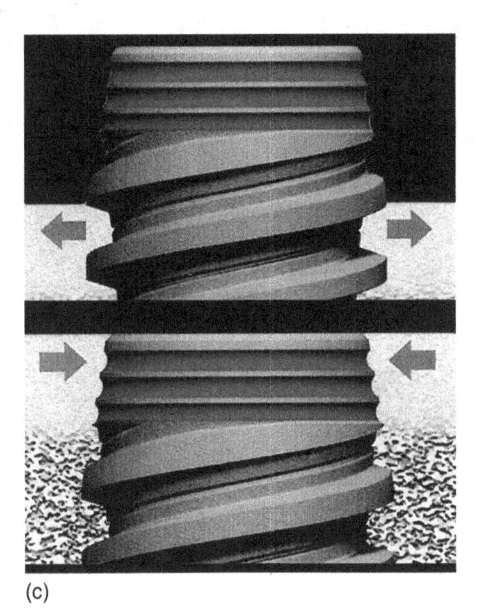

(c)

Figure 6.6 (a) A diagrammatic representation of the three different types of implant design. (b) The divergent, parallel, and convergent cervical collars of three different implant designs. (c) The back-tapered coronal design provides additional cervical bone volume for optimal soft tissue support after implant placement. (Courtesy of Nobel Biocare.)

- Among the contributing factors over which the private practitioner has control is proper treatment planning to ensure the right number and the correct positioning of implants. The bone volume of the implant site should allow ideal positioning of the implant, which is the cornerstone of esthetic success.
- Determination of the right number and correct positioning of implants facilitates proper restoration and occlusal adjustment, thus greatly diminishing the human contribution to crestal bone loss (Marincola *et al.*, 2009).
- The implant should be inserted in an optimal three-dimensional (3D) implant position and orientation, either manually or using a surgical guide, and the following rules should always be respected:
  - Mesiodistal position: 1.5–2.0 mm between a tooth and an implant, and 3 mm between adjacent implants; 3.5–4.5 mm between the upper central incisors (Figs 6.7a–c).
  - Buccolingual position: 2–3 mm inside from the line joining the adjacent gingival margins (Figs 6.7d–f).

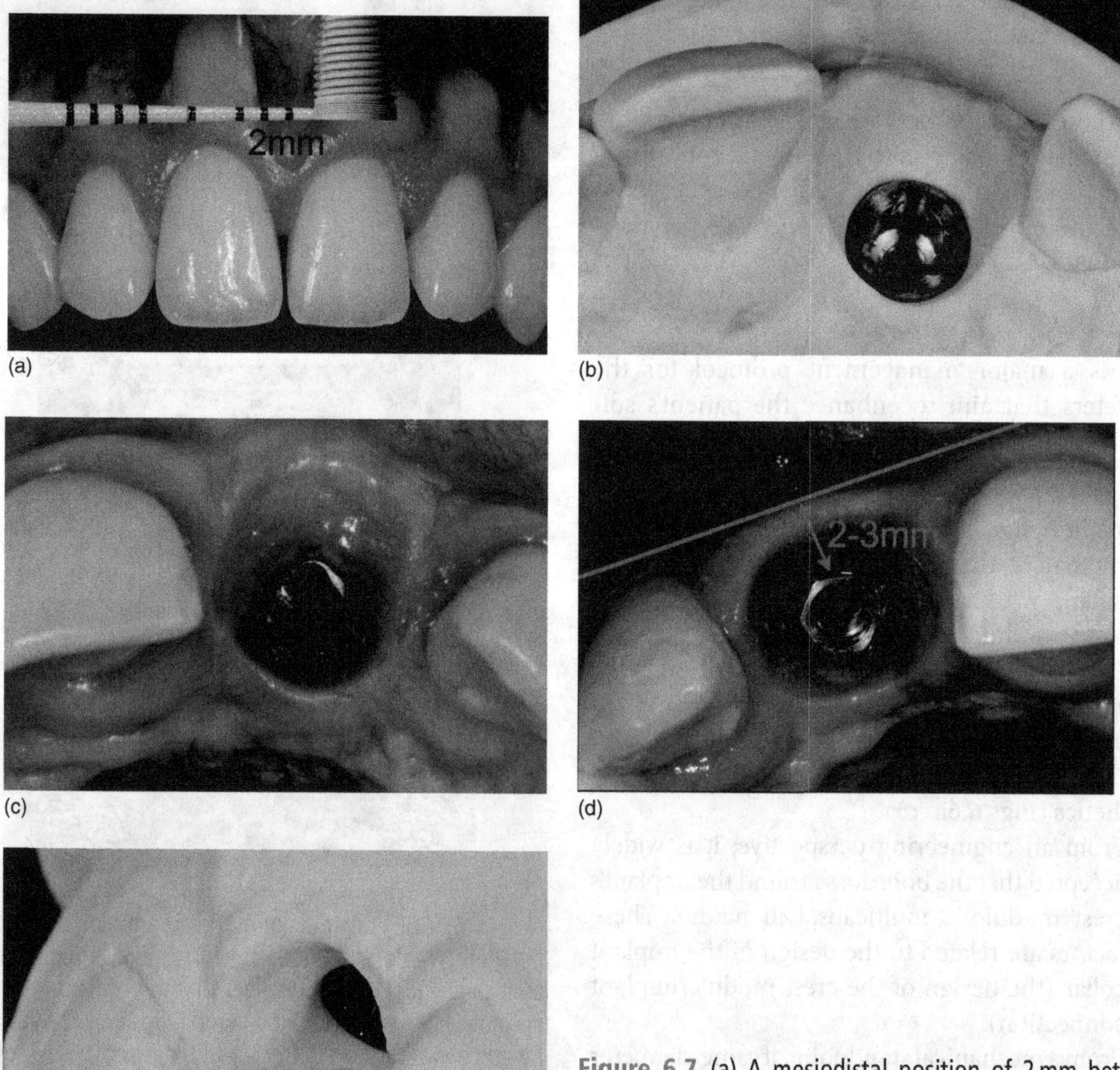

Figure 6.7 (a) A mesiodistal position of 2 mm between the tooth and the implant. (b) The mesiodistal position on the cast model (occlusal view). (c) The mesiodistal position on the patient (occlusal view). (d) A bucco-palatal position of 2–3 mm from the gingival line of the adjacent teeth. (e) The bucco-palatal position on the cast model (left view).

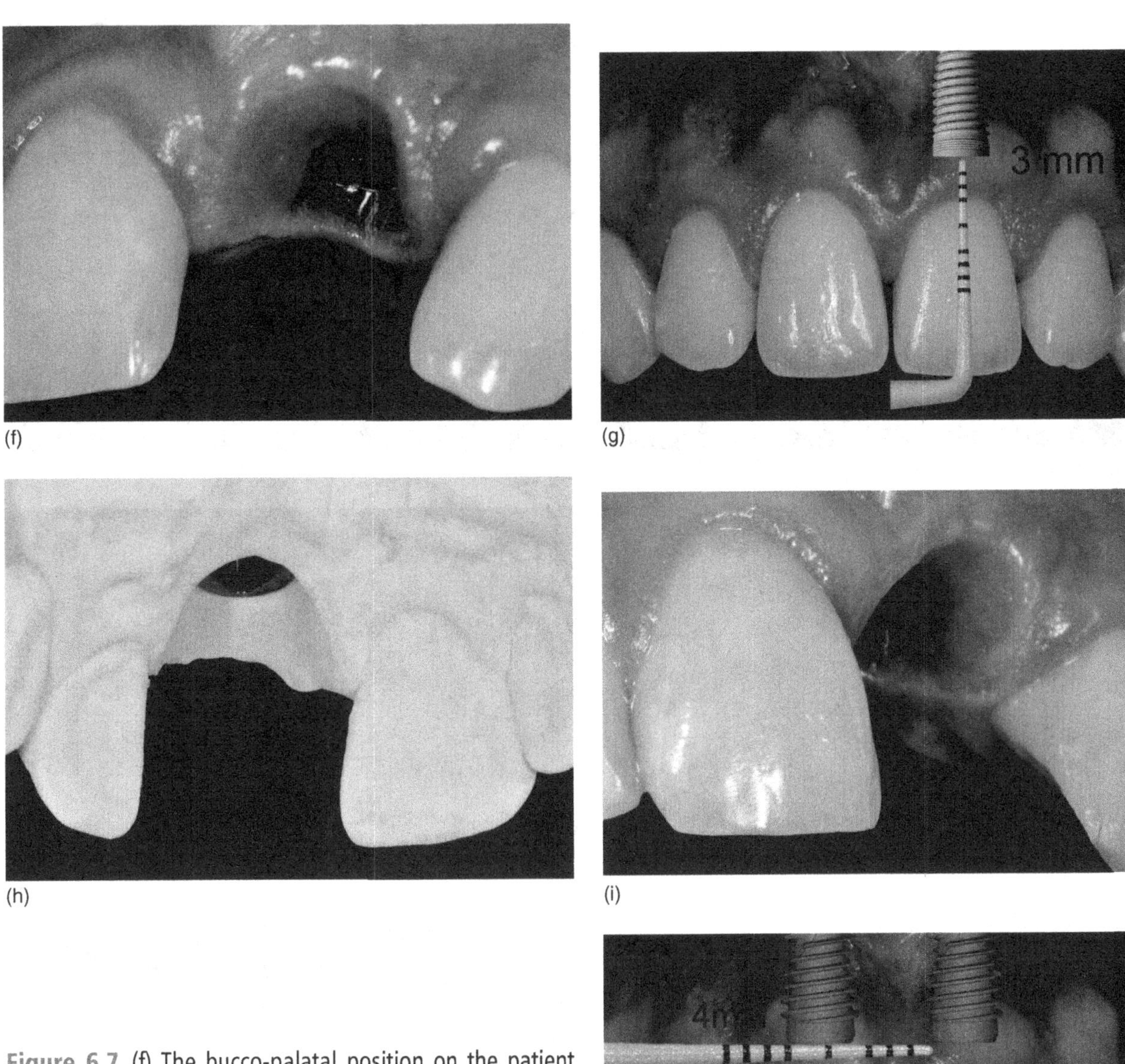

Figure 6.7 (f) The bucco-palatal position on the patient (left view). (g) An apico-coronal position of 3 mm from the gingival margin to the implant platform. (h) The apico-coronal position on the cast model (palatal view). (i) The apico-coronal position on the patient (right view). (j) An interproximal distance of 4.0–4.5 mm between two adjacent implants for the two maxillary central incisors. (Figures (b), (e), and (h) courtesy of Mr. G.M. Etienne, Pulnoy, France.)

  - Apico-coronal position: 3 mm apically from the gingival margin of the implant site (Figs 6.7g–j).
- Factors affecting the esthetic outcome are the implant location, the horizontal buccal size gap, and the thickness of the buccal wall.
- The tridimensional implant position and angulation induces the emergence profile, the architecture of the peri-implant soft tissue, the level of the scalloped gingival margins and the interdental papillae (Saadoun and Le Gall, 1992).
- From a clinical point of view, implants installed into extraction sockets – either manually or using a surgical guide – by means of a model-based (Figs 6.8a–f) or computer-based approach should be utilized to facilitate extreme precision with regard to implant placement. The use of digital instrumentation

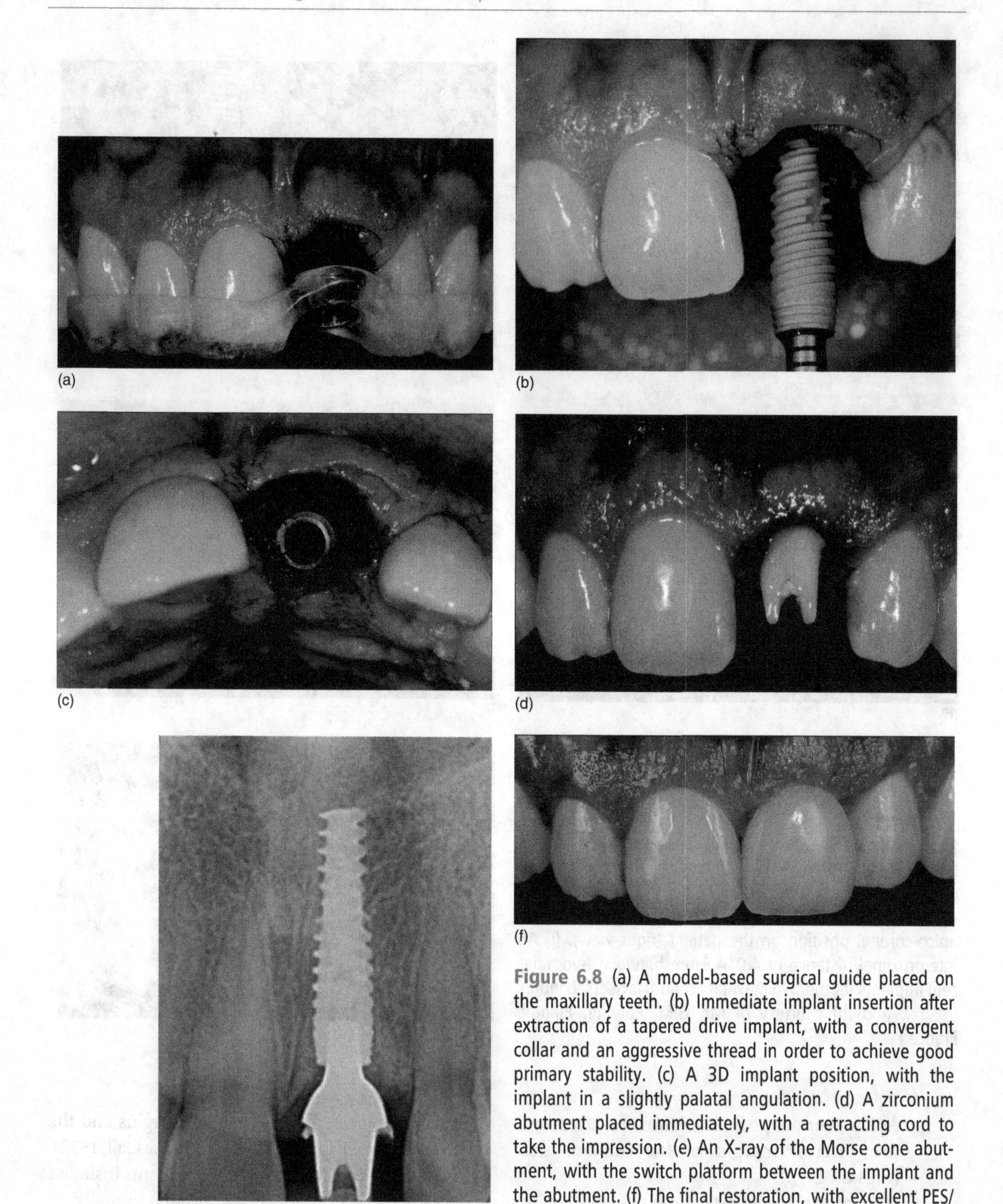

Figure 6.8 (a) A model-based surgical guide placed on the maxillary teeth. (b) Immediate implant insertion after extraction of a tapered drive implant, with a convergent collar and an aggressive thread in order to achieve good primary stability. (c) A 3D implant position, with the implant in a slightly palatal angulation. (d) A zirconium abutment placed immediately, with a retracting cord to take the impression. (e) An X-ray of the Morse cone abutment, with the switch platform between the implant and the abutment. (f) The final restoration, with excellent PES/WES. (Courtesy of Dr. M. Groisman, Rio de Janeiro, Brazil.)

based on 3D imaging has brought new dimensions to implant therapy:

- The buccal cervical implant collar should not go beyond a line joining the buccal enamel convexity of the adjacent teeth; nor should it go beyond 3 mm from a line joining the two cemento-enamel junctions (CEJs).
- Any buccal positioning of the implant will definitely thin out the remaining buccal cortical plate. This is why it is important to place a smaller implant in a slightly more palatal position, to prevent this phenomenon from occurring.
- In a study by Chen *et al.* (2007), when implant shoulder was placed buccally in the fresh extraction socket, three times more soft tissue recession occurred. Therefore, the implant should be positioned palatally, and 1 mm apically to the buccal crest.
- It is imperative, in the esthetic area, to place the implant slightly palatally for a 2–3 mm of buccal bone crest to remain present or to be established. The buccal/implant gap is always grafted (S. Leziy, pers. comm., 2010). Therefore, when implants are placed palatally, the buccal gap of > 2 mm should be filled with bone, exposing less implant on the buccal aspect.
- In sites with thick bony walls (> 1 mm), more bone fill occurs if the gap is < 2 mm.
- Age and smoking negatively affect bone fill (Paolantonio *et al.*, 2001; Tomasi *et al.*, 2010).
- The implant should be positioned approximately 1 mm deeper than the level of the buccal alveolar crest, and in a lingual/palatal position in relation to the center of the alveolus, in order to reduce or eliminate exposure above the alveolar crest of the endosseous (rough) portion of the implant (Caneva *et al.*, 2010).
- More apically positioned implants suffer less implant exposure buccally.

3. *Prosthetic design* – the Morse cone, platform switching, conical connection, and the curvy abutment profile (Figs 6.9a–g):
   - The microgap in the implant/abutment connection exists naturally in the two-part implant system. In most cases, it is susceptible to microbial seeding and micromovements between the parts during clinical occlusal function.
   - Both the microgap and micromovements may lead to localized bacterial inflammation and associated crestal bone loss if the microgap is within a minimum distance, less than 5 mm, from the alveolar crest (Deporter *et al.*, 2008). Therefore, the connection between the implant and the abutment should ideally be biomechanically resistant. Furthermore, the implant/abutment connection is the point of concentration for all the functional stresses. This will induce micro-disconnection, which causes the seal to deteriorate.
   - It is necessary to ensure a good seal in this connection to prevent micromovements, because any leak at the interface between the implant and the abutment will be prejudicial to the health of the biological width (Maeda *et al.*, 2007).
   - This seal will depend on some specific mechanical considerations:
     - Indexation is achieved by a passive hexagon resting in continuity with an active cone, preventing implant deformation.
     - Platform switching is obtained by having an abutment diameter that is smaller than the implant diameter.
     - Resistance is achieved by the friction of the abutment as it enters the implant (a Morse cone with an angle of 2–3° or a cone with 5.2° of conicity). The purpose of this type of internal connection is to spread out the loading of the transversal forces.
     - Anti-rotation is realized by friction between two cones with 15° and 3° conicity.
     - The friction decreases the space between the internal connection and the prosthetic abutment. Consequently, the dispersion of the occlusal forces on the implant's internal surfaces decreases the microgap.

Only a Morse cone connection can create a seal compatible with a healthy biological width and prevent crestal bone loss (Puchades-Roman *et al.*, 2000).

The maintenance of the marginal bone is crucial both from a functional as well as an esthetic point of view. Preserving the marginal bone levels and establishing the biological width at the abutment

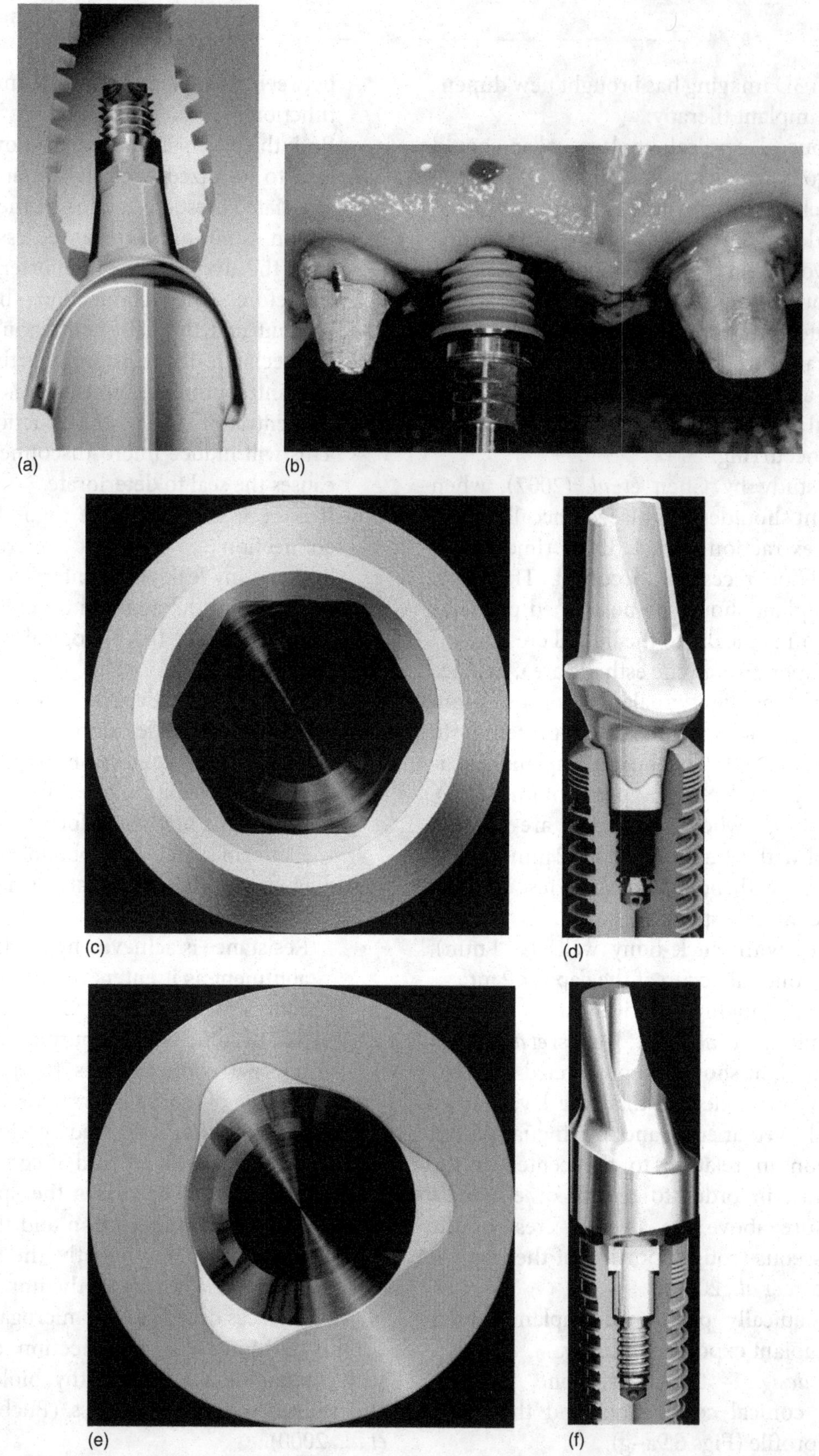

Figure 6.9 (a) A Morse cone abutment in the Neodent Drive® implant guarantees the seal connection and the thickness of the peri-implant tissue. (b) The Biomet Prevail® implant, which allows the switch platform to enhance the soft tissue thickness. (c) The NobelReplace™ conical connection hex platform, which provides a strong seal connection with a maximum peri-implant tissue volume. (d) The strong and tight fit of the NobelReplace™ internal conical connection abutment. (e) The NobelReplace™ three-lobe platform shift, which improves the esthetic appearance of the soft tissue. (f) Nobel Abutment® built-in platform shifting with an internal tri-channel connection. (Figures c–f courtesy of Nobel Biocare.)

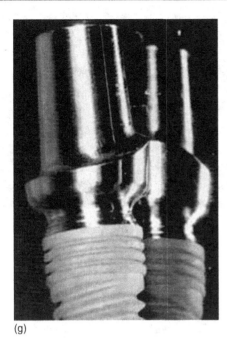

(g)

Figure 6.9 (g) The Nobel Curvy™ abutment on a NobelReplace™ implant increases the subgingival tissue volume.

level are really all about ensuring the right stimulation of the bone and promoting healthy soft tissue (see Fig. 6.7f). Therefore, healthy soft tissue and well-maintained marginal bone are interdependent. The one cannot exist without the other, because while it is vital that the soft tissue protects the bone, the bone must also be maintained to help support the soft tissue - a necessary symbiosis.

Peri-implant mucosa thickness

The acquisition of a significant buccal bone volume alone has, with time, proved to be insufficient to maintain ideal gingival architecture. In fact, it is recommended to systematically boost the initial gingival biotype by adding a connective tissue graft, no matter what the thickness and quality of the soft tissue at the outset (Figs 6.10a–i).

Reinforcement of the peri-implant gingiva to thicken and stabilize it is mostly done by adding connective tissue in the form of a free connective graft with a coronally advanced flap, or combined with the pedicle flap, according to the initial clinical situation and the surgical protocol, in order to prevent any risk of gingival recession (Degorce, 2009).

The absence of keratinized gingiva - or the presence of a limited amount, with regard to both thickness and height - increases bacterial plaque accumulation and induces secondary bone resorption and marginal gingival recession. Therefore, a soft tissue graft to increase the quality and quantity of keratinized gingiva permits the control of plaque accumulation and limits tissue inflammation, which will directly minimize crestal bone resorption and peri-implant soft tissue recession (Rompen, 2011).

Because of the fact that cementum in natural teeth is more preferable than implant titanium, and that there is no more vascularization from the periodontal ligaments, a contraction of 66% of the graft has been observed at 6 months (Bukhardt *et al.*, 2008).

Lastly, it is necessary to create an optimal concave submergence profile using a temporary crown and to wait long enough (a minimum of 3–6 months) to attain maturation and stability of the soft tissue, before taking the final impression and making the final restoration (Small and Tarnow, 2000; Leziy and Miller, 2008a).

Alveolar ridge preservation and augmentation after extraction and implant placement are achieved by:

- Bone grafting:
  - an autogenous graft alone
  - an autogenous graft combined with an allograft or a xenograft
  - slowly resorbing xenograft material.
- A connective tissue graft:
  - an autogenous CT graft
  - an allograft membrane
  - a xenograft membrane.

Regeneration of the bone crest and/or soft tissue should re-create the ideal morphological conditions and reestablish the initial contour, as it existed before bone loss (Poitras, 2003; Kan *et al.*, 2005). Whatever is done, tissue contraction will occur after implant exposition and restoration. The recession process is most pronounced in the first 6 months.

The severity of the tissue recession depends on the morphology and nature of the adjacent structures:

- thick keratinized tissue shows less recession
- a large amount of attached gingiva shows less recession
- an alumina/titanium abutment allows for normal soft tissue integration, and
- a gold alloy may not impede tissue loss (Touati *et al.*, 2008).

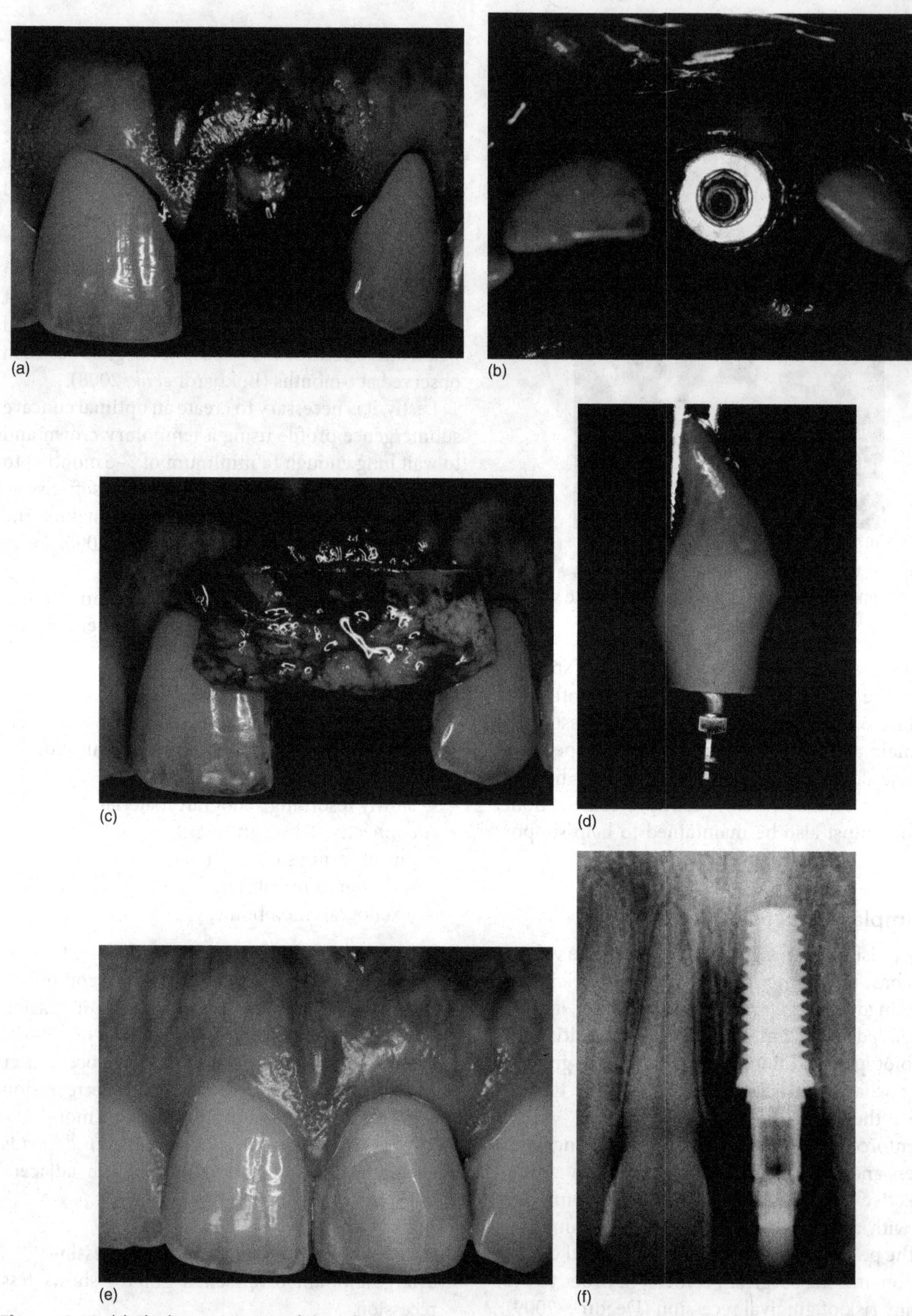

Figure 6.10 (a) Flapless extraction of the left central incisor root. (b) An occlusal view of a Biomet Prevail® implant in a slightly palatal position. (c) A connective tissue graft exposed before insertion in the buccal pouch. (d) An immediate temporary crown with a concave submergence profile. (e) The clinical aspect of the peri-implant soft tissue 3 months after surgery. (f) A retro-alveolar X-ray of the implant with a switch-platform abutment.

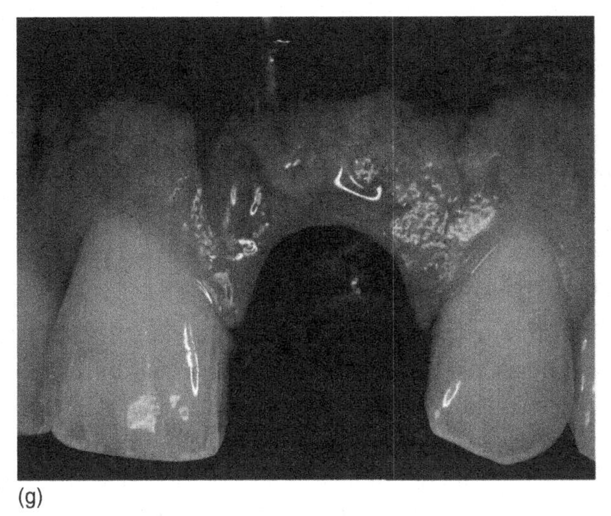

(g)

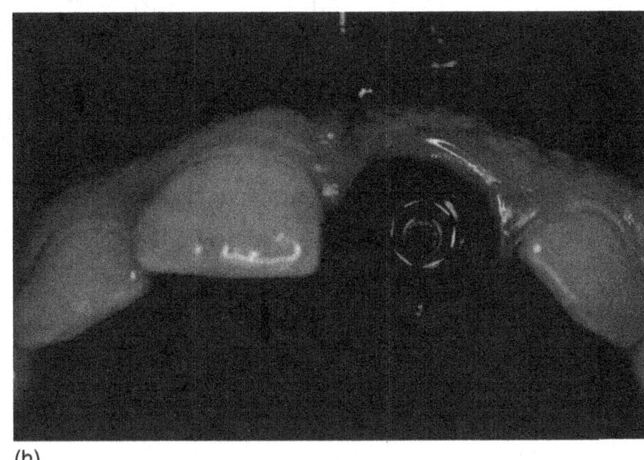

(h)

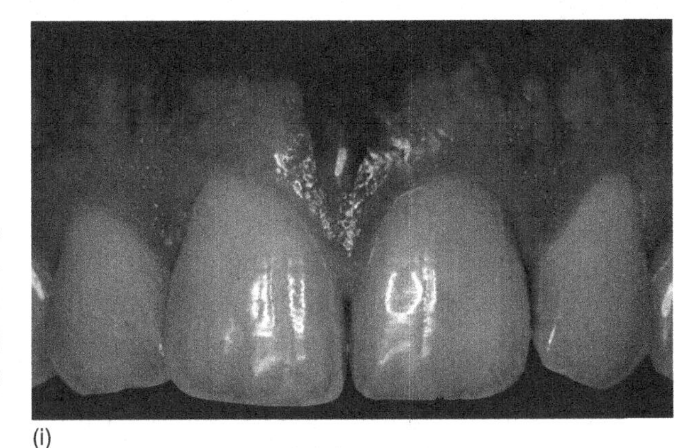

(i)

Figure 6.10 (g) The buccal/proximal contour of the peri-implant soft tissue after removal of the the temporary crown. (h) An occlusal view of the buccal bulk and thickness of the peri-implant soft tissue. (i) The final ceramic implant restoration, with a coronal level of the gingival contour. (Courtesy of Dr. T. Degorce, Tours, France.)

In implant therapy, there are certain prerequisites that must be respected in order to guarantee a long-lasting esthetic outcome. These factors are the preservation of the marginal bone level and the health and stability of the peri-implant soft tissue. However, the clinician should be aware of the fact that marginal bone loss might not influence or impair the esthetic result. This could be attributed, among other causes, to the biotype thickness (Livin *et al.*, 2005).

All peri-implant mucogingival techniques come from basic and current periodontal surgery. Peri-implant recession can be prevented in overbuilding the site by adding bone on the buccal cortical plate before, or in conjunction with, implant placement and by the addition of connective tissue grafts. From an esthetic point of view, the stability of soft tissues may be improved through the use of a connective tissue graft (Cornelini *et al.*, 2008). A connective tissue graft optimizes the esthetic result by preserving the bone level, improving soft tissue fixation, and preventing gingival recession (Mathews, 2000).

It is advisable to use the socket seal epithelial-connective gingival graft (Landsberg, 1997) to seal the extraction socket, protect the allograft material, and improve the biotype. Grafting to seal a socket is preferential to flap advancement because it does not change the mucogingival junction position and it simultaneously enhances soft tissue quality.

A palatal connective tissue graft of 1.5–2.0 mm thickness is frequently used in order to preserve the implant site morphology, increase the gingival thickness, change the gingival biotype, enhance the facial contour of this zone, resolve the facial concavity, and ensure long-term stability, all of which are essential to an esthetic final restoration.

Many techniques have been described to increase the quality and quantity of the peri-implant soft tissue (Rompen, 2011):

- the pedicle flap: the lateral or roll procedure
- the epithelium-connective graft
- the subepithelium-connective graft

- an alveolar graft of frozen dried skin:
  - human dermal allogenic substitutes (AlloDerm®), or
  - porclin xenograft collagen membrane (Mucograft®).

In order to improve and/or increase the marginal soft tissue contour, and to resolve the facial concavity, which influences the final esthetic result of the restoration, it is recommended to use a palatal connective tissue graft and adopt a minimally invasive approach (Becker *et al.*, 2005).

Timing of the connective tissue graft and of implant placement

There are several modalities of connective tissue graft to take into consideration, depending on the implant environment and on the clinical situation.

This graft may be done at any of the following moments: at the time of extraction, without implant placement, using a bone graft (BG) or guided bone regeneration (GBR); at the time of extraction, with implant placement, using a tunneling/saddle procedure; before or during implant exposition; after implant exposition, with or without the roll technique; after placement of the temporary crown or final restoration; and, finally, following buccal implant positioning complications. A connective tissue graft optimizes the esthetic result by preserving the bone level, maintaining long-term soft tissue thickness and stability, and preventing peri-implant gingival recession (Salama, 2011).

Some examples of connective tissue grafts performed using different timings in relation to implant placement are detailed below.

At the time of extraction, prior to implant placement

When site preservation becomes insufficient to maintain the alveolar ridge anatomy at an esthetic site, surgical restoration of the hard and soft tissue components is required at the time of implantation. Therefore, if the integrity of the osseous housing is compromised by coronal dehiscence or limited keratinized gingiva following either the extraction or the drilling, a two-stage approach is necessary to restore the site (Figs 6.11a–t).

An allograft or xenograft, with a membrane and an overlying connective tissue graft, before implant placement, is used to improve the buccal thickness. The use of barrier membranes has been recommended to obtain bone regeneration and to prevent soft tissue growth in the alveolar socket. However, there are several clinical complications that occur when using nonresorbable barrier membranes, such as bacterial colonization and infection, which can lead to failure of the bone graft and/or implant. The connective tissue graft seems to prevent these complications induced by the use of synthetic barrier membranes and, at the same time, it improves the local metabolic environment of the superficial soft

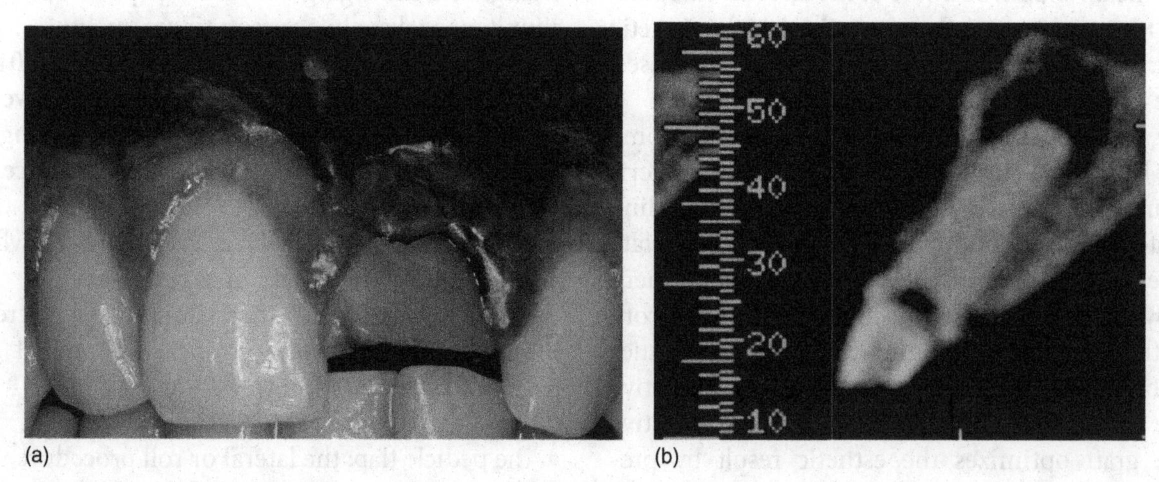

Figure 6.11 (a) A broken left incisor on a patient with a thin biotype. (b) A CT scan of the left central incisor, with a very thin cortical plate and no apical bone.

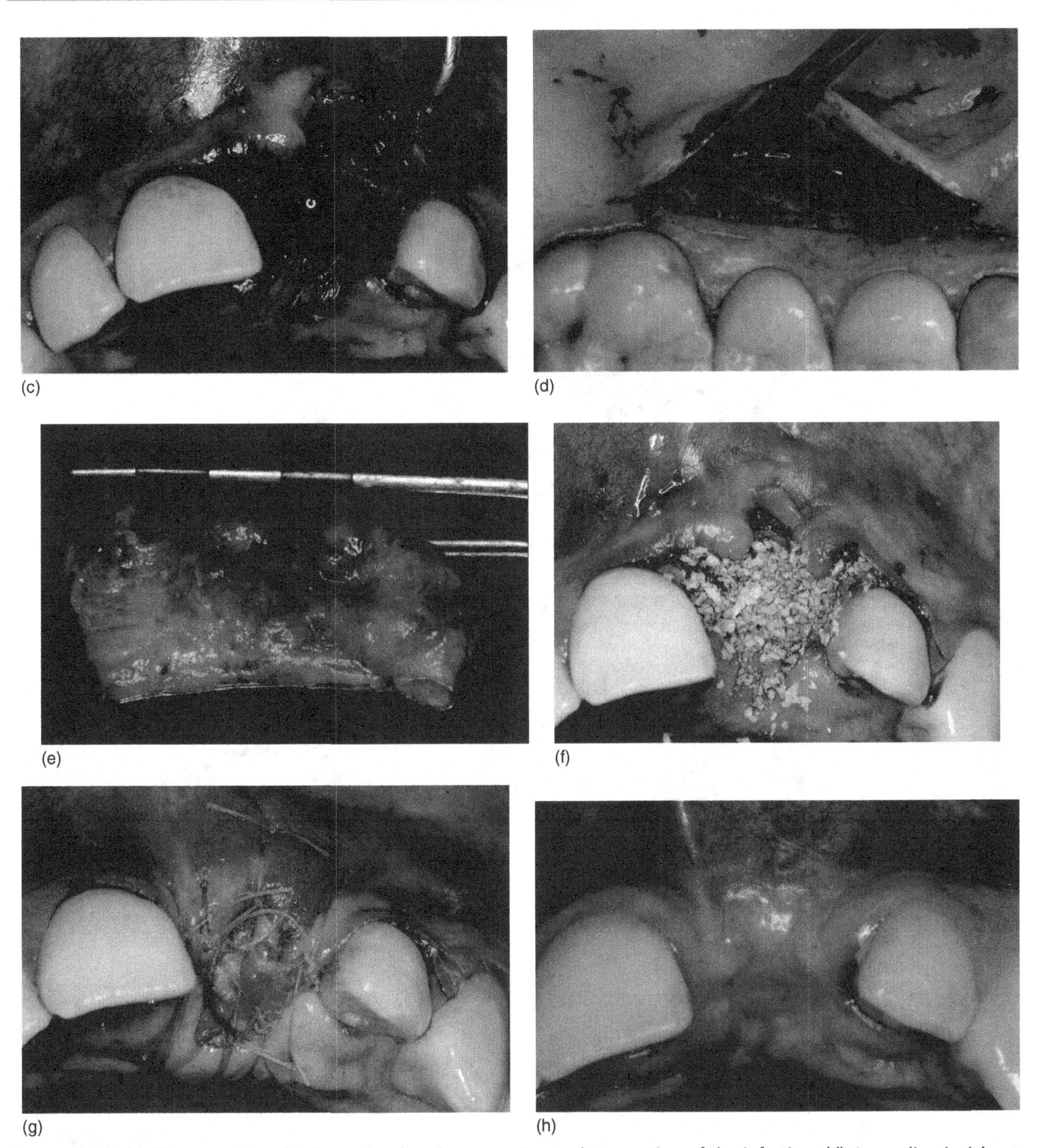

Figure 6.11 (c) The extraction site 2 weeks after the extraction and evacuation of the infection. (d) A one-line incision to harvest the connective tissue graft. (e) The optimal thickness and length of the connective tissue graft (CTG); the palatal harvesting site is immediately sutured using buccal sling sutures. (f) The alveolar socket is filled with a Bio-Oss® allograft and covered with BioGuide®. (g) The CTG is inserted in the buccal pouch, over the graft and under the palatal flap. (h) Crest occlusal view of soft and hard tissue healing 3 months after surgery.

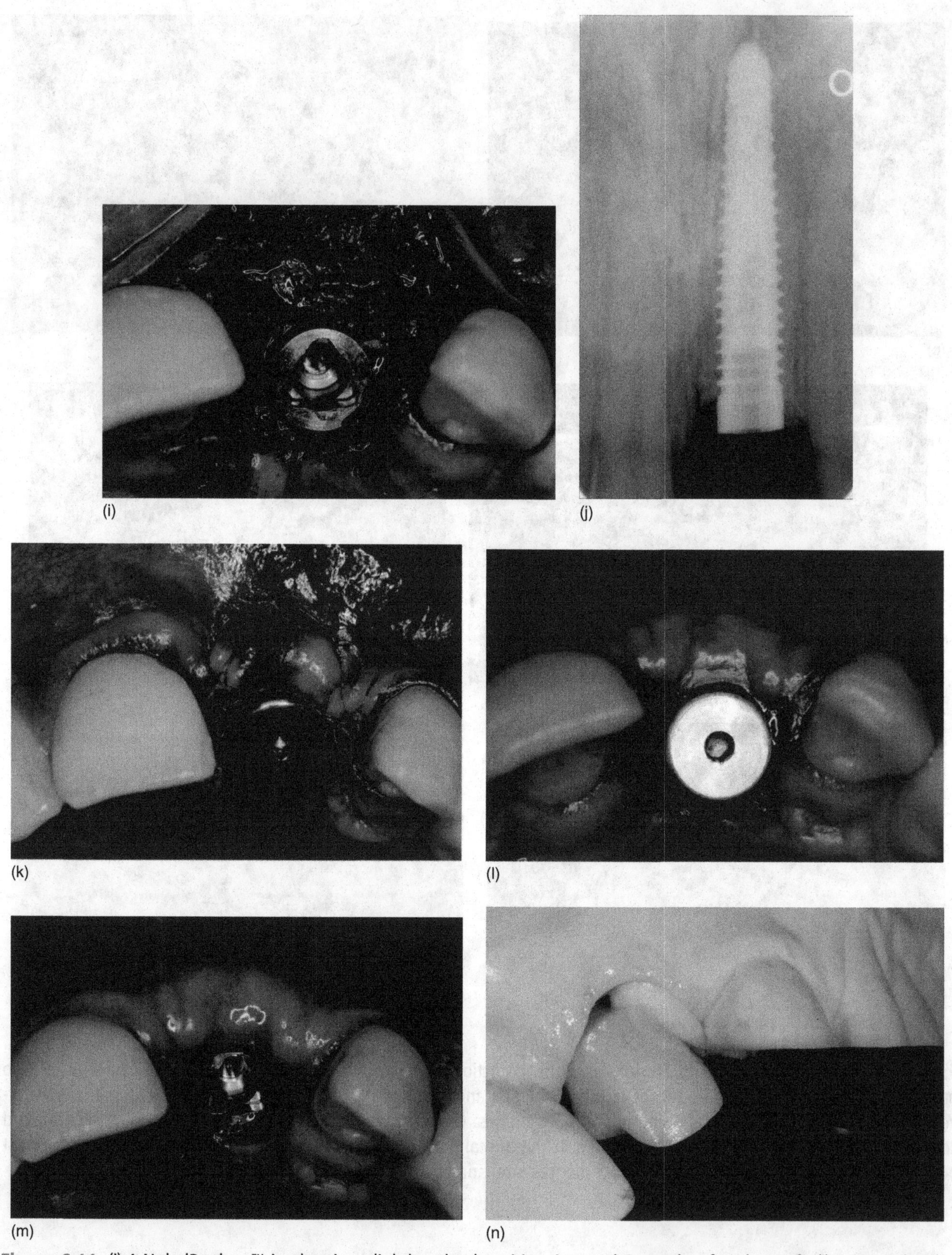

Figure 6.11 (i) A NobelReplace™ implant in a slightly palatal position, inserted 6 months after the graft. (j) A retro-alveolar X-ray of the NobelReplace™ Groovy implant. (k) A palatal roll flap procedure was used to increase the buccal contour. (l) The soft tissue aspect 4 weeks later, with the healing abutment. (m) Ongoing maturation of the excess of soft tissue after removal of the healing abutment. (n) Adding ceramic on the zirconium abutment after remodeling of the gingival contour on the cast.

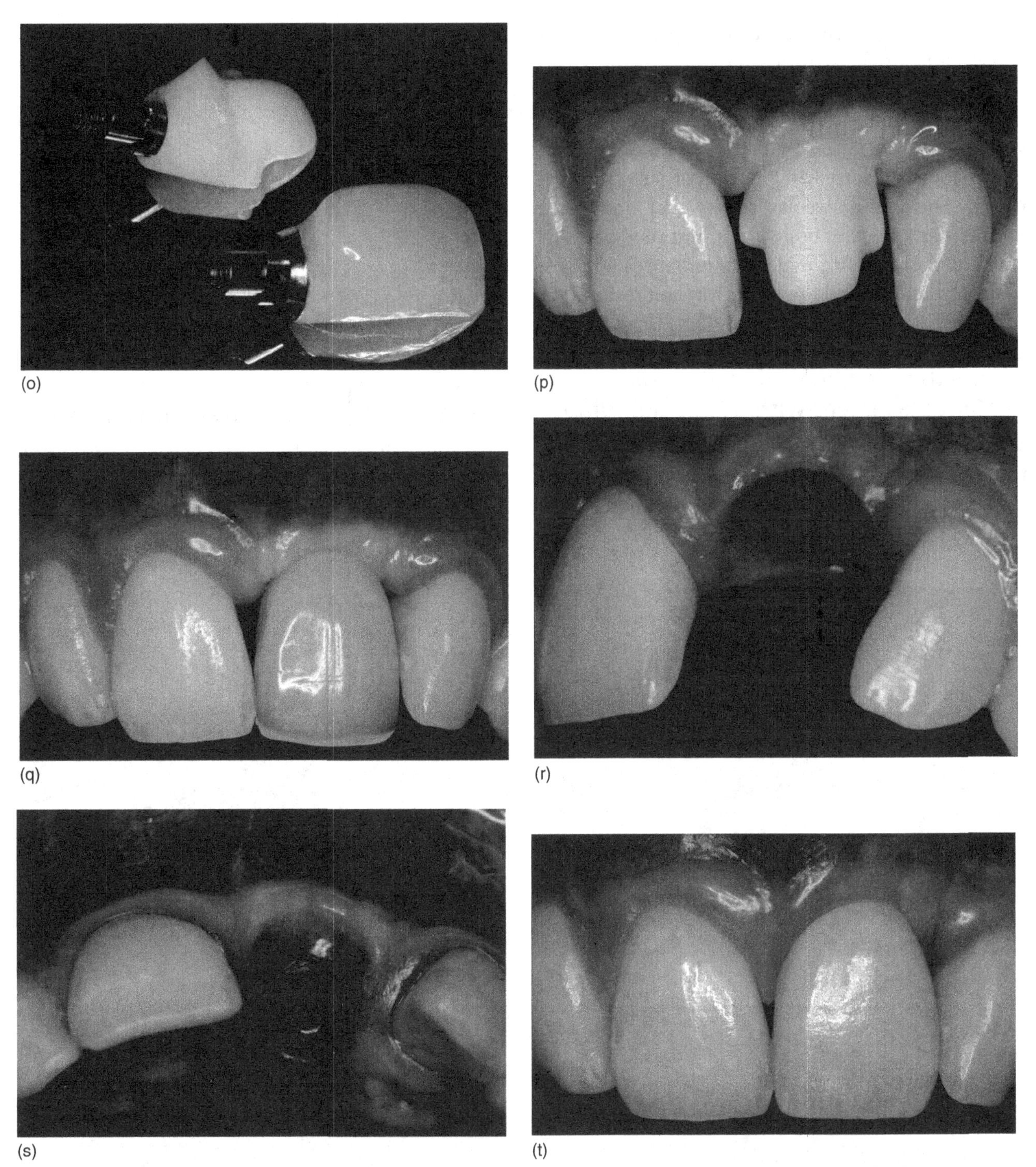

Figure 6.11 (o) A zirconium monoblock screwed abutment crown and a concave temporary crown. (p) The first trial of the screw-type zirconium monoblock abutment. (q) The initial placement of the screw-type monoblock first temporary crown. (r) A buccal view of the gingival contour 4 weeks post-op, after removal of the second temporary crown, with a harmonious vertical contour. (s) An occlusal view showing the new harmonious and thick gingival contour after 6 months. (t) The final implant restoration 36 months after tooth extraction. (Figures (n) and (o) courtesy of Mr. J.M. Etienne, laboratory technician, Pulnoy, France.)

tissues, thus preserving, and increasing the quality and quantity of, the keratinized tissues.

The interposition before implant placement of a large, thick autogenous connective tissue graft for site preservation immediately following extraction of the tooth (inserted in the buccal subperiosteal pouch, above the alveolar socket and under the palatal flap) with a bone graft improves and/or changes the tissue biotype and enhances the soft tissue esthetic around the future implant restoration (Caplanis, 2008).

After extraction, in conjunction with implant placement with a tunneling flap

Soft tissue recession is minimized by enhancing the volume of the labial margins and the interproximal papillae, and this technique enhances the clinician's ability to design and sculpt the soft tissue contour around the soft tissue graft (Landsberg, 1997, 2008). This could be done in a different way, as follows:

- By combining, after extraction and immediate implant placement, a bone graft over the implant with a regenerative membrane. The membrane will be then covered with a connective tissue graft (Figs 6.12a–h).
- By using a rolled pedicle connective graft in conjunction with implant placement and a healing abutment (Figs 6.13a–f).
- By placing implants in fresh extraction sites, an immediate subepithelial connective tissue graft (Figs 6.14a–i), sutured in the buccal pouch, was shown to be a valid treatment procedure that

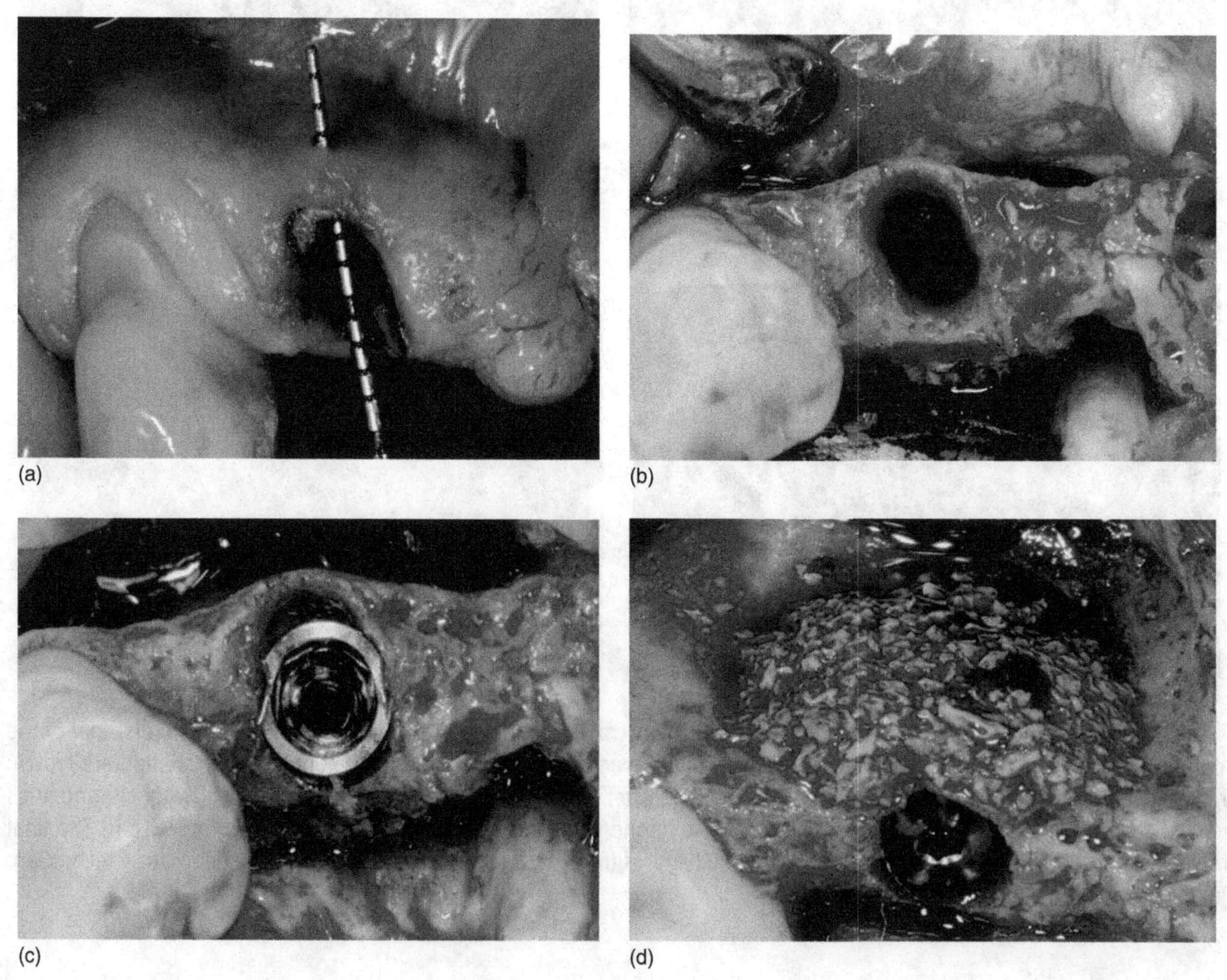

Figure 6.12 (a) Perforation of buccal tissue after tooth extraction. (b) The cleaned alveolar socket after flap elevation. (c) Immediate implant placement. (d) Bio-Oss® filling the dehiscence and fenestration on the buccal cortical plate

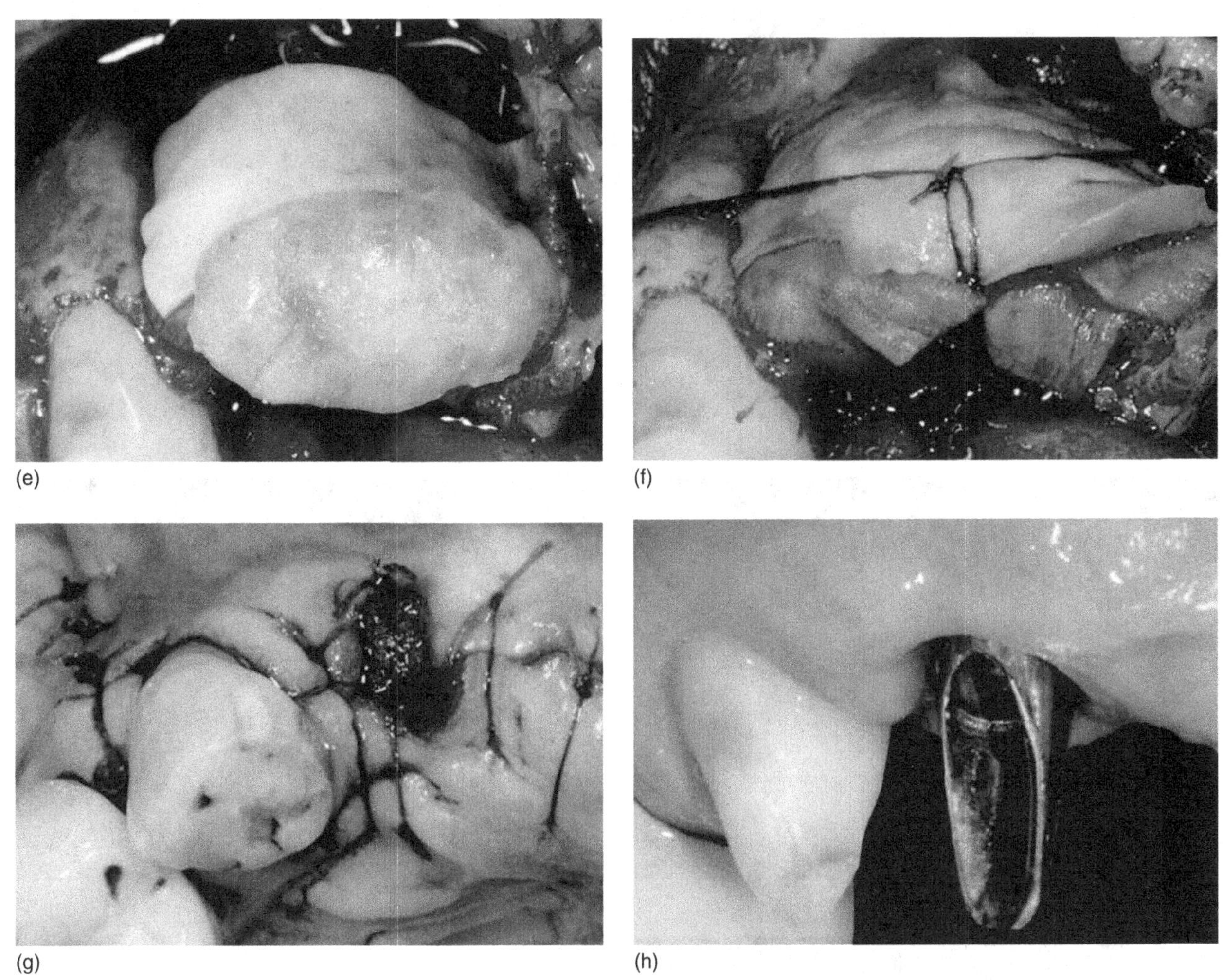

Figure 6.12 (e) The BioGuide® on the Bio-Oss® and connective tissue graft on the membrane will be stabilized through partial thickness dissection (f) with resorbable sutures. (g) The flap is sutured over the implant and the GBR and CTG. (h) The bulky appearance of the soft tissue, with the implant abutment. (Courtesy of Dr. T. Testori, Como, Italy.)

produces esthetically predictable results for the treatment of nonsalvageable teeth (Covani *et al.*, 2007).

Immediately after implant placement in a mature edentulous site, a connective tissue graft placed on top of the cover screw will increase the thickness, and the vertical and buccal contours, and also prevent the implant from leaving a grayish shadow (Jovanovic *et al.*, 1999). Whatever is done, tissue contraction will occur after implant exposition and restoration in the first 3–6 months. At its highest point, the gingival margin will lose 0.61 mm, and the interdental papillae will retract by an average of 0.37 mm (Grunder, 1999).

The technique of immediate loading of implants following tooth extraction, associated with grafting of a connective-bone sliver harvested from the maxillary tuberosity, promotes acceleration of bone repair for the implant and graft, and minimizes the number of surgical procedures. The connective-bone sliver not only restores the lost vestibular bone plate but also impedes cell competition between the hard and soft tissues, thereby promoting effective bone and gingival healing.

Before or after implant exposition with or without the roll technique

In order to compensate for recession, thick, keratinized palatal tissue should always be positioned buccally before surgery (Figs 6.15a–d) or at the second stage of surgery (Figs 6.15e–g), to increase the amount of facial keratinized gingiva and improve the soft tissue contour (Grunder *et al.*, 2005). This

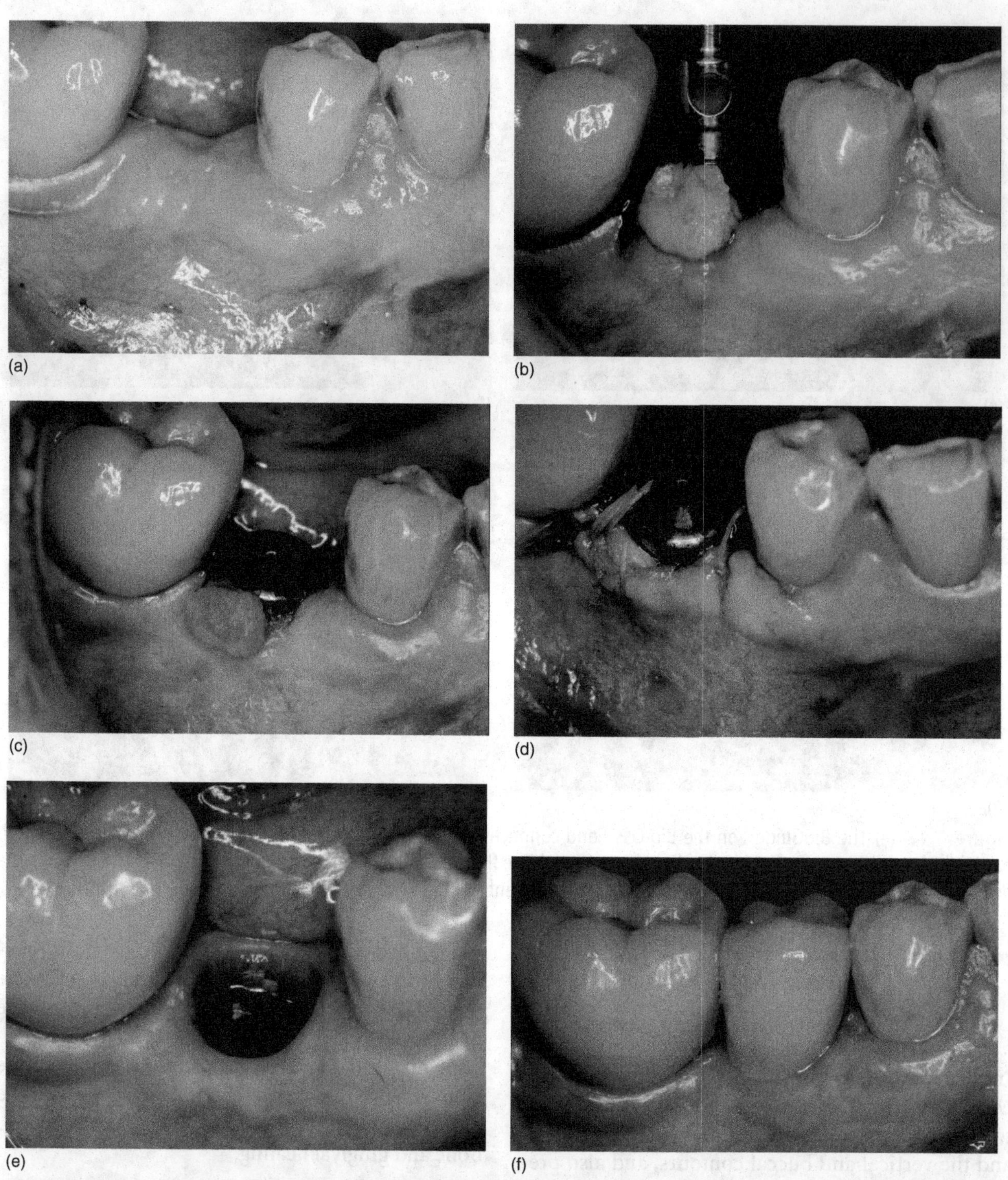

Figure 6.13 (a) A deformed ridge after lower second premolar extraction. (b) Tissue-punching round the buccal pedicle flap during preparation of the implant site. (c) The healing abutment in place after removal of the buccal flap epithelium. (d) The buccal flap is rolled into the buccal pouch. (e) The appearance of the bulky ridge 2 months later, with the healing abutment. (f) The scalloped appearance of the gingival margin without the healing abutment.

is accomplished by making a more lingually oriented crestal incision, elevating the buccal flap, and securing it in such a way that it remains on the labial aspect of the placed healing abutment. Any exposed bone will be covered during tissue granulation.

In a study by Martins da Rosa *et al.* (2009), a connective-bone sliver graft from the maxillary tuberosity was indicated for recovery of the vestibular bone cortex of the damaged fresh socket and covering of the exposed threads of the implant, and it increased the thickness and quality of the gingiva. In combination with the coronal repositioning of a gingival flap, correction of the gingival recession was enabled.

After temporary crown or final restoration

At implant insertion and temporization, or after final restoration (Figs 6.16a–d), a connective tissue graft, harvested from the palatal aspect, is placed into the subperiosteal buccal tunnel. The microflap elevator is used to create a buccal pouch. A long suture needle is then used to penetrate at the

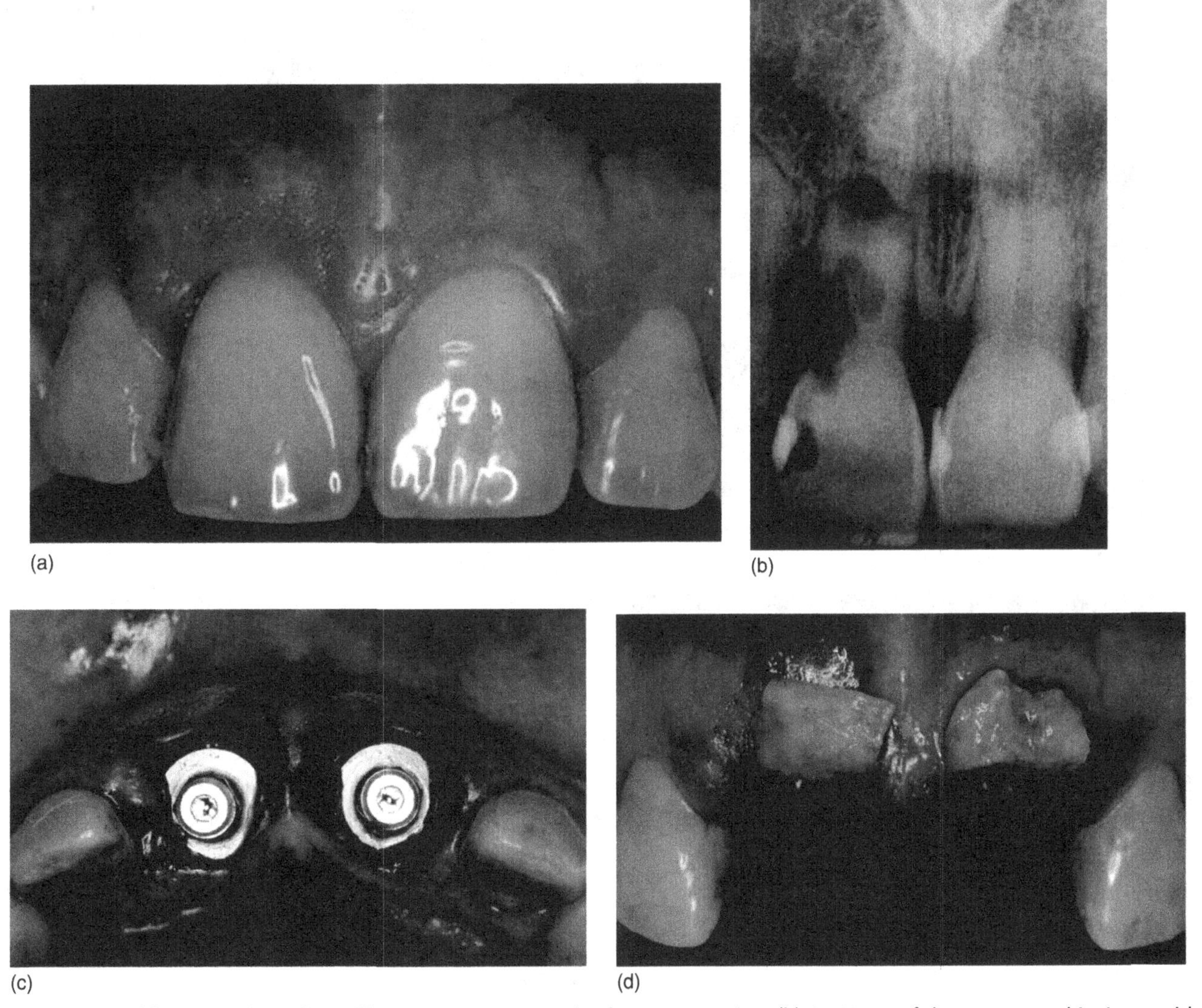

Figure 6.14 (a) A loose lateral maxillary incisor, as a result of root resorption. (b) An X-ray of the two central incisors with internal root resorption. (c) The right implant in a slightly palatal position compared to the left central incisor, which will be extracted after the implant is placed, and then the left implant placed immediately, in a slightly palatal position. (d) After the insertion of allograft into the buccal gap, two pieces of CTG from the tuberosity are submerged in the buccal pouch of the adjacent implant and sutured.

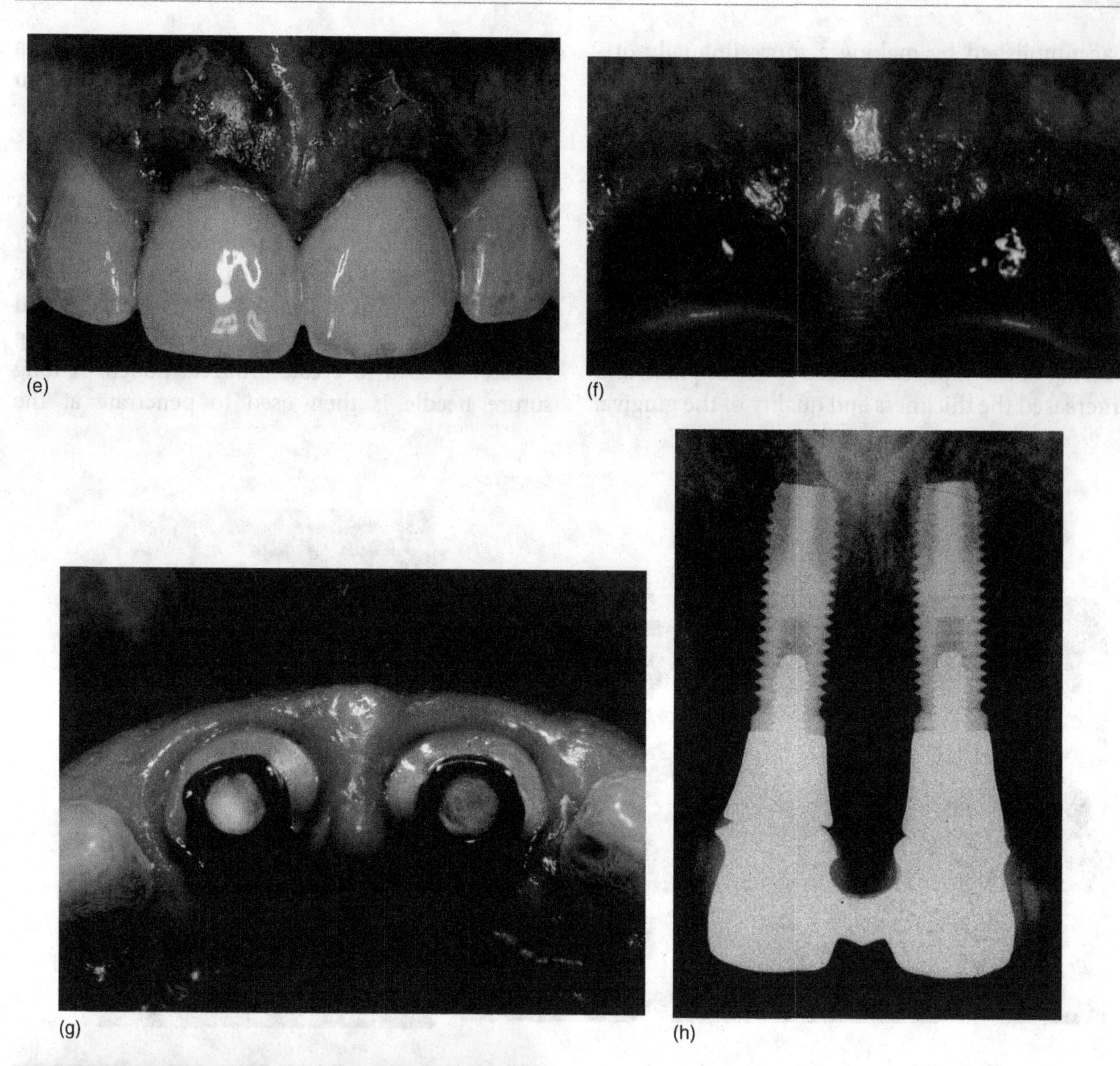

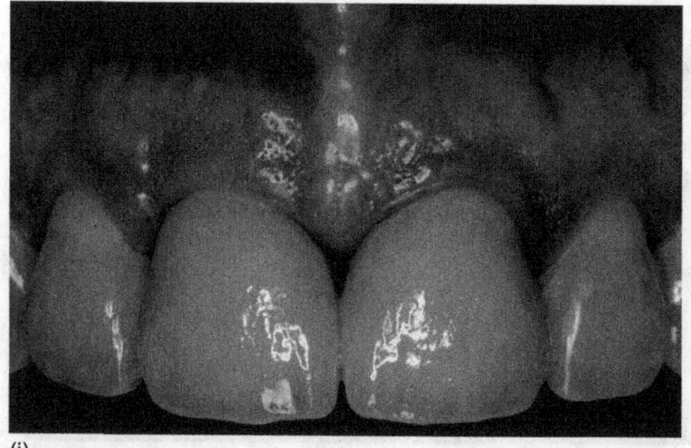

Figure 6.14 (e) The bulky gingival aspect of the splinted temporary crown, 1 week after insertion. (f) The gingival aspect of the implant site 3 months after removal of the crowns. (g) An occlusal view of the ceramometal abutment, which is respecting the emergence profile. (h) A retro-alveolar X-ray of the two splinted implant restorations. (i) The final aspect: adjacent ceramic implant restorations and a satisfactory gingival contour. (Courtesy of Dr. T. Degorce, Tours, France.)

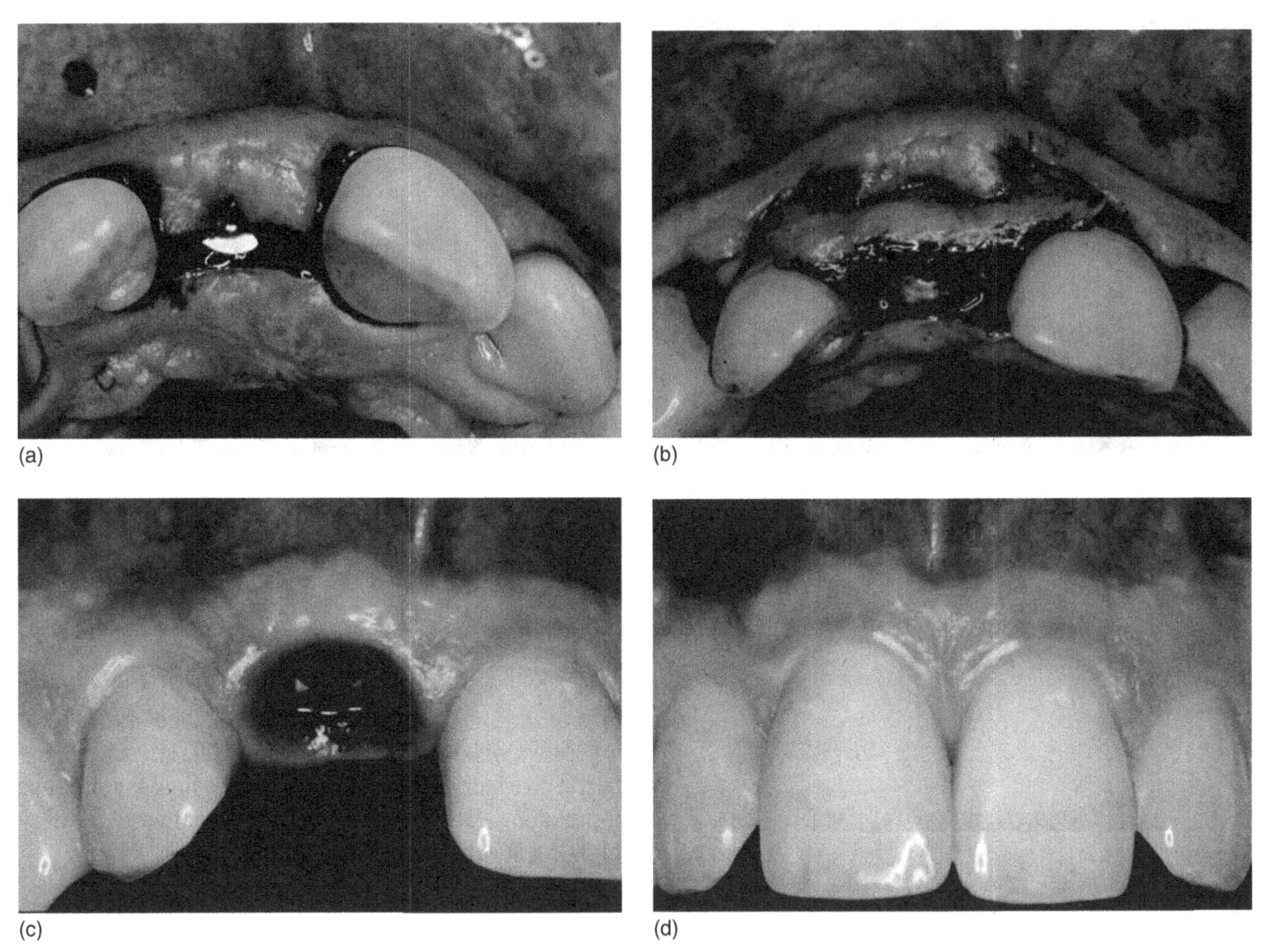

Figure 6.15 (a) A palatal incision combined with a buccal sulcular incision. (b) A mini-flap elevation allows insertion of the CTG. (c) The clinical appearance of the peri-implant soft tissue 3 months before the taking of impressions for the implant. (d) The ceramic implant restoration, with an optimal ridge, marginal and large papilla contour.

mesio-apical line angle of the pouch, to capture the mesial part of the connective tissue graft, which is pulled inside the mesial pouch and sutured. Afterwards, the distal part of the connective tissue graft is pulled and sutured into the distal pouch using the same procedure with another needle. The flap is advanced coronally so that the buccal margin is 2 mm coronal to the adjacent teeth gingival margin. It is then sutured to be adapted against the temporary or final restoration crown (Kinsel and Capoferri, 2008).

After 3 months of healing, there is an increase in the thickness of the gingival margin, and the connective tissue grafts will increase the long-term stability of the gingival margin and improve tissue management throughout the provisional and final restorative treatment phases, which will directly enhance the thickness of the gingiva. The definitive implant restoration appears to emerge from the soft tissue rather than resting on top (Saadoun, 2006).

Platelet-rich fibrin (PRF) can be considered as an autologous healing biomaterial, incorporating, in a matrix of autologous fibrin, a high percentage of leucocytes, platelets, and growth factors obtained from a simple blood sample drawn from the patient at the time of the surgical procedure.

Platelet-rich fibrin contains growth factors such as PDGF, TGFB, IGF, and VEGF, and provides accelerated healing of superficial and bone tissues, the development of good neo-angiogenesis, and faster wound healing.

The blood sample is treated with a single centrifugation, in a specific centrifuge, without any blood manipulation, anticoagulant, bovine thrombin,

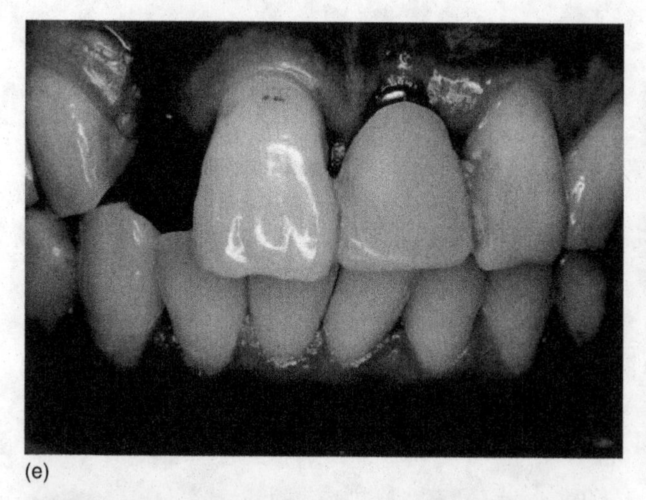

(e)

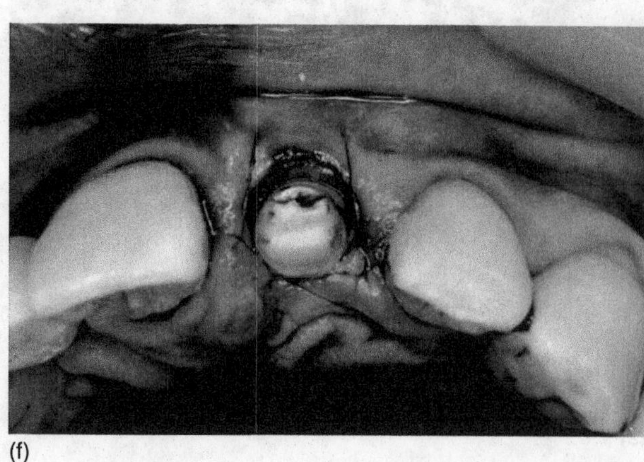

(f)

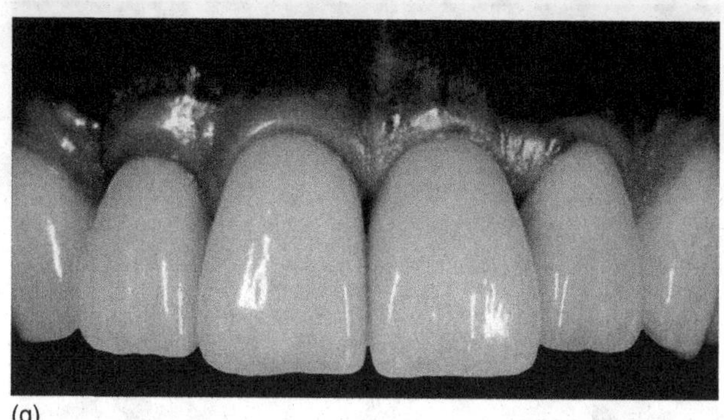

(g)

Figure 6.15 (e) A compromised buccal ridge after implant exposition, with healing abutments. (f) A CTG inserted into the buccal pouch of each implant site. (g) The final four ceramic restorations, with harmonious gingival contours. (Courtesy of Dr. M. Suzuki, Tokyo, Japan.)

sodium nitrate, or calcium chloride. At the end of the centrifugation process, three distinct factions are found:

- a deeper-level part containing the red cells
- a superficial part containing platelet-poor plasma, and
- an intermediate fraction including the platelet-rich fibrin clot, which is then, after compression, used as a platelet-rich fibrin membrane.

The platelet-rich fibrin membrane is more elastic and consistent than the platelet-concentrated clot traditionally obtained in some plasma-rich platelet (PRP) protocols and can be employed in several clinical situations (Saadoun, 2006; Simonpieri *et al.*, 2011).

The presence of leukocytes (containing PDGF and VEGF) and the absence of manipulation, differentiate platelet-rich fibrin from other more complex platelet-concentration protocols.

The platelet cytokines, and especially PDGF, RGFB-1, and IGF, are gradually released during physiological resorption of the fibrin matrix (Figs 6.16e–j). This allows the healing process to be protected from external injuries. The gradual release of cytokines indeed appears to play a regulatory role in the inflammatory phenomena within the graft (Del Corso, 2008).

Neovessels grow inside fibrin: following tissue injury, under normal conditions, the patient's fibrin is colonized rapidly by inflammatory cells, fibroblasts, and endothelial cells, which remodel it into granulation tissue and subsequently into mature connective tissue.

Used as a membrane, which can also be sutured, the platelet-rich fibrin allows the surgical site to be protected from external injuries and constitutes a matrix for faster healing of the wound edges.

After placement of an over-buccally inclined implant

Gingival recession tends to form more frequently in this situation, thereby necessitating a longer crown

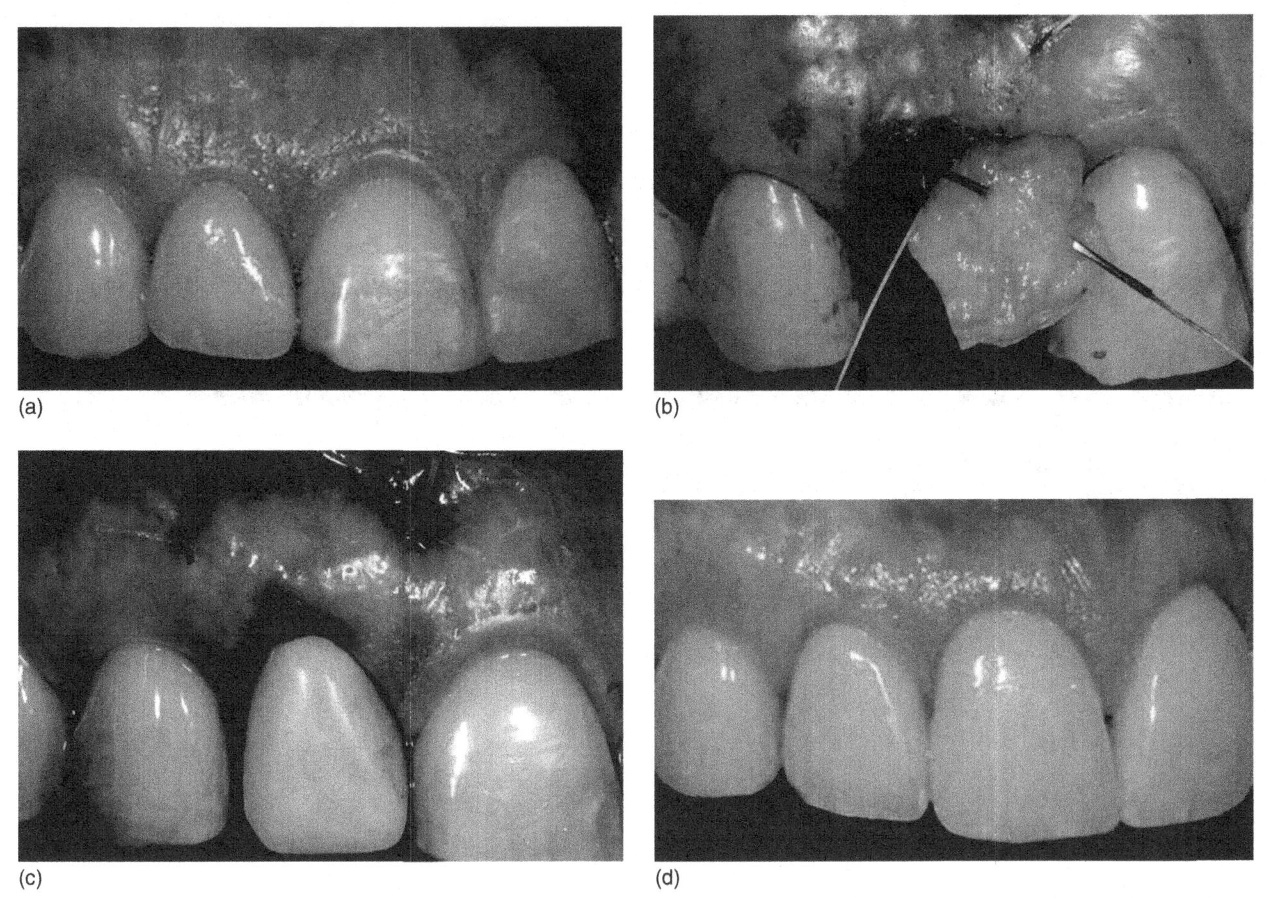

Figure 6.16 (a) A loose lateral incisor with a grayish color will be extracted delicately. (b) An implant is inserted immediately, with a concave subgingival abutment. The mesial part of the CTG is pulled inside the mesial pouch, and then the distal part of the CTG is pulled into the distal pouch, using another needle. (c) The implant provisional restoration is cemented and is surrounded by a thick gingival margin. Note the bulky facial aspect. (d) Laminate veneers on the three teeth adjacent to the implant restoration, showing an optimal papilla height and gingival margin contour. (Courtesy of Dr. A. Pinto, Paris, France.)

restoration. This provides a less pleasing esthetic outcome. In some cases, it is possible to resolve this problem by combining several mucogingival surgeries (connective grafts and coronally advanced flaps). These procedures are concomitant with the removal of the old abutment and restoration, which are replaced by new ones with a submarginal concave submergence profile (Figs 6.17a–h).

The connective tissue graft and pontics

When multiple implants are to be placed in the anterior esthetic zone, treatment planning becomes a real challenge for the clinician. The prosthetically derived rules for the distance between the remaining bone crest level and the contact point restoration, as discussed above, will determine the choice between inserting adjacent implants or strategic implant placement combined with pontics (Tarnow *et al.*, 2003).

The use of pontics rather than adjacent implants to replace the two central incisors poses its own challenge (Spear, 1999). As is the case between adjacent implants, the concern in this instance is the papilla between the adjacent pontics. The difference, however, is that when pontics are used, it can almost be guaranteed that interproximal crestal bone between the extracted central incisors will resorb, creating a flat bony ridge and a subsequent loss of papillary height. This is due to the absence of a bone-stabilizing presence, such as an implant adjacent to a tooth.

It is, however, possible to significantly augment the soft tissue between pontics above the flattened osseous crest (i.e., by an average of 6.6 mm). This is

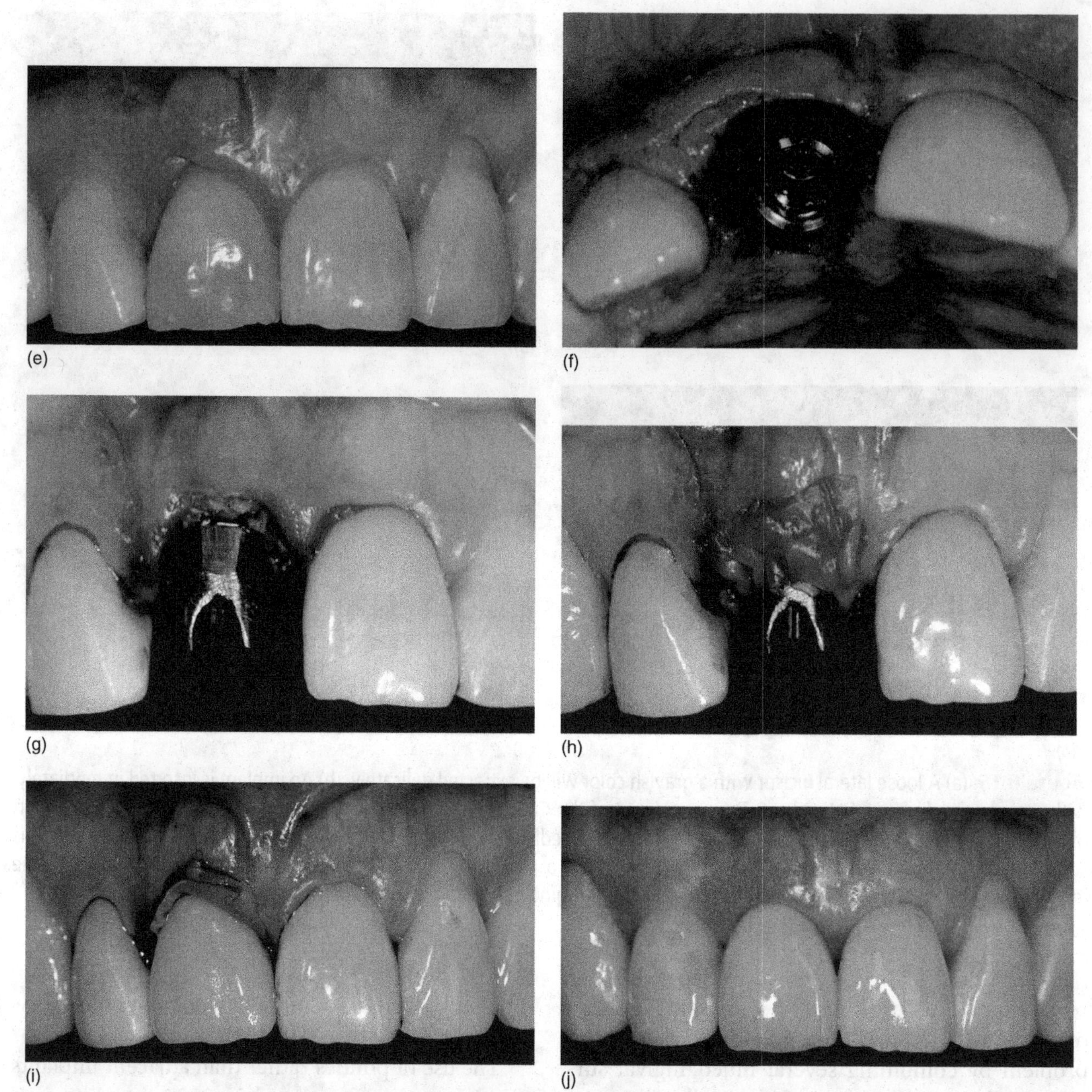

Figure 6.16 (e) Internal root resorption on the right maxillary incisor, with discoloration on this thin gingival biotype. (f) The implant is placed immediately in a slightly palatal position to leave a buccal macrogap, and the abutment is fixed on the implant. (g) Xenograft mixed with L-PRF membrane pieces is inserted into the gap. (h) An L-PRF membrane is plugged into the gap, below the buccal pouch. (i) The temporary crown formed from the initial tooth is placed over the PRF membrane, which will take 2 weeks to heal. (j) The final ceramic implant restoration, with a harmonious gingival contour, one year. (Courtesy of Dr. M. Del Corso, Turin, Italy.)

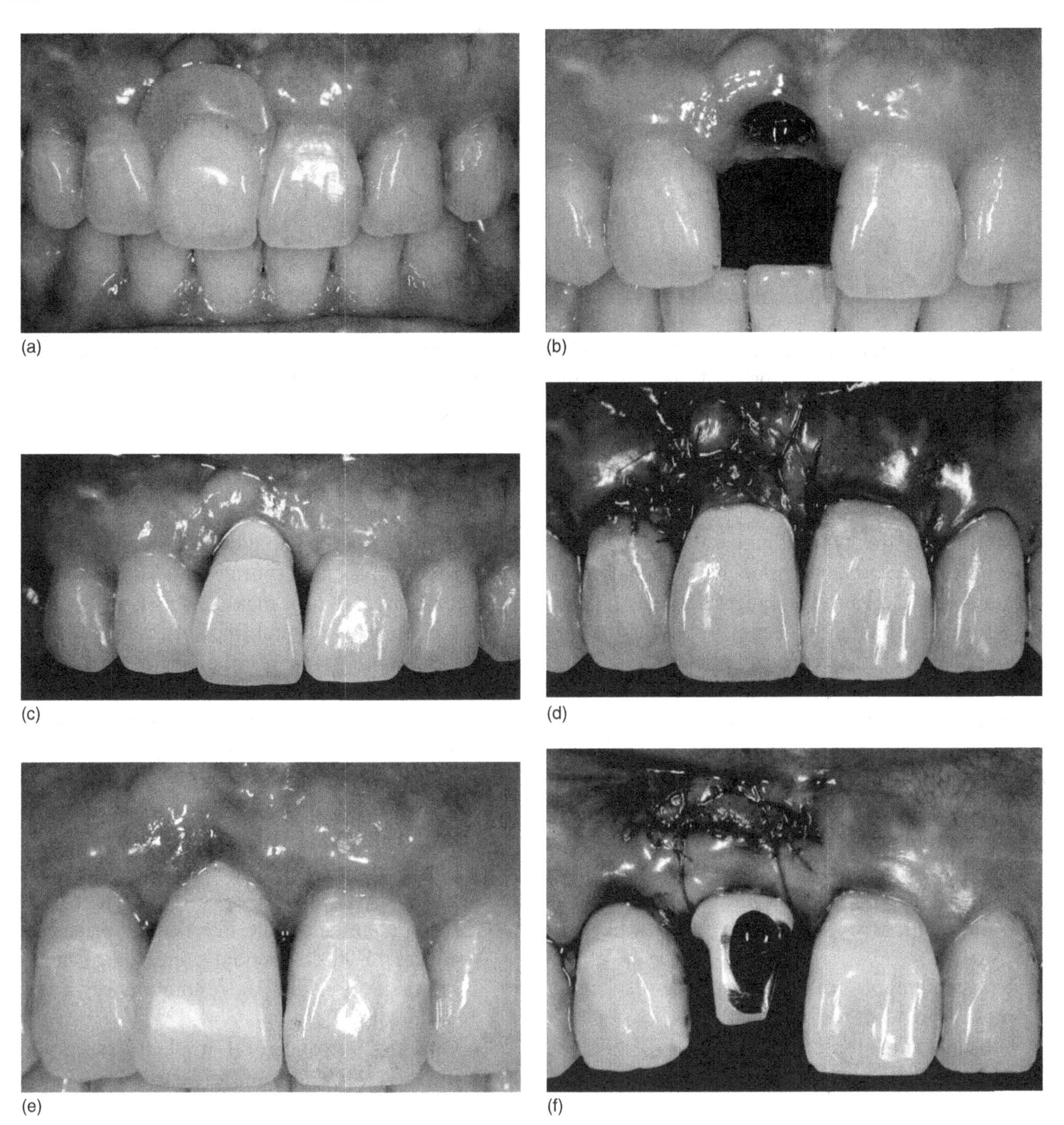

Figure 6.17 (a) An implant restoration with buccal pink porcelain, to hide the gingival recession. (b) Significant loss of buccal soft tissue due to overly buccal implant angulation. (c) A new ceramometal abutment with a concave submergence profile and supragingival margin, with a new temporary crown. (d) A submerged connective tissue graft with a coronally advanced flap on the abutment. (e) Healing 6 weeks post-op, with some coronal gain of the gingival margin on the abutment. (f) An apically submerged CTG with a new coronally advanced flap.

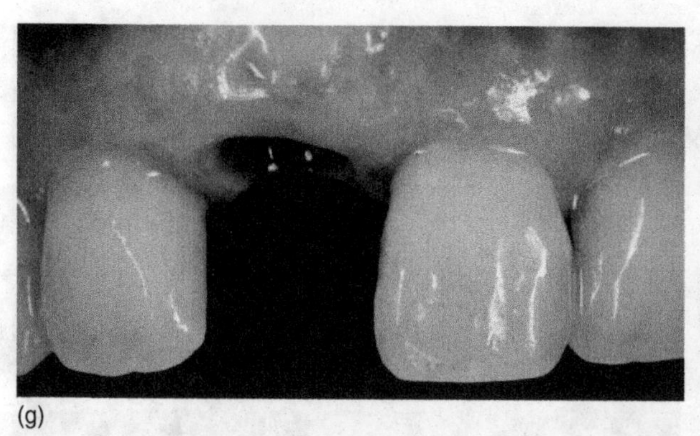
(g)

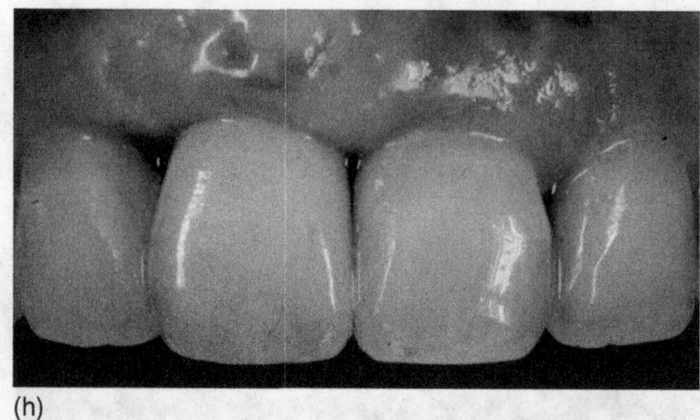
(h)

Figure 6.17 (g) The gingival aspect of the peri-implant soft tissue with coronal gain before the taking of the impression. (h) The final ceramic restoration, with a harmonious gingival contour and buccal convexity. (Courtesy of Dr. M. Suzuki and Dr. M. Yamazaki, Tokyo, Japan.)

in contrast to the typical mucosal tissue height above the interproximal bone between adjacent implants which, on average, ranges between 2.3 mm and 3.5 mm. Ultimately, it becomes possible to have a papilla between the central pontics that is 3 mm more coronal than a papilla between adjacent implants for the same interproximal crest location and achieve optimal esthetic results (Spear, 2008). Therefore, it is sometimes more recommended biologically to use a pontic rather than an adjacent implant restoration.

There are some clinical indications regarding when and when not to combine implant restorations and pontics:

a. Replacement of two maxillary incisors – two implant-adjacent restorations:
   - to close the interdental space
   - to prevent the dark space between the restorations, and
   - to maintain the symmetry between the adjacent teeth.
b. Replacement of one central maxillary incisor and one lateral incisor – one central implant restoration and one lateral pontic restoration:
   - to help the papillae to recuperate, and
   - to maintain the symmetry with the contralateral side.
c. Replacement of one maxillary lateral incisor and one canine – one canine implant restoration and one lateral pontic restoration (Figs 6.18a–c):
   - to maintain the papillae, and
   - to obtain a subtle symmetry.
d. Replacement of four maxillary incisors:
   - Option 1: two lateral implant restorations plus two central pontic restorations (optimal papilla result, limited biomechanical resistance). Unfavorable relationships between the residual edentulous ridge, pontic, and gingival papillae may compromise the definitive result of a restoration. Kim *et al.* (2009) described a unique pontic design, as well as the application of pressure during insertion of the pontic, to achieve proper tissue displacement (Figs 6.18d–k). Controlled pressure enhances the interdental papillae and creates the illusion of pontics emerging from the soft tissue, providing the restoration with a natural-looking effect.
   - Option 2: two central implant restorations plus two lateral pontic restorations (short central papilla result, optimal biomechanical resistance).
   - Option 3: four implant restorations (a short papilla result between the adjacent restorations, normal papilla height adjacent to the teeth – this option is limited to isolated clinical situations) (Figs 6.19a–h).
e. Replacement of four mandibular incisors:
   - Two lateral implant restorations plus two central pontic restorations (predictable esthetic and biomechanical results).
f. Replacement of six anterior teeth – four maxillary incisors and two cuspids:

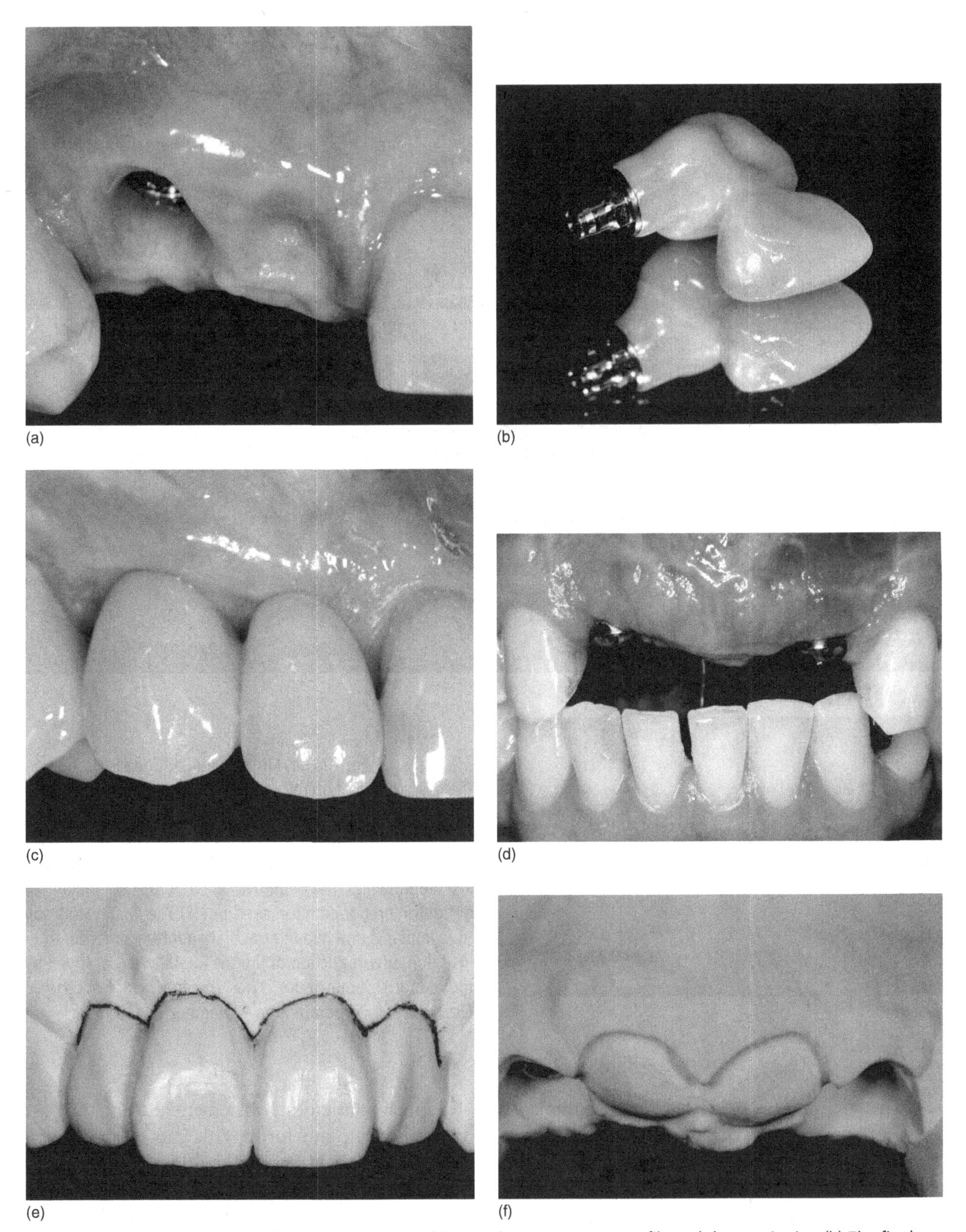

Figure 6.18 (a) An optimal soft tissue contour around the implant emergence profile and the pontic site. (b) The final two-unit restoration, with an implant restoration on the cuspid and a pontic on the lateral. (c) Zirconium restorations in place, with harmonious gingival contours. (Courtesy of Dr. T. Degorce, Tours, France.) (d) The intra-oral situation, with implant healing abutments on the maxillary lateral incisors. (e) The sulcus area marked on the cast model with a pencil prior to removal of the waxing. (f) The scored pontic area after removal of the wax-up and of the healing abutment on the model.

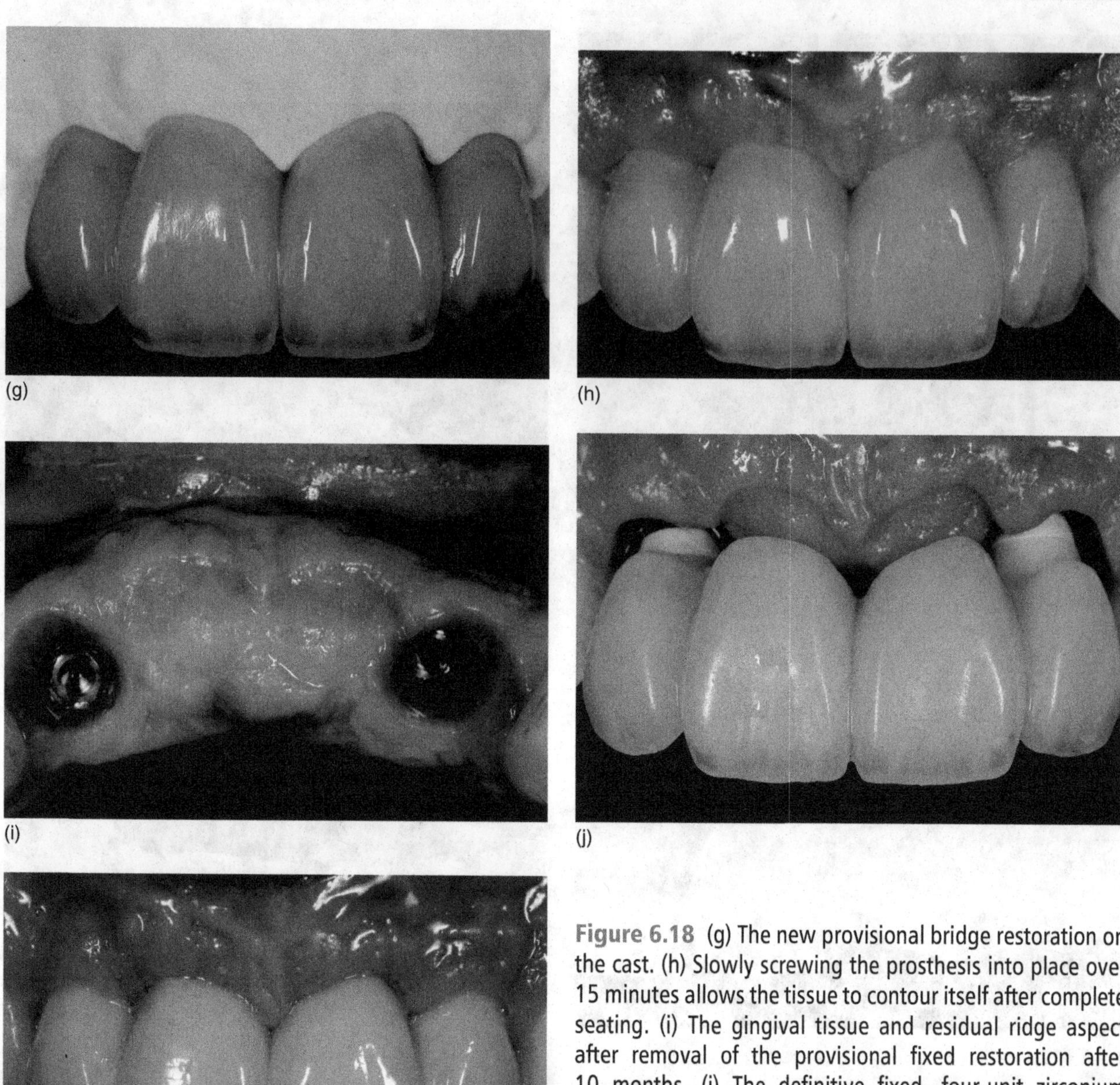

Figure 6.18 (g) The new provisional bridge restoration on the cast. (h) Slowly screwing the prosthesis into place over 15 minutes allows the tissue to contour itself after complete seating. (i) The gingival tissue and residual ridge aspect after removal of the provisional fixed restoration after 10 months. (j) The definitive fixed, four-unit zirconium bridges in preparation for insertion. (k) The final restoration (two implants and two intermediary pontics) 3 months after insertion. (Reproduction of figures (d)–(k) was approved by the Editorial Council for *The Journal of Prosthetic Dentistry*, Incorporated, on November 30, 2011.)

- The best option would be to have two implants on the cuspids to regenerate the papillae from the adjacent bicuspids, two pontics on the lateral to obtain optimal soft tissue control, and two implants on the central incisors to maintain the symmetry.

Proper pontic design is essential to guiding soft tissue healing and form. This can be done using fixed or removable partial dentures. The goal is to create the illusion that the pontic emerges from the tissue as would a natural tooth. Edentulous ridge sites can be modified to enhance the ridge form

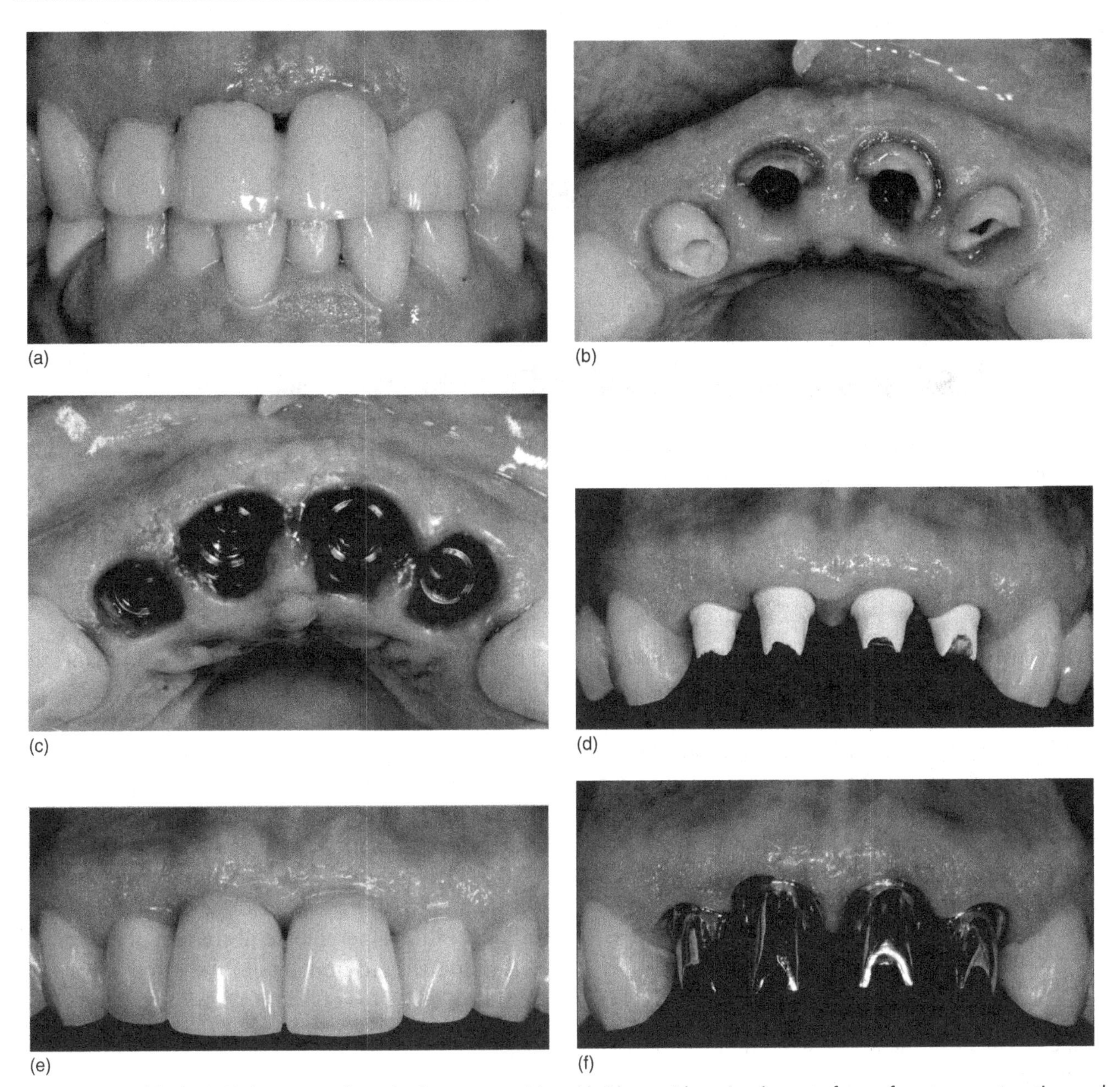

Figure 6.19 (a) The initial presentation of a former transitional bridge, with an inadequate form of contour restoration and an irregular gingival margin. (b) The aspect of the four anterior roots before removal of the bridge. (c) After root removal with limited bony defect, immediate placement of implants in an optimal 3D position (for the laterals, a narrow diameter of 3.25 mm; for the centrals, a regular diameter of 4.1 mm). (d) The clinical aspect of the immediate temporary abutments that were placed after surgery, after 1 month of tissue maturation. (e) Immediate temporary crowns at 1 month, after tissue maturation. (f) Four gold abutments screwed into the implants.

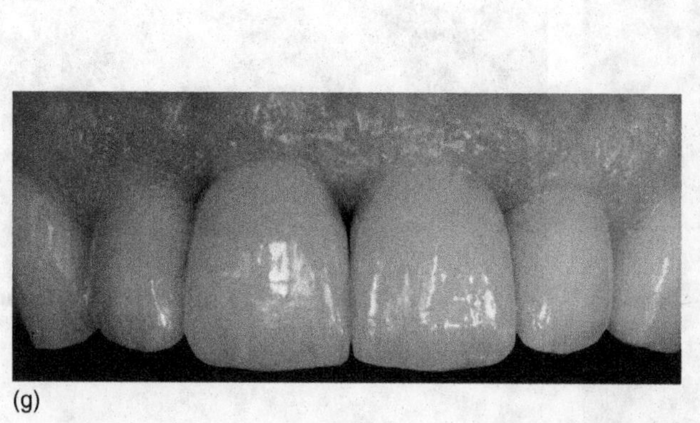
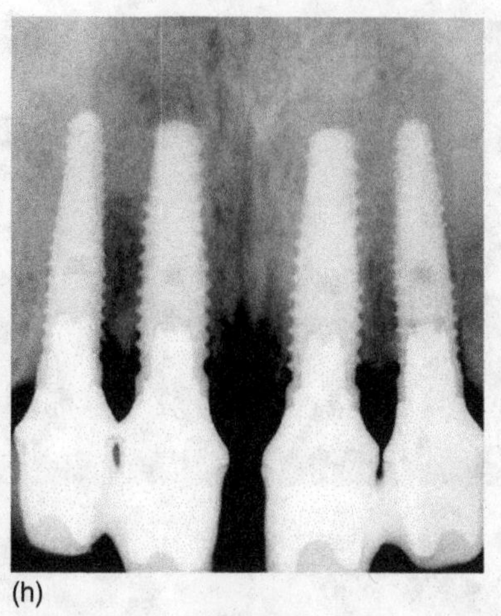

(g) (h)

Figure 6.19 (g) Four ceramic restorations with an optimal soft tissue contour, and with an optimal marginal gingival contour and papilla height, and excellent PES/WES (facial view). (h) Postoperative X-rays showing the excellent interproximal bone peak of the four incisor implant restorations and excellent PES/WES (facial view) at 6 months. (Courtesy of Dr. C. Landsberg, surgeon, Dr. E. Sawdayee, restorative dentist, and Mr. R. Lahav, laboratory technician, Tel Aviv, Israel.)

architecturally, allowing the clinician to convert a flat ridge into a sculpted or anatomical form. But the placement of immediate strategic implants after multiple extractions, with immediate loading (Figs 6.19i–o), can create the appearance of an intimate relationship between the ridge and the overlying pontic (Mitrani *et al.*, 1999).

Such illusions can be achieved through the following surgical and prosthetic steps:

- Soft tissue removal, and if necessary, bone removal, with burs or other resective tools.
- Avoidance of tissue removal or reshaping on the facial aspect of the pontic site. Removal of tissue in this region will compromise the esthetic result and is difficult to repair.
- No tissue removal beyond the depth and palatal aspect of the pontic site.
- Properly designed provisional restorations that allow the clinician to move or push tissue into the desired position. In fact, tissues do not grow; they are simply relocated (Bichacho and Landsberg, 1994).

The influence of the abutment, and of the temporary and final restorations

The implant/abutment connection complex plays an important role in peri-implant tissue stability. The interface between the bone, the implant, the abutment connection, and the gingiva is the most difficult zone to manage and the most important to consider in the esthetic area. In order to preserve and to maintain this interface with a high degree of predictability, it should be considered before placement of the implant (Salama, 2011).

The interactions of the various components in this complex, and their relationship to each other, influence the shape, color, and contour of the critical soft tissue around implants in the esthetic zone. In addition, each type of custom abutment has its own respective influence on the soft tissue (Goldenberg, 2011).

Once the implant is osseointegrated, a variety of prosthetic factors can alter the stability of peri-implant tissues. Prosthetic requirements (such as an ideal position for a prosthetic restoration) and biological imperatives (such as tissue stability) rule all implant treatments. The thickness of the soft tissue should be sufficient around the implant collar, and can be achieved naturally in the thick biotype; but in the thin biotype, this is achieved surgically with a subepithelial connective tissue graft and prosthetically using a platform-switching design or a concave implant abutment (Baumgarten *et al.*, 2005; Gardner, 2005; Lazzara and Porter, 2006; Rompen *et al.*, 2007).

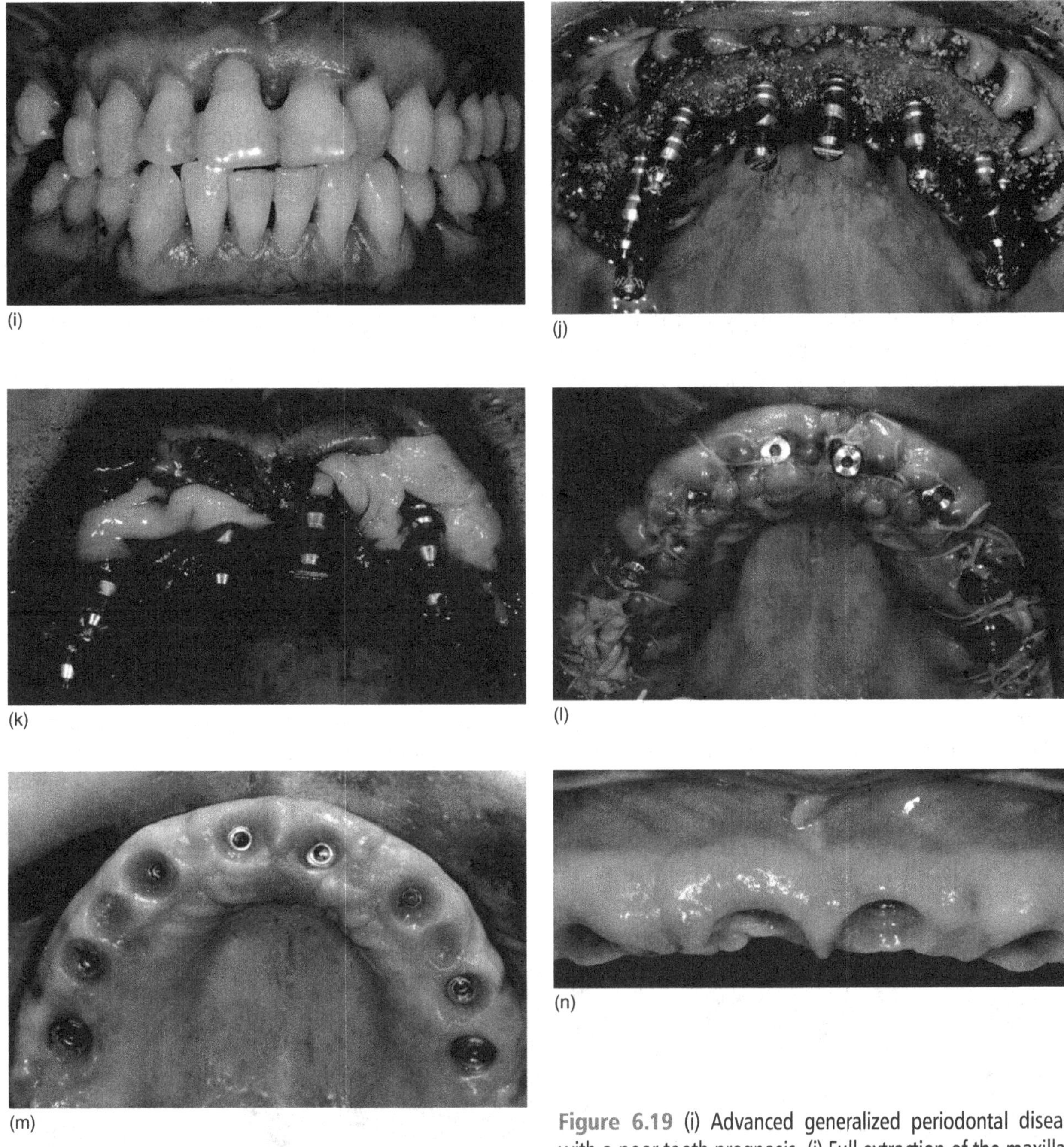

(i) (j) (k) (l) (m) (n)

(o)

Figure 6.19 (i) Advanced generalized periodontal disease with a poor tooth prognosis. (j) Full extraction of the maxillary teeth followed by the immediate placement of eight strategic 3D implants. (k) L-PRF triple-layer membranes covering the xenograft material to remodel the maxillary ridge. (l) Healing of soft tissue at 3 days, showing the healing abutments and accelerated tissue maturation. (m) Healing at 6 months after implant osseointegration, with optimal peri-implant and pontic site soft tissue maturation. (n) The facial clinical aspect after removal of the temporary bridge and implant abutments, showing the harmonious marginal soft tissue contour and papillae. (o) The final full implant maxillary ceramometal bridge restoration 3 years later, with an esthetic marginal contour and papilla height. (Courtesy of Dr. M. Del Corso, Turin, Italy.)

Abutment selection

Changes in abutment design – for example, the use of an abutment that has a concavity in the subgingival region, coupled with platform switching – are made to enhance soft tissue stability and to protect underlying bone.

The provisionalization phase should be done meticulously to build harmony between the teeth/implant restoration and the soft tissue. A more recent provisionalization strategy in the esthetic zone is to place a final abutment at the time of surgery. Newly available, prefabricated zirconium abutments allow the surgeon or restoring dentist to complete any modifications chairside and allow the clinician to place, and torque to 35 N cm, a final zirconia abutment at the time of surgery or following a period of integration (Figs 6.20a, b). Placement of a final abutment at the temporary crown phase encourages the earlier onset of soft tissue maturation and renders any major detachment of the abutment/implant/tissue seal unnecessary when the final restoration phase is undertaken.

The subgingival margin of the modifiable, prefabricated, zirconium abutment positively impacts tissue health due to its superior biocompatibility and its potential to help in positioning the cement line coronally. It also yields a more esthetic result in the gingival margin, because of the white color of the material (Rimondini *et al*., 2002).

The smoother surface of the zirconium compared to machined titanium limits plaque formation and is vital for obtaining a good correlation between the soft tissue and the implant, and an esthetic result (Tetè *et al*., 2009). Rotational load fatigue testing performance on zirconium abutments is dependent on the abutment diameter. According to Nguyen *et al*. (2009), failure modes vary according to the characteristics of the system design.

In general, in the early postsurgical period, the provisional restoration margin is kept in a supragingival position, with subsequent apical positioning following soft tissue integration, maturation, and stability (Figs 6.20c, d).

The crown form or prefabricated shell is relined with acrylic and indexed intra-orally over a prefabricated zirconium abutment, but finished extra-orally. The temporary crown is then cemented onto the abutment at the time of surgery (Leziy and Miller, 2008b).

The zirconium abutment has an optimal biocompatibility and the capacity to to impede the formation of bacterial biofilm. However, it is important not to polish the concave subgingival surface, in order to obtain better epithelial adhesion (Leziy and Miller, 2008b).

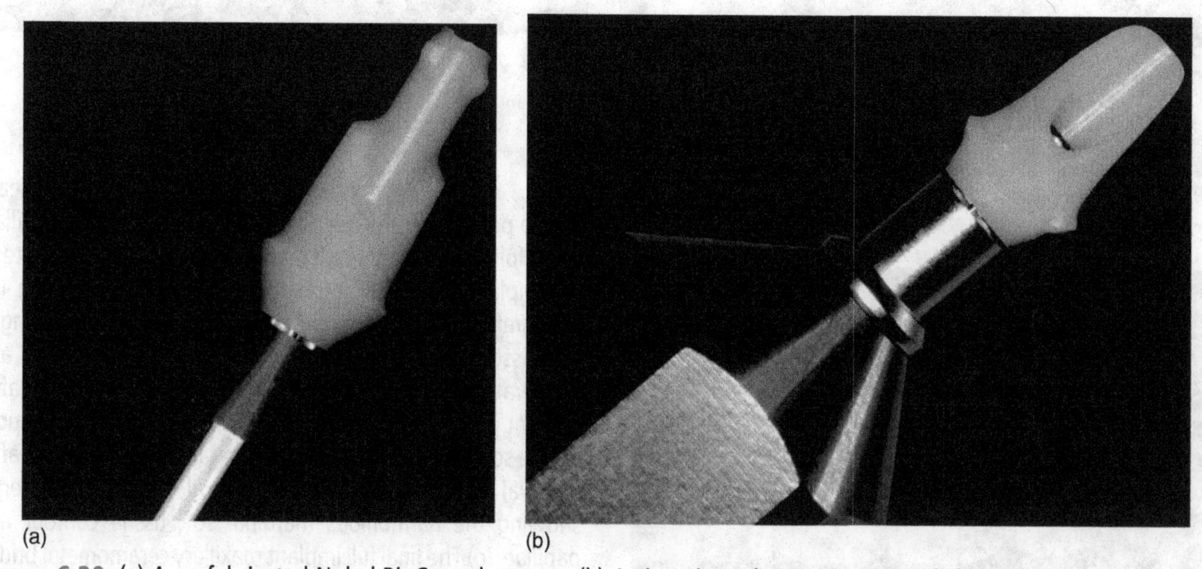

(a) (b)

Figure 6.20 (a) A prefabricated Nobel BioCare abutment. (b) A zirconium abutment prepared chairside.

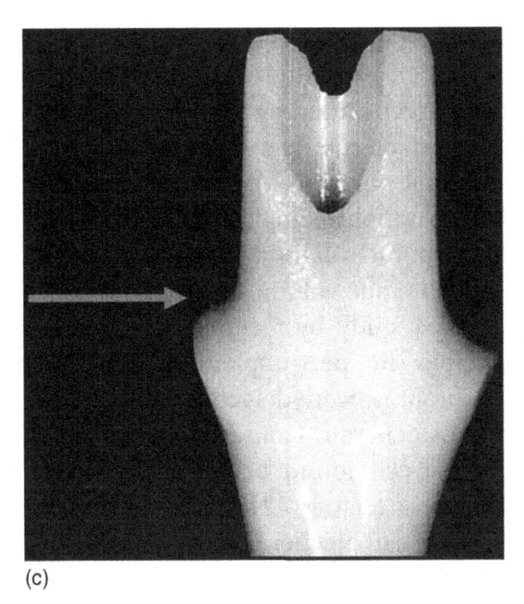
(c)

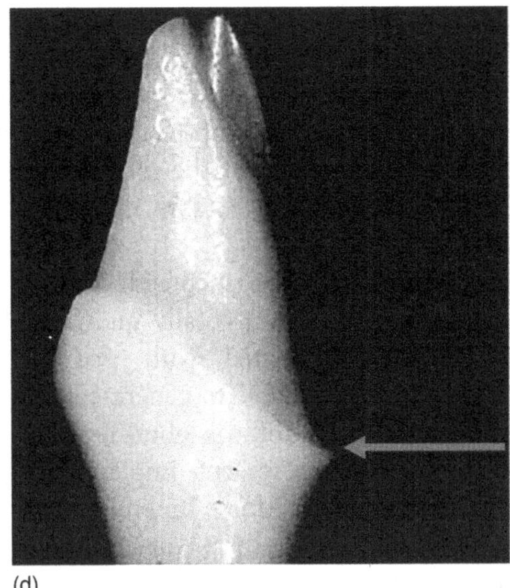
(d)

Figure 6.20 (c) The final abutment before insertion, with a concave submergence profile (frontal view). (d) The final abutment before insertion, with a concave submergence profile (proximal view) and the precise finishing line located below the implant gingival margin.

Connection procedures

Repeated connections and disconnections of healing or implant abutments at different stages of surgery or prosthetic execution are the cause of the trauma of soft tissue attachment, which results in disruption of the bond between the epithelial attachment and the connective tissue, and in bacterial colonization that induces bone resorption, followed, in thin gingival biotypes, by gingival recession (Abrahamsson *et al.*, 1997). Repeated placement and removal of transmucosal components can potentially contribute to increased crestal ridge remodeling and an apical movement of the connective tissue/epithelial complex (Abrahamsson *et al.*, 2003). These subtle bone changes in turn can negatively impact soft tissue stability.

Immediate prosthetic immobilization of the abutment prevents any micromovement or cervical bone resorption, and maintains the horizontal component of the biological width, by thickening the connective tissue and ensuring better isolation of the microgap (Touati *et al.*, 2005).

Avoiding the removal and replacement of prosthetic components would offer significant advantages by enhancing soft tissue stability through diminished crestal ridge remodeling. This would be particularly important in the restoration of adjacent implants, where clinicians are challenged to conserve optimal papilla anatomy in the inter-implant region (Leziy and Miller, 2008a).

Therefore, it is important to reduce or minimize the number of connections and disconnections of the different components by loading the implant abutment at the first stage of surgery whenever possible.

Micromovements of the implant abutment and microgap infiltration

Most two-piece implant systems feature a microgap which allows bacterial infiltration at this level and on the screw connecting the abutment and the implant, inducing peri-implant crestal bone loss (Ericsson *et al.*, 1995).

The inevitable gap between the implant and the abutment seems to play a role in biological adaptation, while the location of the microgap seems to be the determining factor rather than its size: moving the microgap more apically seems to lead to greater bone resorption, even with very well-fitting components.

In addition, it is important that the process of regeneration of the biological width takes place without any disturbance, and without micromovements and micro-leakage in the abutment/implant connection, since this will disrupt the healing process and compromise the long-term result. The rigidity of the connection between the implant and the pillar is a crucial factor. The long-term stability of the marginal bone depends on the mechanical stress generated by the implant, notably around its collar.

The external hexagon, long considered an archetypal connection, does not totally guarantee this stability and is associated with possible prosthetic problems that are liable to generate bone resorption (i.e., unscrewing of the abutment, or fracturing of the screw). Some internal implant connections, which integrate a Morse-tapered cone, seem to not only stabilize the implant/abutment relation, but also seal out bacterial colonization (Norton, 2006).

Zipprich *et al.* (2007) recorded the interface of the implant/abutment connection using a high-speed digital camera and measured it radiographically. The results showed that under simulated clinical conditions, complex mechanisms are responsible for the presence or absence of micromovements. All reversible implant/abutment connections (flat to flat, without self-locking internal joints) exhibit micromovements because of the elastic plastic deformation of the connecting screw between the abutment and the implant (Figs 6.21a, b).

Precision self-locking conical connections (in the presence of a steep cone angle and a precisely fitting abutment) cannot be tilted by an extra-oral force and show no micromovement (Figs 6.21c–e).

The potential clinical relevance of the results of Zipprich *et al.*'s study rests on the fact that the pumping effect caused by the micromovements plays an important role in crestal bone resorption. At the implant platform, the crestal bone is contaminated by a nonphysiological fluid. The extent of bone resorption is delimited by the radius of the contaminated tissue volume (Fig. 6.21f).

In a study by Canullo *et al.* (2011), individual trends in peri-implant bone resorption, after 36 months, were detected and paralleled by immunohistochemical and clinical findings. Correlations have been found between Bi-glycans and tumor necrosis factor (TNF) and bone resorption. The individual biochemical bone pattern (Bi-glycans/TNF-α) seems to affect the dimensions of the peri-implant bone resorption.

The tight conical connection is designed to preserve the crestal bone through the reduction of micromovements, as well as micro-leaks on the implant/pillar interface, and this leads to a better pink esthetic.

To prevent this bacterial phenomenon, in other implant systems the implant/abutment junction has been moved away from the bone toward the center, using an abutment with a diameter smaller than that of a regular implant. Hence there are predictable ways in which the clinician can achieve better soft tissue health around the implant.

The osseous tissue around the neck of the implant is preserved in its entirety. Hence the clinician is able to obtain a natural-looking restoration with a

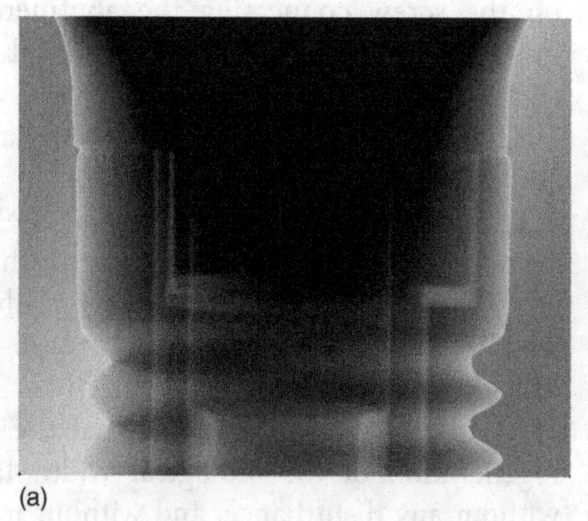

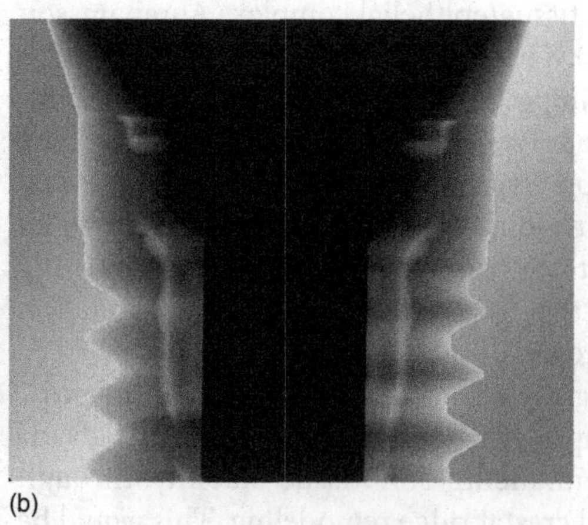

Figure 6.21 (a) NobelReplace™, 4.3 mm: connection without self-locking, and a flat-to-flat interface with a polygon. The binding screw is coated and has an initial torque of 35 N cm. (b) Biomet Certain®, 4 mm: connection without self-locking, and a flat-to-flat interface with a hexagon. The binding screw is of gold platinum alloy with an initial torque of 20 N cm.

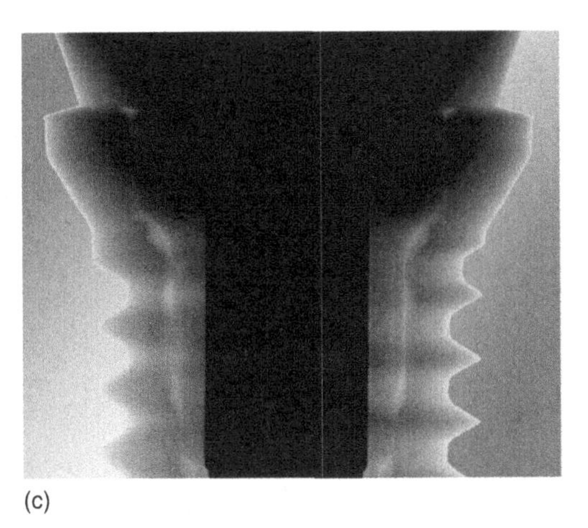
(c)

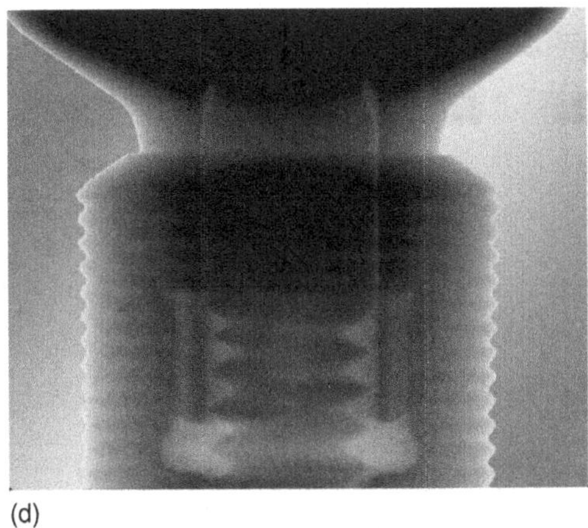
(d)

Figure 6.21 (c) Biomet 3i Certain® Prevail®, 4–4.5 mm: connection without self-locking. Platform-switching, internal flat-to-flat interface with a hexagon. The binding screw is of gold–platinum alloy, with an initial torque of 20 N cm. (d) Astra Tech®, 4 mm: self-locking connection and a conical interface with a cone angle of 11°. The initial torque for the binding screw is 20 N cm. (e) Ankylos®, 4.5 mm: self-locking connection and a conical interface with a cone angle of 5.71°. The initial torque for the binding screw is 15 N cm.

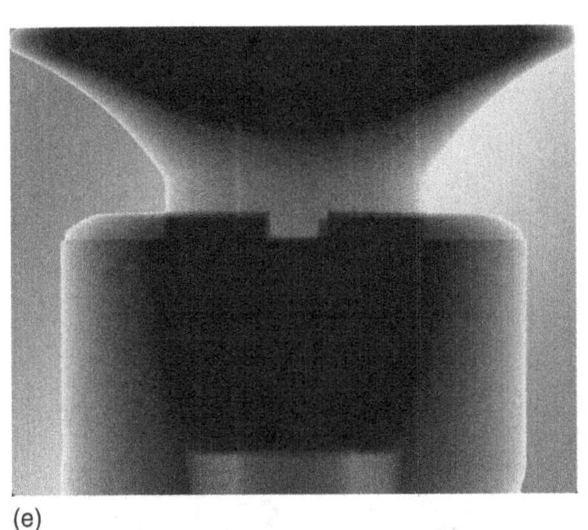
(e)

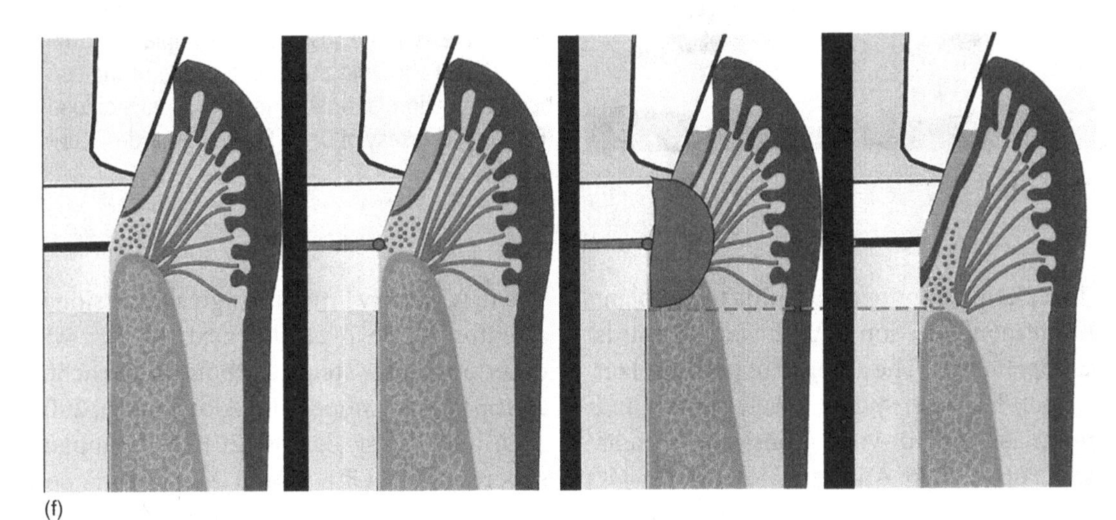
(f)

Figure 6.21 (f) The implant/abutment microgap with a pumping effect in the presence of micromovement. (Figures (a) to (f) courtesy of Mr. H. Zipprich and colleagues, Germany.)

healthy soft tissue architecture, thus obviating the need for the patient to undergo grafting procedures (Pozzi, 2011).

Switch platform concept

The smaller diameter of the prosthetic abutment compared with a wider implant platform is called the "switch platform," and will result in a smaller abutment compared to the diameter of the implant. This concept, known as "platform switching," results in an implant/abutment connection that is further away from the edge of the implant; this limits the resorptive influence of micromovements and inflammatory infiltration.

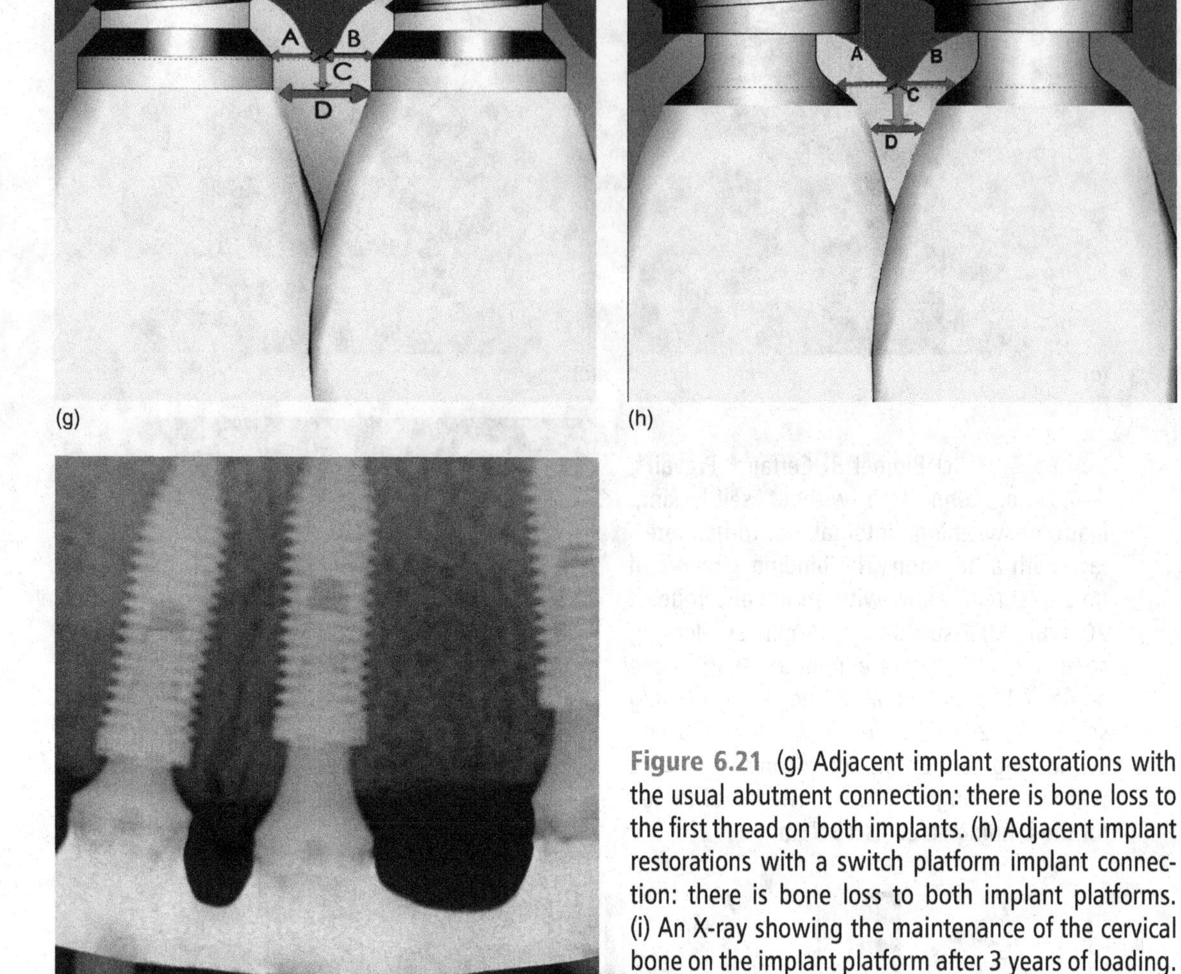

Figure 6.21 (g) Adjacent implant restorations with the usual abutment connection: there is bone loss to the first thread on both implants. (h) Adjacent implant restorations with a switch platform implant connection: there is bone loss to both implant platforms. (i) An X-ray showing the maintenance of the cervical bone on the implant platform after 3 years of loading. (Figure (i) courtesy of Dr. S. Rocha Bernardes, Curitiba, Brazil.)

The switch platform connection shifts the implant perimeter/abutment junction (IAJ) inward, towards the central implant axis. The absence of peri-implant bone resorption has been systematically proven and the technique seems to yield consistent results (Lazzara and Porter, 2006; Atieh *et al.*, 2010).

Therefore, among implantologists, there is an evolving consensus that appears to favor an internal Morse-tapered cone used in conjunction with platform switching, which seems to be a judicious choice in order to limit peri-implant crestal bone resorption and to preserve sustainable, soft tissue esthetic results (Figs 6.21 g–i).

Further research on the Morse-tapered cone connection has uniformly shown that peri-implant marginal bone resorption reaches 0.4 mm after 1 year, with very limited gingival recession, and then remains stable over the next 4 years, whereas in other implant systems the bone loss reaches 1.5 mm after 5 years (Cooper and Albrektsson, 2008).

In a study by Barros (2010), an implant placed subcrestally (SCL), with a Morse cone connection on adjacent implants, restored immediately using the platform-shifting protocol and with a distance of 3 mm between the contact point and the crestal bone tip, yielded lower indices of crestal bone resorption when compared with implants placed equicrestally (ECL).

The peak of crestal bone found between implants placed subcrestally could positively influence the treatment of esthetic areas. When using a switch platform, inter-implant distances of 2 and 3 mm did

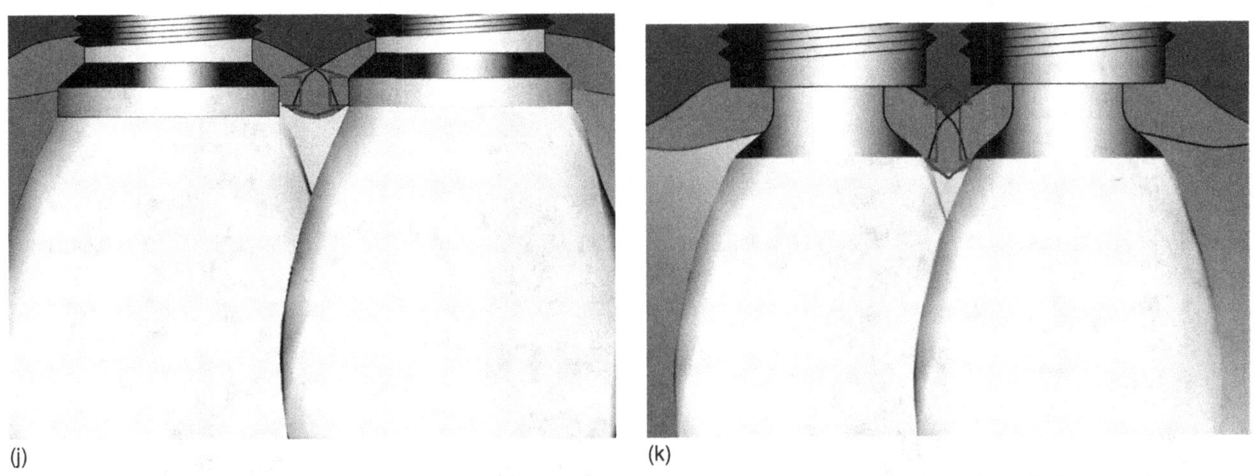

(j) (k)

Figure 6.21 (j) The decreased inter-implant distance with the usual abutment connection: there is increased bone loss beyond the first thread. (k) The decreased inter-implant distance with the switch platform/implant connection: there is limited bone loss at the platform. (Figures (g)–(k) courtesy of Dr. A. Pinto, Paris, France.)

not significantly affect the crestal bone resorption or any other parameter that was evaluated (Figs 6.21j, k).

The results of a bacterial study by Canullo *et al.* (2010) reveal similar histological characteristics at 4 years: they reported the extent of the inflamed connective tissue, the microvascular density and the collagen content of peri-implant soft tissue biopsies taken from implants restored with a platform-matched or a platform-switched interface.

Canullo *et al.* (2010) suggest that the difference in bone crest resorption between implants restored with platform switching compared to traditionally restored implants is not associated with differences in the peri-implant microbiota. The data could not support the hypothesis that the difference in bone crest resorption between implants restored with platform switching compared to a traditional approach was associated with a different composition of the peri-implant biofilm. Consequently, bone crest resorption is not considered to be influenced by the submucosal implant microbiota.

In addition, a recent biomechanical analysis by Schroetenboer *et al.* (2008) demonstrated a shift of the stress concentration area away from the cervical bone/implant interface when smaller-diameter implant abutments were used. When the concept of platform switching was applied by decreasing the abutment diameter, less stress was translated to the crestal bone in the microthread and smooth-neck groups. Platform switching reduced stress to a greater degree in the microthread model compared to the smooth-neck model.

Therefore, moving the microgap inward to shift the implant/abutment junction, effectively switching the morphology of the platform, potentially reduces crestal bone loss, preserves implant bone levels and, therefore, maintains the peri-implant soft tissue level and prevents soft tissue recession. Implants restored with matching wide-diameter prosthetic components show a more statistically significant difference in marginal bone loss than implants restored with platform-switched ones.

In a recent study (Canullo *et al.*, 2010), after a follow-up period of 33 months with an implant abutment that was 3.8 mm in diameter and different increasing implant diameters (Figs 6.22a, b), the mean marginal bone losses were as follows:

- 1.48±0.42 mm for the control group – implant Ø3.8 mm (no switch platform)
- 0.99±0.42 mm for test group 1 – implant Ø4.3 mm
- 0.87±0.43 mm for test group 2 – implant Ø4.8 mm
- 0.64±0.32 mm for test group 3 – implant Ø5.5 mm

The marginal bone loss in the test and control groups ranged from 0.5 to 0.99 mm and 0.19 to 1.67 mm, respectively. The findings of the study suggested the following:

- The extent of the inward shifting was inversely proportional to the amount of marginal bone loss. The marginal bone loss decreased from

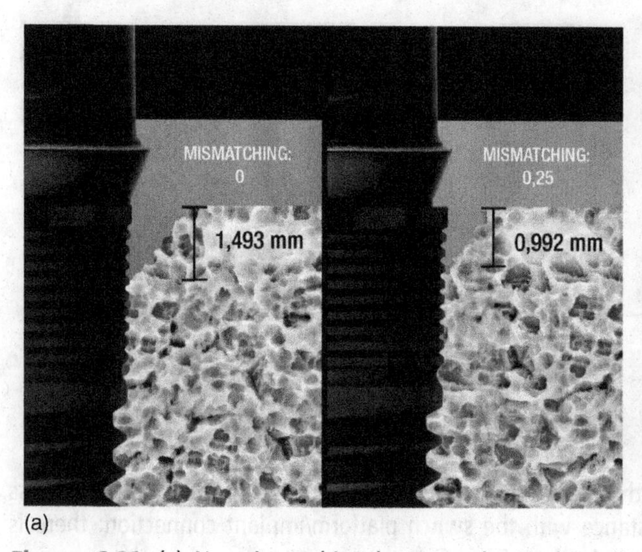

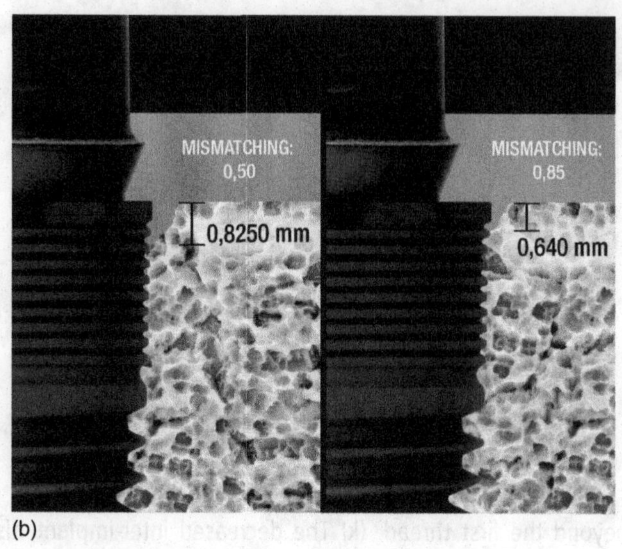

(a) (b)

Figure 6.22 (a) No mismatching between the implant diameter and the abutment, with a bone loss of 1.5 mm; and mismatching of 0.25 mm, with a bone loss of around 1 mm. (b) Mismatching of 0.5 mm and 0.85 mm between the implant diameter and the abutment: with bone losses of around 0.82 mm and 0.65 mm, respectively. (Images of global dental implant reproduced with permission from Canullo *et al*., 2010.)

1.5 mm in the control group, with no mismatching, to 0.65 mm in the test group, with mismatching of 0.85 mm (the implant diameter of 5.5 mm minus the abutment diameter of 3.8 mm equals 1.7 mm which, divided by 2, equals 0.85 mm).

- The meta-analysis concluded that marginal bone loss around the platform-switched (PS) implants was significantly less than around platform-matched (PM) implants.
- The marginal bone level alterations could be related to the extent of the implant/abutment mismatching.
- The marginal bone levels were better maintained at implants restored using the platform-switching concept.
- The degree of marginal bone loss resorption is inversely related to the extent of the implant/abutment mismatching.

The results reveal that the inward shift of the IAJ platform switching can be considered a desirable morphological feature that may prevent horizontal saucerization and preserve vertical crestal bone levels (Figs 6.22c, d). In terms of failure rates, implants with or without platform switching performed similarly (Canullo *et al*., 2010). This concept not only reduces the risk of peri-implantitis in the future, but also has the benefit in the esthetic zone of providing better soft tissue support (Cappiello *et al*., 2008).

Tabata *et al*. (2011) found that platform switching led to an improved biomechanical stress distribution in peri-implant bone tissue. Oblique loads resulted in higher stress concentration than axial loads for all models. The wide-diameter implant had a large influence in reducing stress values in the implant systems.

The early events leading to the establishment of the biological width and the soft tissue characteristics could differ between platform-matched and platform-switched implants, which could explain the favorable marginal change in the bone level around platform-switched implants, compared to platform-matched implants.

In a study by Estafanous *et al*. (2011), the horizontal offset of platform switching had two results:

- It increased the surface area to which the soft tissue could become attached. Therefore, the crestal resorption needed to establish a biological width was decreased in comparison to the matched implant and abutment diameters.
- It increased the distance between the implant/abutment junction and the adjacent bone, which, in turn, limited the resorption effect of the

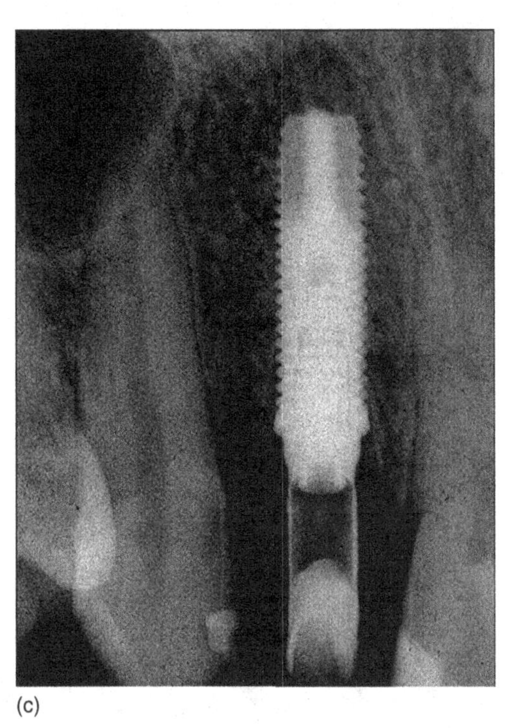

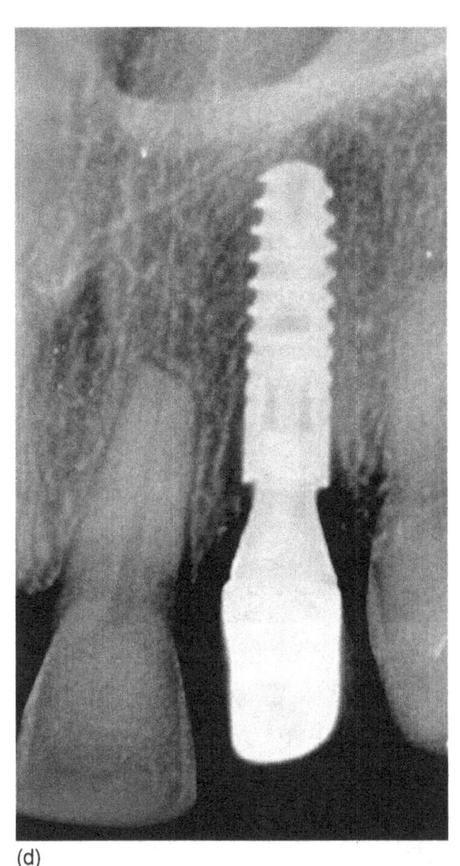

(c) (d)

Figure 6.22 (c) The Biomet Prevail® switch platform implant with an abutment: there is no significant bone loss. (d) The Ankylos® implant with the switch platform abutment: bone on the platform.

implant/abutment junction, associated with the inflammatory cell infiltrate.

Once the biological width was established, the differences in the soft tissue characteristics were no longer noticeable (Canullo *et al.*, 2011).

Platform switching presents several advantages:

- the supracrestal fibers are above the bone
- the implant/abutment interface is located away from the bone
- has an effect on the inter-implant distance and on the inter-implant bone crest height
- it increases the horizontal component of the biological width
- it induces maintenance of the horizontal and vertical height of the mesiodistal papilla
- it decreases cervical bone resorption to the usual minimum amount of bone loss as far as the first thread of the implant.

Most authors today agree that the reduced circumferential bone loss achieved with platform switching preserves soft tissue levels (Figs 6.23a–i), which may lead to more predictable esthetic results (Landolt and Blatz, 2008; Vigolo and Givani, 2009; Atieh *et al.*, 2010; Cocchetto *et al.*, 2010; Huynh-Ba *et al.*, 2010).

The esthetics and stability of the marginal peri-implant mucosa are essential. This vertical stability guarantees better preservation of the crestal bone and gingival margin toward which a biological space of 3–4 mm will regenerate. The 3D volume of this mucosal barrier – and in particular the connective tissue – plays a primary role in the protection of the crestal bone and in the prevention of bone resorption and/or marginal recession.

Prosthetic abutment profile

To retain the soft and hard tissues around the implant abutment, the transmucosal connection of the implant abutment design should be narrow, concave, and not oversized or divergent. This profile induces a thicker, more stable, and tighter peri-implant mucosa (Rompen *et al.*, 2007). Two

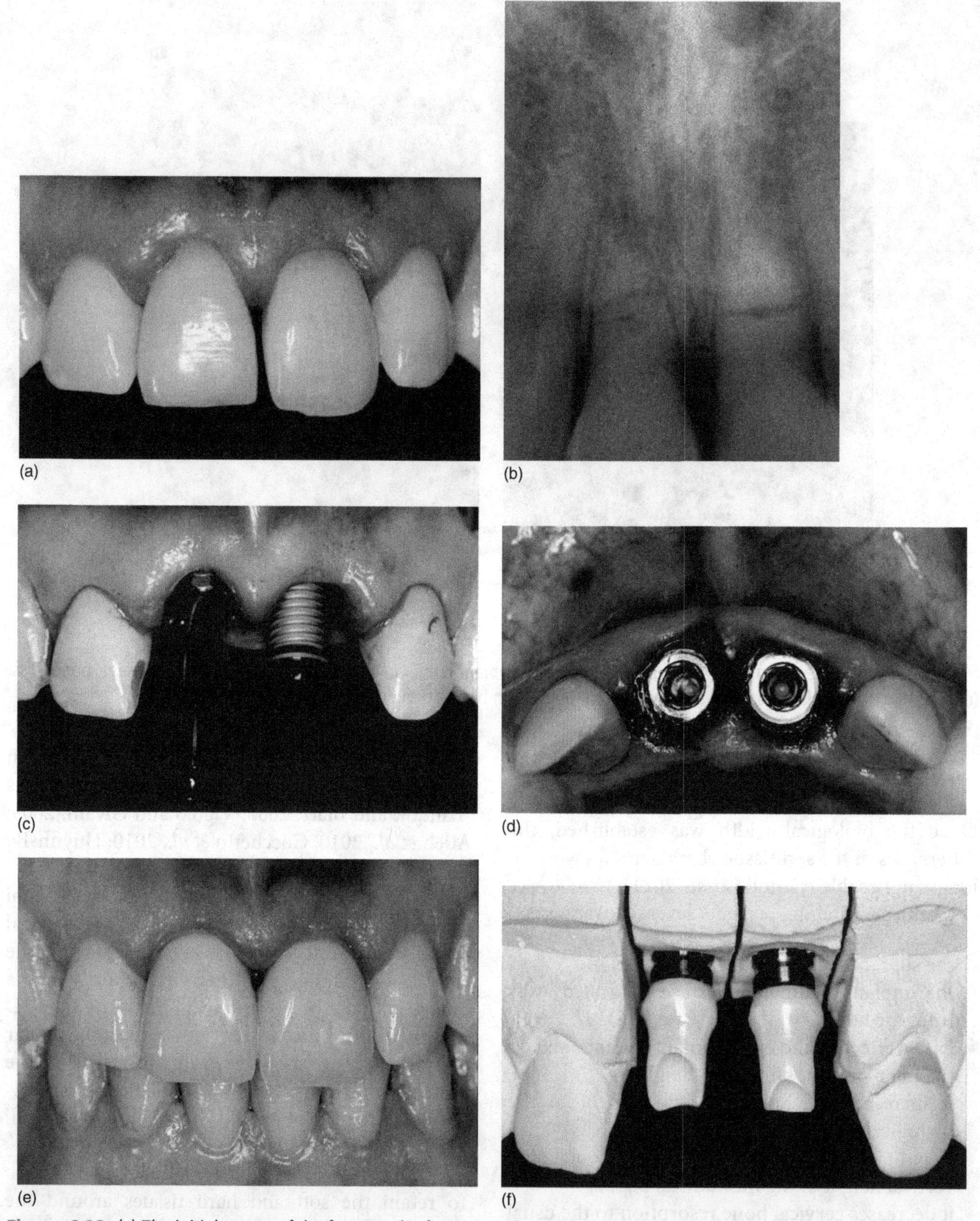

Figure 6.23 (a) The initial aspect of the front teeth after an accident. (b) An X-ray showing the mid-root fracture of the two central incisors. (c) Insertion of the left Biomet Prevail® implant, guided by the right orientation pin. (d) The two implants are placed slightly palatally and a bone graft is plugged into the buccal gap. (e) The immediate temporary bridge, without any functional contact. An X-ray is taken to check that the implant is correctly positioned and that the abutment fits perfectly. (f) The frontal view of the zirconium abutment on the model cast.

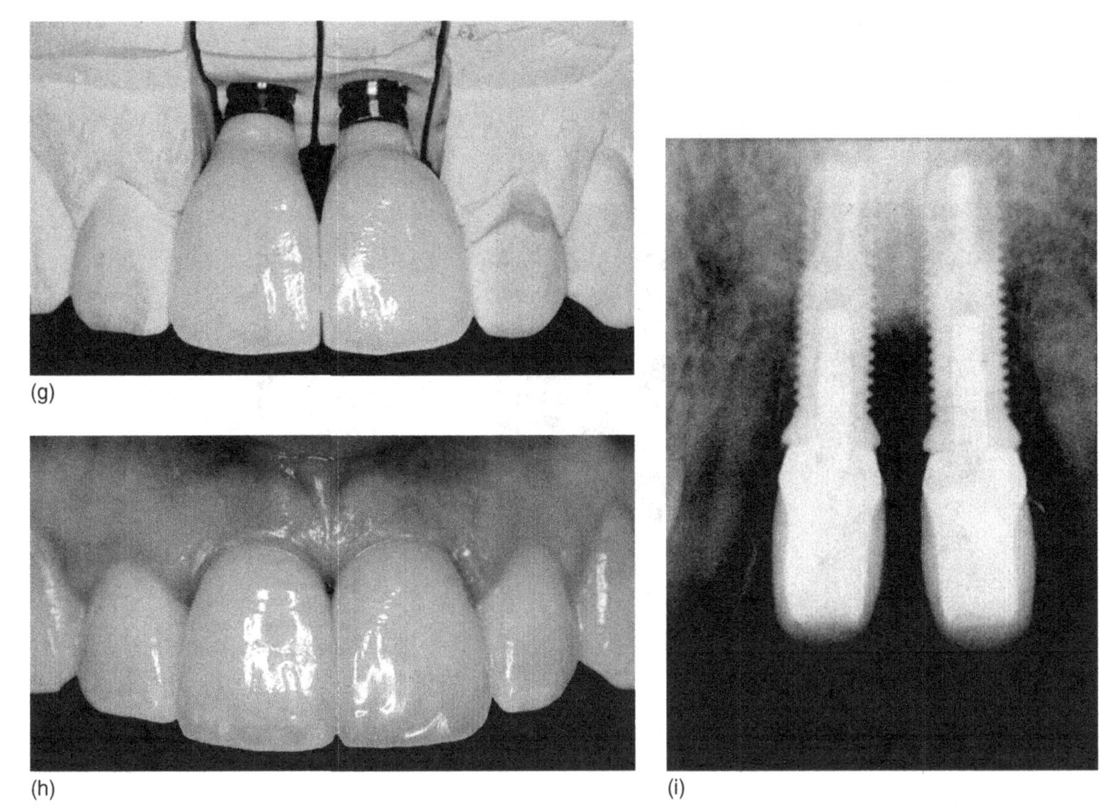

Figure 6.23 (g) The flat emergence profile of the two ceramic crown units fitted into the abutments. (h) The final restorations, with a harmonious gingival contour, correct papillae on the distal sides adjacent to the teeth, and a high papilla between the two central incisors. (i) An X-ray of the restoration 1 year later, showing that the bone has remained at the switch platform level. (Courtesy of Dr. F. Chiche, Paris, France.)

Table 6.2 Conventional and curvy abutment design

Conventional abutment design	Curvy abutment design
Buccal marginal recession: • in 80% of cases • 0.5–1.5 mm • vertical gain 0%	Buccal marginal recession: • in 5% of cases • always less than 0.5 mm • vertical stability in 25% of cases • vertical gain in 70% of cases

prosthetic abutment architectures contribute to the thickness of the peri-implant tissue: the platform switching concept and the concave curvy abutment.

These two abutments increase the volume of connective tissue, the former by inwardly displacing the cervical limit of the abutment in comparison to the platform (Lazzara and Porter, 1988), while the latter has a concave transmucosal profile (Rompen *et al.*, 2003).

The smaller diameter of the supracrestal prosthetic abutment compared with the implant platform, called the switch platform and the concave curvy abutment, allows for the possibility of changing the vertical biological space into a horizontal and a vertical component, maintaining the same total biological dimensions. This profile induces a thicker, more stable, and tighter peri-implant mucosa (Rompen *et al.*, 2007).

In a comparative study between conventional abutment design and curvy abutment design (see Fig. 6.9 g and Table 6.2; see also Figs 6.24a, b), a significant difference was found between

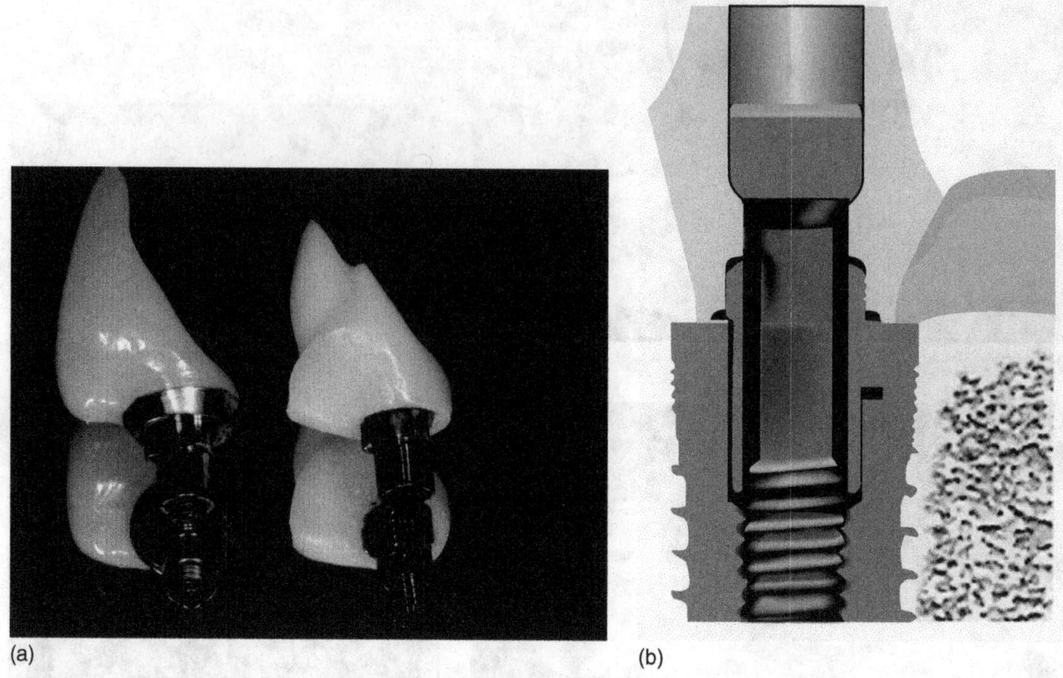

Figure 6.24 (a) Subgingival concave design and supragingival convex design of the temporary and final restorations. (b) The built-in platform shifting will improve the soft tissue thickness and volume to provide natural-looking esthetics.

the vertical amounts of gingival recession (Touati *et al.*, 2008).

When the connection increases the seal between the implant and the abutment (as with the Morse cone), the result is a thicker gingival mucosa with less inflammatory infiltration and less micromovement, which plays a protective role for the peri-implant crestal bone and gingival margin levels.

Provisional and final restoration

Preparation of an implant site with adequate soft and hard tissue support, combined with proper positioning of a smaller or concave abutment on the implant restorative platform, enhances the potential for a successful esthetic restoration (Figs 6.25a–j).

Provisionalization is definitely the most important step in promoting an optimal tissue form around implants. The provisional implant restoration plays an essential role in the anterior sector in the preservation or the shaping and formation of peri-implant tissues and in its biological dynamism. Developing the tissue form using interim restorations provides distinct advantages for the restorative dentist, technician, and patient. Whether it is started prior to implant placement (ridge preservation), in immediate implant placement and restoration, or in delayed implant placement with or without loading protocols, provisionalization ultimately defines the final final peri-implant soft tissue contour.

The esthetics of maxillary anterior crowns on single natural teeth is one of the most difficult challenges in restorative dentistry. The challenge of fabricating a crown on an implant abutment is even greater. The implant diameter and cross-section rarely match the anatomy of the root of an anterior tooth. Consequently, the esthetics of a single implant crown in the cervical zone needs to accommodate an implant with a circular cross-section, while balancing the biological and esthetic parameters. A dilemma is faced when developing the restoration form from the circular shape normally found at the platform of an implant to the full contours to replicate the shape of a natural tooth crown around the cemento-enamel junction level. To a certain extent, the diameter of the placed implants is influenced by the available volume of labial bone and the interproximal distance (Van Dooren, 2000).

For any implant restoration in the anterior area, the temporary crown phase is an important prerequisite. A screwed temporary crown allows an adequate emergence profile to be realized and provides

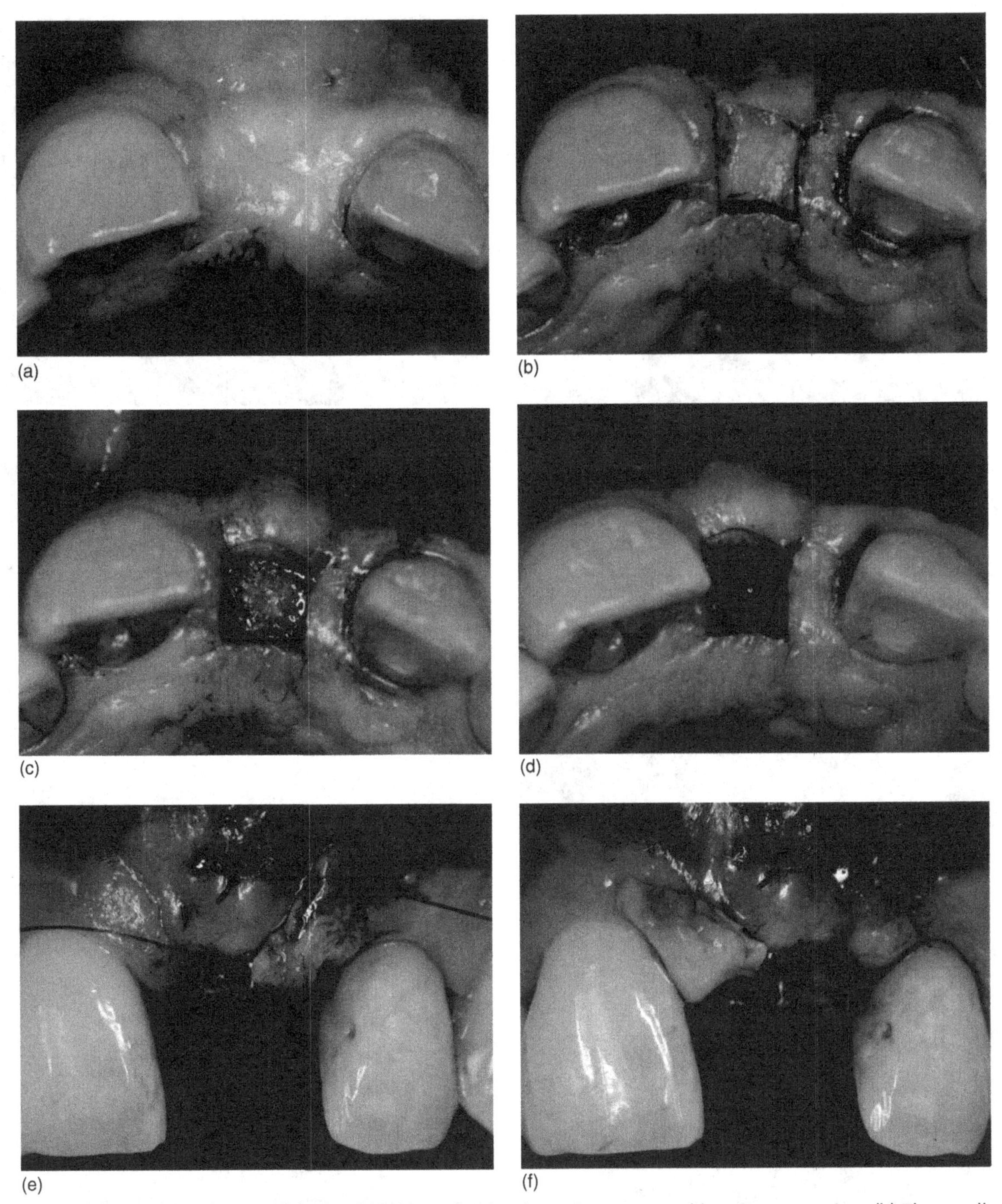

Figure 6.25 (a) An occlusal view of the healed ridge after implant placement and bone regeneration. (b) The small palatal pedicle flap is designed to preserve the adjacent papillae. (c) After removal of the epithelium, the palatal pedicle is rolled and sutured inside the buccal pouch. (d) Implant exposition, showing the placement in the correct 3D position. (e) A connective tissue graft from the tuberosity is presented on the distal site. (f) then inserted and sutured into the distal buccal pouch, another piece of connective tissue graft is then inserted and sutured into the mesial buccal pouch.

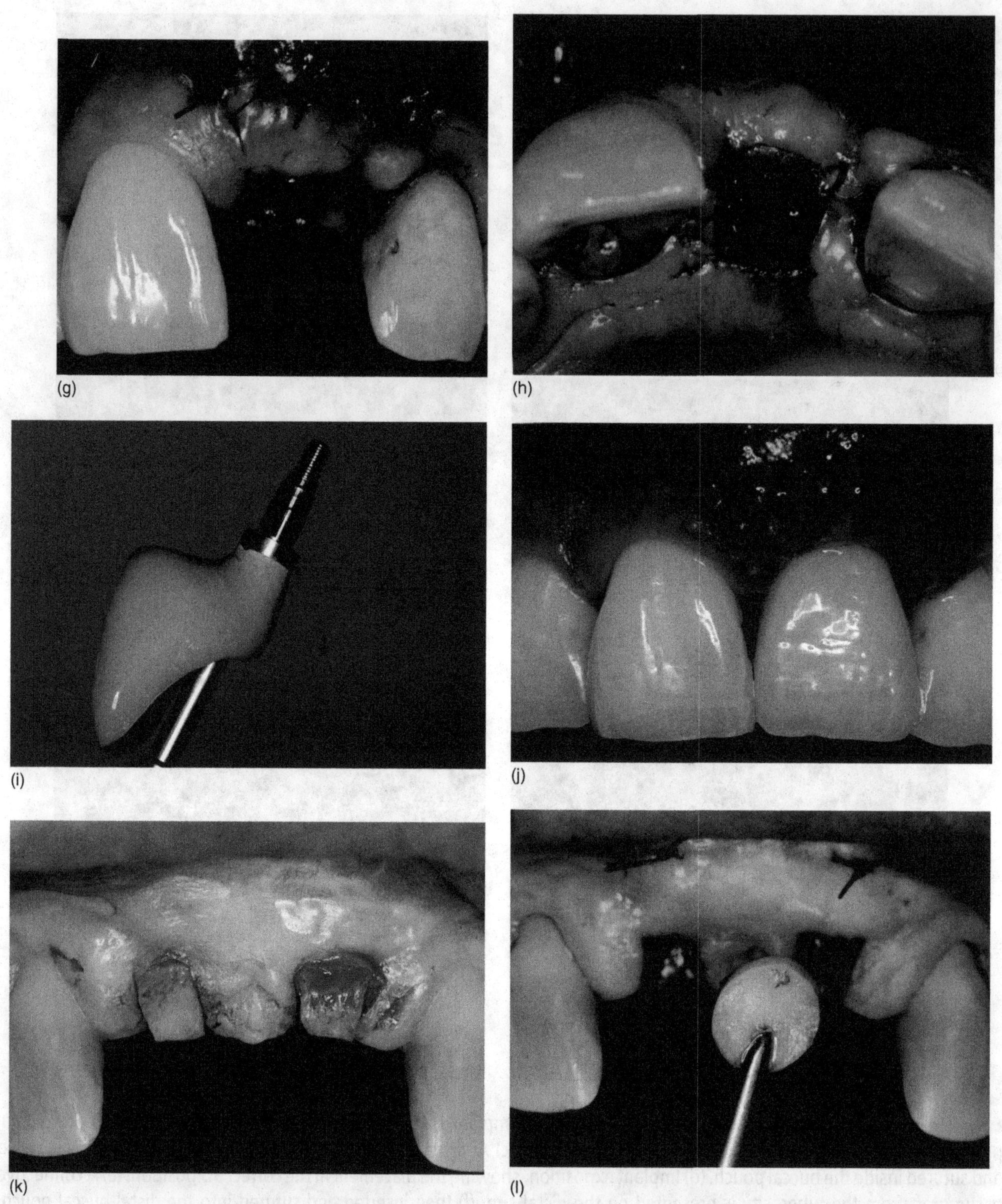

Figure 6.25 (g) A buccal view of the convex soft tissue contour after a combined palatal pedicle flap and the mesiodistal CTG. (h) An occlusal view of the soft tissue contour after the combined palatal pedicle flap and the mesiodistal connective tissue graft. (i) A concave temporary crown about to be screwed into the implant. (j) The temporary crown in place, with a harmonious gingival and proximal contour, after 2 weeks' healing. (k) After the placement of two central incisors implants, and bone regeneration that has been carried out previously, the double palatal pedicle flaps on the healed ridge are designed to preserve the central interdental incisor papilla. The pedicle flaps are then sutured buccally (l) and a tuberosity CTG is then plugged and sutured under the central incisor interdental papilla pouch

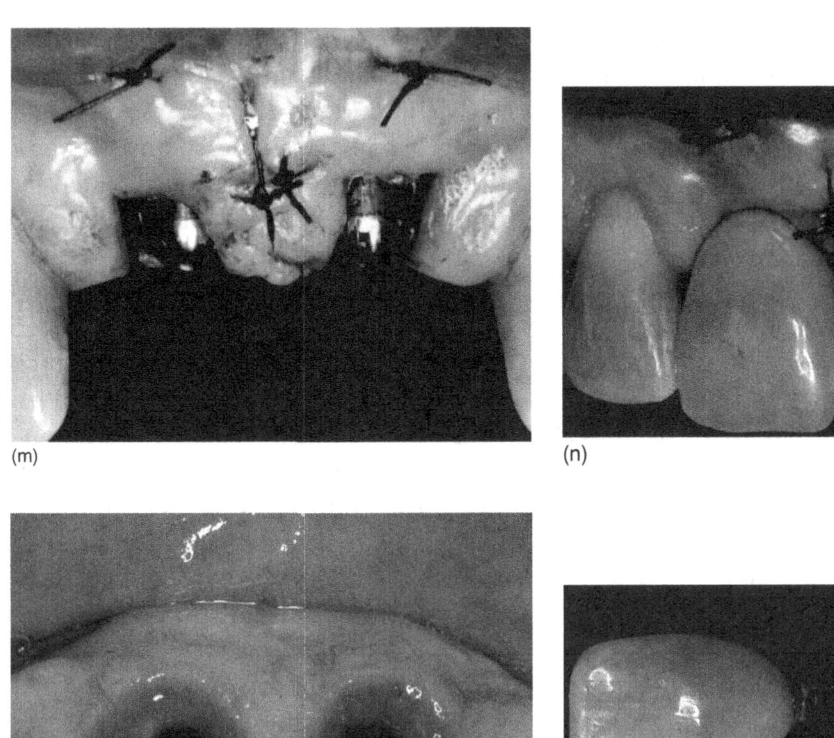

(m) (n)

(o) (p)

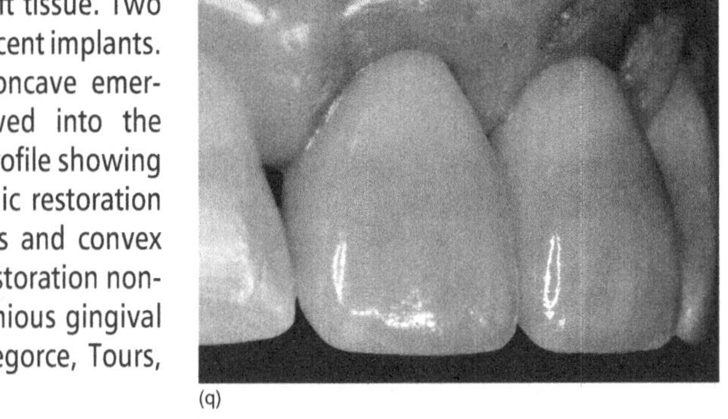

(q)

Figure 6.25 (m), to raise and thicken the soft tissue. Two healing abutments are then placed on the adjacent implants. (n) Two temporary acrylic crowns with a concave emergence profile are then immediately screwed into the implant. (o) Occlusal view of the emergence profile showing thick peri-implant soft tissue. (p) Final ceramic restoration with particular concave submergence profiles and convex supragingival profiles. (q) The final ceramic restoration non-splinted in place 3 months later, with harmonious gingival and proximal contours. (Courtesy of Dr. T. Degorce, Tours, France.)

for a better connection of the final abutment. The optimal implant position gives the clinician and laboratory technician a sufficient buccal surface for the 3 mm emergence profile, in order to leave 0.8 mm of thickness for the abutment, to prevent any risk of fracture (Leziy and Miller, 2008a).

The optimal soft tissue integration in implant restorations is influenced by two interfaces, between:

- the implant collar and the bone, and
- the abutment and the soft tissue.

Consequently, a large increase in diameter from the fixture head to the crown needs to be accommodated by the abutment and the overlying crown (Van Dooren, 2000). In comparison to natural teeth, peri-implant tissues have a reduced capacity to withstand manipulation during retraction and such procedures are often significantly traumatic for the peri-implant mucosa.

Laceration of the sulcular epithelium during the taking of impressions may cause breakdown and ulceration, with delayed healing, loss of attachment, and a significant risk of permanent recession (Bennani and Vaudoin, 2000). Therefore, any manipulation of the peri-implant soft tissue should be done as delicately as possible.

A NobelProcera™ restoration should have a concave submergence profile to decrease the buccal marginal pressure, with a convex facial profile at 3 mm. This will maintain the tonicity and contour of the marginal gingiva.

Consequently, the provisional restoration serves the primary purpose of maximizing the volume of the surrounding soft tissue both facially and coronally (the flatter or more concave the emergence profile, the more the buccal gingiva will move coronally, and the greater the interproximal convexity may be, which will compress the papilla, stimulating it to shift coronally). Convex proximal surfaces will increase the papilla height (Bichacho and Lansberg, 1994). Subsequent precise movement of the gingival margin will be obtained, maintained, and stabilized before the definitive implant or ceramic restoration is used (Figs 6.25k–q).

The histological specificity of the peri-implant soft tissue could enable the practitioner to re-develop the optimal gingival contour and thickness, and the reformation of the interproximal papillae, by working carefully for a few weeks or months on the temporary crown, either indirectly, on the emergence profile of the cast, or directly on the patient.

A concave submergence profile for the final abutment and a ceramic restoration with a natural convexity at the cemento-enamel junction level, especially in the thin biotype, will reinforce the thickness of the peri-implant gingival margin, maintain the gingival tonicity, and contribute to a harmonious gingival level with the adjacent teeth.

In a thick biotype, a concave submergence profile is realized on the abutment and a flat submergence profile is achieved on the ceramic restoration, to ensure gingival tonicity.

Provisionalization is even more critical when the implant-supported restoration involves a pontic site (see the section on "The connective tissue graft and pontics").

It is important that the restorative dentist and dental technician understand that the outline of the facial gingival margin is dictated by the location of the cemento-enamel junction relative to the root surface, and specifically that the convexity or concavity of the outline of the cemento-enamel junction will ultimately determine the gingival frame. A maxillary central incisor tooth, for instance, reveals the facial–distal prominence near the cemento-enamel junction. In the presence of adequate soft tissue, duplication of this convex outline in the definitive crown moves the facial gingiva into a position that emulates the gingival zenith in the natural dentition. To facilitate this goal, the cemento-enamel junction convexity of the provisional restoration is placed more incisally than the desired final gingival margin. The facial contour of the provisional crown is adjusted to promote coronal migration of the soft tissue by increasing the root subgingival concavity apical to the cemento-enamel junction. By modifying the position of the proximal contact points proximal to the crown, and by increasing the length of the contact areas, the height of the interdental papillae can be positively influenced (Blatz *et al.*, 1999).

Deliberate control of crown contours and the line angles helps to complete the illusion by shaping the gingival interdental papillae and mimicking the immaculate design of natural teeth (Prato *et al.*, 2004). Six weeks to 3 months later, the facial soft tissue will migrate into a more coronal position (Kinsel and Capoferri, 2008).

In conclusion, it is necessary to create an optimal emergence profile using the temporary crown and to wait for a minimum of 3–6 months to obtain maturation and stability of the soft tissue before taking the final impression and making the final restoration (Small and Tarnow, 2000). The result of these carefully orchestrated and often subtle alterations of the temporary crown in an implant-supported permanent crown should always be in visual harmony with the surrounding dentition. The refinement of the soft tissue architecture by careful provisionalization is a crucial step that simplifies the ultimate restorative phase (see Figs 6.11l–t).

A variation on the conventional methods, immediate provisionalization, or placement of a temporary crown at the time of implant placement, refines the soft tissue emergence profile at an early stage by judicious contouring of the provisional restoration rather than by defining the position of the final free gingival margin (Bashutski and Wang, 2008).

Finally, the definitive restoration is typically delivered following a 4–6 month provisionalization phase. In a study by Kinsel and Capoferri (2008), the successful restoration of the missing single central incisor was a compilation of the implant team's collaborative skills.

As for the cement line and preparation, it should be ideally kept flush with the level of the soft tissue margin at surgery, but it may later be extended to lie 0.5–1.0 mm subgingivally following implant integration (Leziy and Miller, 2008a). Coronal movement of the finishing line preparation facilitates the cementation process and avoids cement entrapment (Agar *et al.*, 1997).

In a study by Wilson (2009), excess dental cement was associated with signs of peri-implant disease in the majority (81%) of cases. Clinical and endoscopic signs of peri-implant disease were absent in 74% of the test implants after the removal of excess cement.

Recommendations for the main prosthetic steps are shown in Box 6.1.

Box 6.1 Prosthetic recommendations

- Place the final abutment as soon as possible.
- A customized abutment with juxta-gingival limits is to be preferred.
- Reduce the need for repeated abutment reconnections and/or disconnections.
- Prevent chemical contamination due to the laboratory procedures.
- Avoid subgingival resin injection, and cement from the provisional or final restoration.
- Guide the soft tissue by means of the temporary crown.
- Wait for stability of the peri-implant soft tissue before taking the final impression.

Note that the final restoration is a replica of the temporary one, but made of a different material.

The management of artificial soft tissue

In spite of the recent developments in periodontal and peri-implant surgical regenerative procedures, it is still a challenge to completely and predictably reestablish the hard and soft tissue contours in cases with 3D ridge deficiencies.

During smiling, the treated site may reveal a vertical deficiency of tissue. The only treatment possible today to treat such an inter-implant defect is either to proceed with segmental distraction of the osseous block with the implants and the mucosa, or to add a prosthetic pink supplement, which, although it is a restorative solution, remains a biological compromise.

Recent articles (Coachman *et al.*, 2010; Bichacho, 2011) have presented a reliable and consistent alternative to prosthetically restored cases with an uncertain surgical outcome, or for those patients who do not want to undergo regenerative surgical procedures (Figs 6.26a–j). The best solution is to install the restoration with only the ceramic part finished, and then add the pink composite resin at a second appointment, after healing of the soft tissue has allowed the patient's hygiene procedure to become established. The innovative hybrid prosthetic gingival restoration makes it possible to predictably achieve an excellent match between the prosthetic and natural gingiva. Understanding the indications and procedures involved with this technique requires a paradigm shift for the whole interdisciplinary team, but with considerable benefits to the patient. When properly planned and executed, the hybrid prosthetic gingival restoration offers predictable functional and esthetic results.

Final remarks

The new peri-implant treatment protocols try to achieve several objectives: a decrease in time, cost, and discomfort for the patient and, in particular, optimization of the esthetic result. Therefore, esthetic success can only be predictable through the development of a systematic approach to treatment and a proper understanding of the parameters that influence the esthetic outcome at the dentogingival junction and the implant restorative interface.

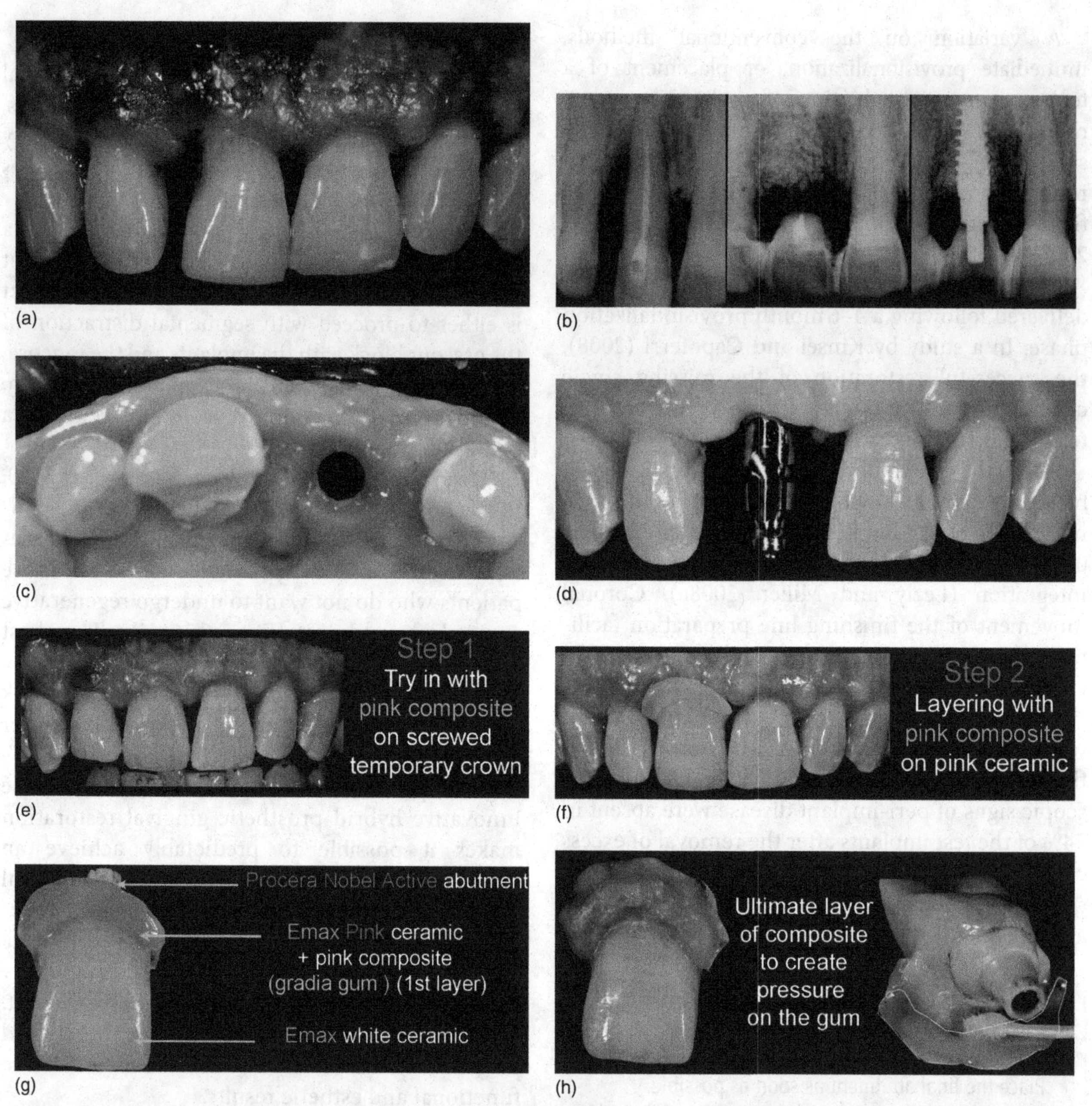

Figure 6.26 (a) The initial consultation for a loose right central incisor with Class IV gingival recession and a large space to the adjacent lateral incisor. (b) Radio-alveolar X-rays before and after extraction, and after implant placement with a bonded bridge. (c) The alveolar soft tissue crest aspect after removal of the implant healing abutment, with a depressed aspect to the alveolar soft tissue crest. (d) The transfer pin for the 3D implant impression. (e) Step 1: a trial fitting with pink composite on a screwed temporary crown. (f) Step 2: layering with pink composite on the pink ceramic. (g) White crown ceramic with pink gingival ceramic and composite gradia gum (first layer). (h) The ultimate layer of composite to create pressure on the gum.

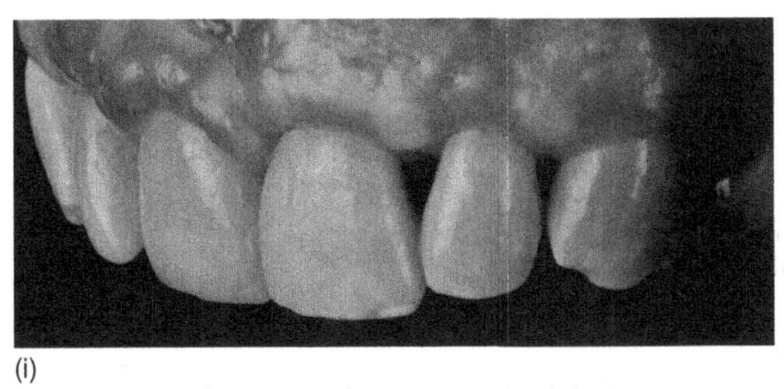
(i)

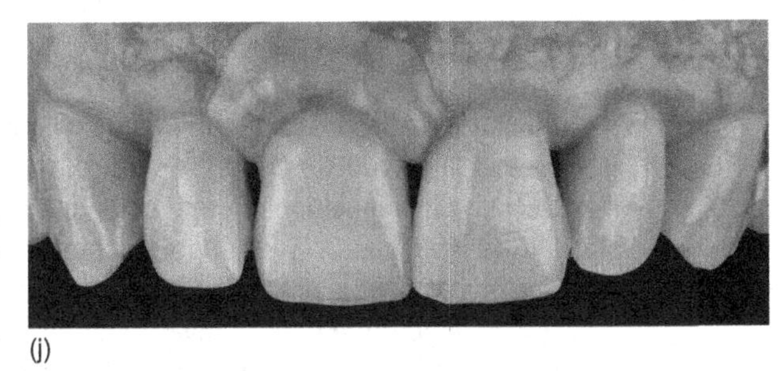
(j)

Figure 6.26 (i) The left clinical aspect of the screwed implant restoration, combining the pink ceramic and composite. This will allow regular hygiene with dental floss. (j) The frontal view of the tooth restoration with a ceramic chip on the left central incisor, with optimal implant crown proportions and harmonized gingival contours. (Courtesy of Dr. S. Koubi, restorative dentist, Marseille, France.)

Box 6.2 Key published works in esthetic implant dentistry

- "Diagnostic five keys" and evaluation of gingival thickness: Kan *et al.* (2003) and Kois (2006).
- Interproximal bone levels between implants, teeth, and pontics 3.5–6 mm: Salama *et al.* (1998).
- The tridimensional implant position: Saadoun and Le Gall (1992). Inter-implant distance > 3 mm: Tarnow *et al.* (2003).
- Immediate implant placement after extraction: Schwartz-Arad and Chaushu (1997), Wörhle (1998), and Saadoun (2002).
- Height of tissue between two adjacent implants 3.4 mm: Salama *et al.* (1998) and Tarnow *et al.* (2003).
- Jumping distance from socket walls to implant surface > 2 mm: Botticelli *et al.* (2003).
- Ridge alteration following extraction and implant placement > 1.5 mm B-L: Araújo and Lindhe (2005) and Becker *et al.* (2005).
- Bundle bone resorption post extraction > 1 mm: Araújo *et al.* (2006).
- Labial bone thickness required for esthetics and tissue maintenance (2 mm): Grunder *et al.* (2005).
- Implant/abutment connection and switch platform: Lazzara and De Porter (2006) and Cannullo *et al.* (2010); curvy abutment: Rompen *et al.* (2007).
- Zirconium abutments only suggested when tissue thickness < 2 mm: Jung *et al.* (2007).
- Crestal bone and tissue maintenance on Laser-Lok® implant surface: Nevins *et al.* (2008).

Implant dentistry has come a long way since 1981 – when the modern therapeutic techniques were introduced by Professor Per-Ingvar Brånemark, after 20 years of research – with great improvements made to achieve initial primary implant stability, improve bone-to-implant contact, and obtain a higher success rate in implant osseointegration. The focus of functional osseointegration has since shifted toward the creation of an esthetic implant restoration that is indistinguishable from natural teeth and is stable over time, through clinical minimally invasive procedures, and in harmony with the biological factors of the peri-implant mucosa.

In the past 20 years, a number of authors have contributed to establishing the scientific basis, as the main key to success in esthetic implant dentistry (Box 6.2).

There is a general consensus that the maintenance of bone around dental implants is one of the most essential features in successful long-term treatment, and that progressive bone loss drastically decreases the survivability of dental implants under occlusal loading (Marincola *et al.*, 2009).

The advantages of minimally invasive surgery in contemporary esthetic implant procedures are highlighted in Box 6.3.

All the factors in Table 6.3 play a key part in the esthetic outcome and the long-term stability of the soft tissue esthetics. Some are related to the patient, and the local anatomical factors, while other are related to the surgical protocol, the implant characteristics, and finally the

Box 6.3 Guidelines for minimally invasive surgery

- Minimize soft and hard tissue trauma by means of flapless surgery.
- Protect the blood supply at the surgical site.
- Decrease manipulation of the prosthetic components.
- Induce immediate tissue support by means of a temporary crown.
- Use biocompatible prosthetic materials.
- Under-contour the transgingival components.
- Move the restoration cement line coronally, but keep it 0.5 mm below the gingival margin.

Table 6.3 Factors influencing the architecture of peri-implant mucosa

Patient-related	Local anatomical factors
• Genetics: healing potential • Metabolic diseases: diabetes, obesity • Poor oral hygiene • Periodontal disease • Smoking, bruxism habits • Excessive alcohol consumption • Mucosal erosive pathology	• Tissue biotype: thick or thin • Biological width weakness • Osseous topography and thickness • Soft tissue AKG: height and width
Surgical protocol	**Implant characteristics**
• Minimal invasive surgery with minimal incisions and tissue elevation, especially around the papillae • Flap or flapless elevation • With or without bone counter-bore • Correct 3D implant placement • Inter-implant and tooth–implant distance • No excessive bone compression • Alveolar microgap and/or ridge: bone graft • Soft tissue management: CTG	• Implant design: platform, collar, body, threads, and apex • Implant surface: smooth or rough • Platform diameter smaller than that of the implant body • Type of connection: Morse cone, Tapered or Conical • Peri-implant biological width and seal
Prosthetic connection/restoration	
• Implant abutment type of connection: – The level of the microgap, micromovement – Reduced manipulation in connection/disconnection of the abutment – Cylindrical, tapered, or Morse conical connection – Flat platform or platform switching • Temporary or final abutment: biomaterial, design, and surface – Temporary or final crown restoration: emergence profile (flat or concave) – The vertical distance between the interproximal bone and the implant restoration contact point – Waiting for peri-implant soft tissue stability before taking the final impression – The final restoration as a replica of the temporary one – Avoidance of excess or cement retention • Functional occlusion with no occlusal overload • The patient's and the professional hygiene maintenance	

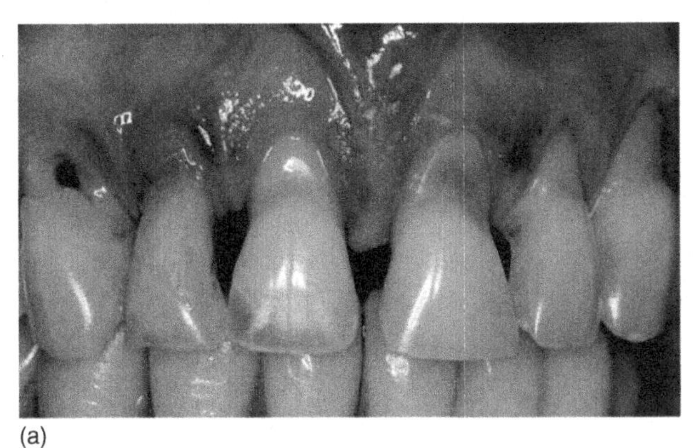
(a)

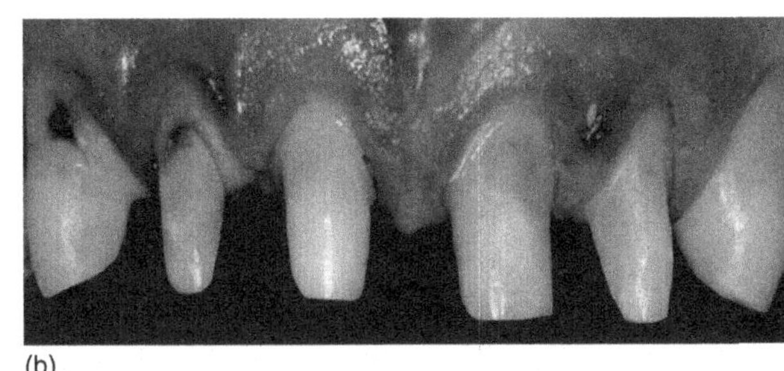
(b)

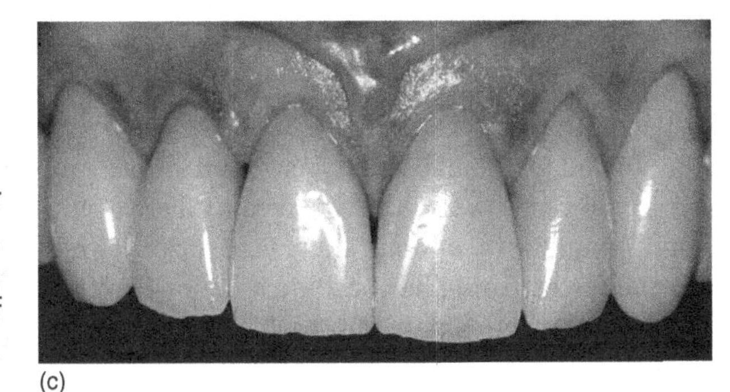
(c)

Figure 6.27 (a) The clinical aspect of the six anterior maxillary teeth after only scaling and root planing. (b) Intrasulcular crown preparation on the root surface, without impinging on the JE. (c) The clinical aspect of the six biocompatible vitro-ceramic e.max® restorations. (Courtesy of Dr. G. Tirlet, Paris, France.)

connection of the implant to the abutment and the restoration.

Long-term esthetic results are the main objective of the more demanding and better-informed patients. The purpose of esthetic implant treatment is to obtain a pleasant aspect of the restoration and correct alignment of the soft tissue: the gingival margin and the papillae. The esthetics of the implant should be biological: osseous and gingival remodeling can be reduced if the biological rules are respected.

The effective management of esthetic peri-implant dentistry depends on:

- a multidisciplinary approach to understanding the various parameters, and
- cooperation between the surgeon, restorative dentist, and laboratory technician.

Each member of the team has the same biological concerns and is aware of the same trends. One could easily say that, today, esthetics in implant therapy is similar to conventional restorative dentistry (Figs 6.27a–c).

7

Conclusion

The perception of beauty continually varies over time. Nowadays, facial beauty is based more on today's "make-up" than on natural beauty. However, in our generation, among the facial criteria of beauty, a perfect smile has become a major feature and offers many advantages for the person wearing the smile.

Every individual has unique facial characteristics, including those of their smiles. According to the definition of esthetics, a smile is something very personal, relating directly to that person's facial structure, gender, style, and character. Esthetic dentists should not be limited or restricted by specific requirements but, rather, should consider them as useful guidelines for creating a smile that best suits that particular patient's personal needs.

Clinicians can no longer content themselves with purely practical procedures. Esthetics must be taken into account in comprehensive oral therapy. Due to this paradigm shift, esthetic dentistry can now deliver increasingly predictable and natural results. Not only that, but a more complete understanding of the components behind an esthetic smile – precise anatomical, functional, and biological integration – has caused clinicians to make achieving this precision a prerequisite for any successful treatment. The latest trends in dentistry tend toward minimally invasive options that will cause the least possible tissue disruption. This is challenging, but well worth the effort.

Therefore, the purpose of modern dentistry is to achieve the best possible result with minimal tissue invasion and time, giving the patient a beautiful smile, with a long-term predictable result, and without prejudicing the integrity of the structure of the remaining teeth (Fig. 7.1). Furthermore, when a smile needs to be redesigned, the clinician should have the competence to evaluate and integrate this smile into the harmony of the face.

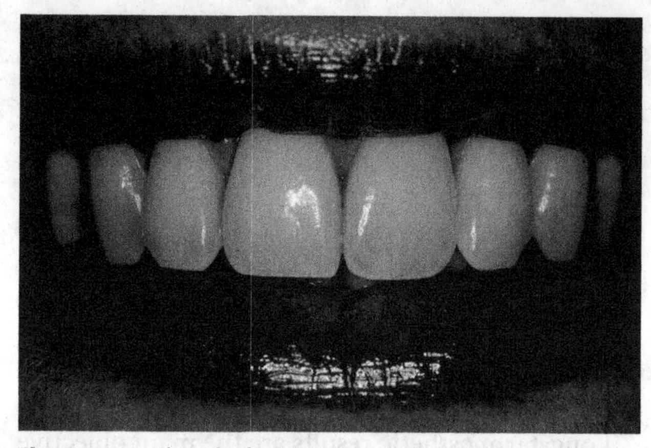

Figure 7.1 The ideal gingival smile of a beautiful young woman.

In order to be esthetically pleasing, a comprehensive oral treatment must take into account both hard and soft tissues, after establishing a proper diagnosis that takes the local and general risk factors into consideration. The highest goal of perio-implantology and restorative dentistry is to achieve – through periodontal plastic surgery, resective (Figs 7.2a, b) or additive (Figs 7.3a–d), and implant surgical and prosthetic manipulation (Figs 7.4a, b) – an esthetic and harmonious gingival

Esthetic Soft Tissue Management of Teeth and Implants, First Edition. André P. Saadoun.

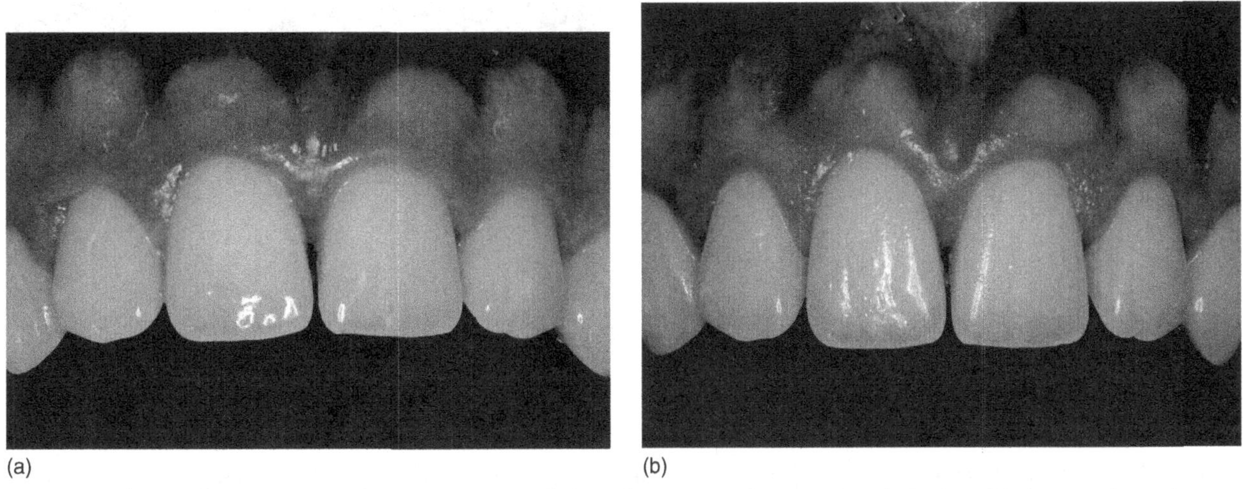

(a) (b)

Figure 7.2 (a) The frontal aspect of a disproportioned clinical crown, with an excess of gingiva. (b) The new frontal aspect, with longer teeth and less gingiva, 12 months after surgery, with a harmonious gingival contour and tooth proportion on the maxillary arch.

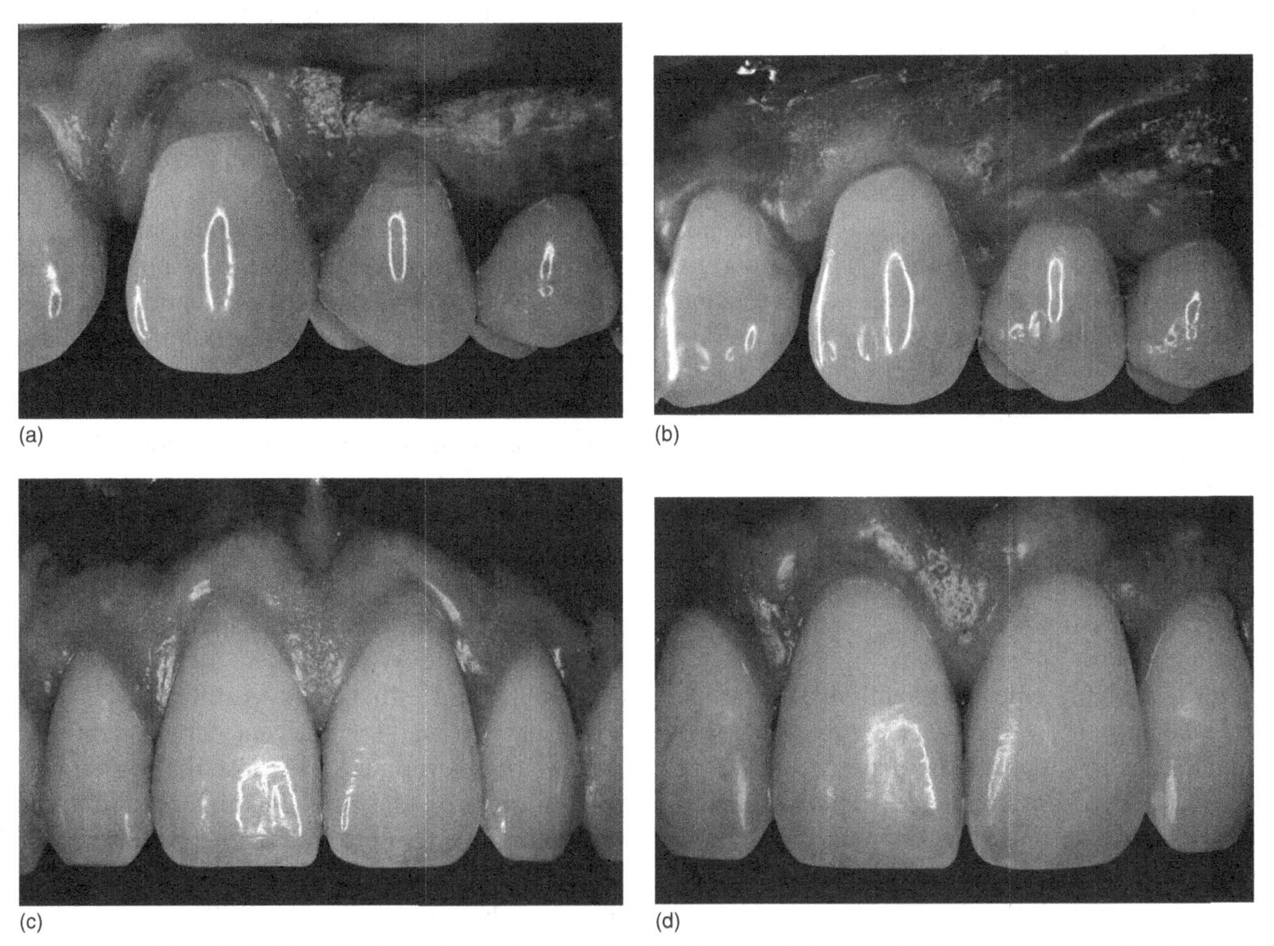

(a) (b) (c) (d)

Figure 7.3 (a) Multiple Class I/II gingival recession combined with enamel abrasion. (b) One-year post-op after Emdogain® treatment, showing full root coverage and slight enamel abrasion. (c) Multiple Class I/II maxillary anterior recessions on a young woman. (d) One year post-op after a tunneling procedure using AlloDerm®.

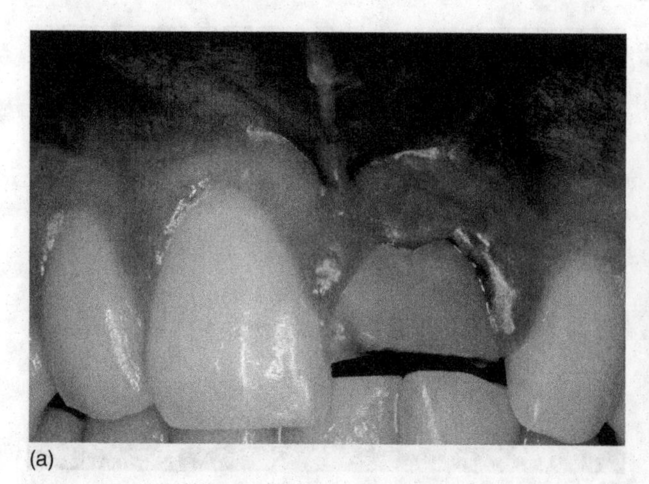
(a)

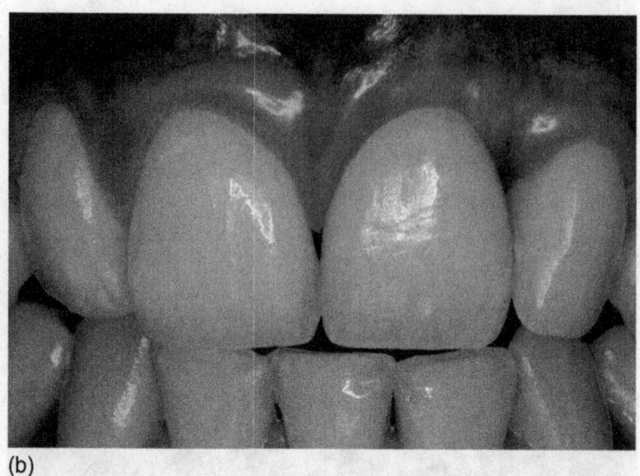
(b)

Figure 7.4 (a) A broken left central incisor after a chronic untreated infection. (b) The final NobelProcera™ restoration, in harmony with the adjacent tooth and gingival contour, at 36 months.

contour around a beautiful restoration. It is not easy to attain this goal; nor is the "how" immediately obvious. Peri-implant esthetic stability is a complex issue, due to the number of factors that have to be taken into account. It is therefore imperative that the esthetics of peri-implant treatments be biologically and scientifically based. Two of the main difficulties to be overcome are the phenomenon of crestal bone loss and the relative fragility of peri-implant soft tissues. However, osseous and mucosal remodeling can be minimized by adhering strictly to the rules of biological physiology. This will prevent bone loss peri-implant recession and lead to long-term esthetic outcomes.

Today, surgeons and restorative dentists have many therapeutic options available to them, but in order to preserve and stabilize the peri-implant bone and mucosa, they must consider the implications of each and choose with care.

Patients show an ever-increasing demand for esthetic tooth replacement, with minimal downtime and inconvenience. The dental profession has responded with innovations that decrease the length of treatment, enhance implant survival rates, preserve soft tissue contours, minimize volume loss, decrease functional stress, achieve esthetic predictability, and improve the psychological aspects for the patient.

Despite the increase of interest in the profession concerning the esthetic integration of implant restorations, the level of scientific proof has been relatively low, which involves only single implants. Therefore, future clinical publications should integrate a more objective analysis of the esthetic result through a scale of evaluation.

In the meantime, it is a prerequisite to evaluate, with precision, the level of complexity of each clinical situation, following a precise protocol, and to correlate each case with the patient's esthetic demands, in order to avoid an esthetic failure.

When selecting appropriate prosthetic procedures and in considering tissue remodeling, it is essential to understand the periodontal implications, the physiology of the biological space, and its reformation around implants, as well as the biocompatibility of the prosthetic components. The esthetic predictability of implant procedures is achieved by respecting these multifactorial biological principles.

Choosing prosthetic procedures wisely is especially important when implants are to be placed in the esthetic zone. When making a comprehensive periodontal and esthetic pre-treatment evaluation of the implant site, the adjacent natural dentition should not be overlooked, because the goal should be to harmonize the two. By thinking about the desired esthetic result from the outset, the clinician can determine the necessary restorative material, abutment design (if applicable), emergence profile, and optimal tissue architecture required to bring it about, which in turn will guide the treatment sequence and protocol required. Then, once an esthetic result is obtained, professional periodontal maintenance and diligent patient home care can ensure the long-term success of the periodontal plastic surgery and dental implants.

The primary role of the clinician is to help patients and guide them in their decision-making process, so that an enlightened consensus about what treatment is needed and which treatment option is best can be obtained. Clinicians can do this by comparing the pros and cons of various treatment options based on data regarding success rates, giving a critical appraisal of the dental literature, and sharing personal clinical experiences.

The new philosophy of implant treatment is: simple, sure, fast, and durable. This philosophy is characterized by a surgical approach that is minimally invasive, with a very biocompatible prosthetic precision guaranteeing the patient's comfort and providing a more natural esthetic.

The objective of any implant treatment is to evaluate the risk factors, do better, and push the clinician to the highest level, always having one major goal in mind: the patient's satisfaction. Today, one can assert that providing an esthetic result is no longer just an option: it has become a clinical imperative, the proof of both biological and functional success.

However, more often than not, an esthetic outcome to their treatment is of the utmost concern to patients. If they know that when the process is over, they will be able to flash a winning smile, they are more able to "grin and bear it." In this day and age, with all of the advances made in all dental specialties, it is no longer necessary to follow the old adage, "function before form." Now, with the help of expert clinicians, patients can have form, function, and esthetic. A sign in one oral surgeon's office says it best: "Smile please!" (Fig. 7.5).

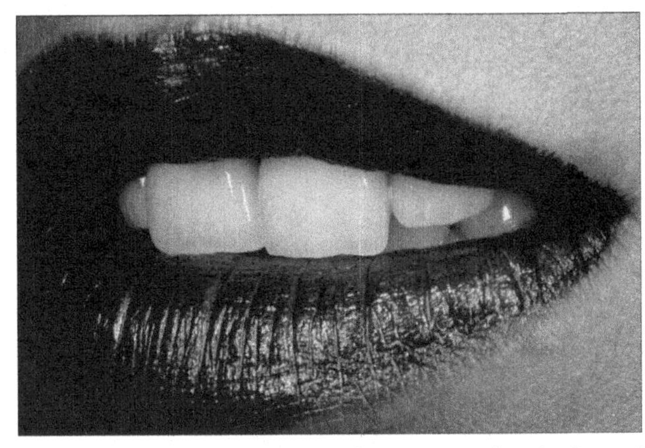

Figure 7.5 Esthetic dentistry changes people's looks and makes them happier.

Do you want your patients to have a film star smile and become absolutely irresistible? The hottest reds of the season, brown or coral lipsticks, shiny glosses, well-chosen make-up, anti-age treatments, plastic surgery – the list goes on. But above all – they must take care of their teeth and gums for life!

The esthetic long-term results become the main objective of our well-informed patients and clinicians: "An esthetic result must be biological and functional, otherwise it is not esthetic." Dentists help to create beautiful smiles, and beautiful smiles change patients' personalities, create happier people, and ultimately make the world a better place.

References

Abrahamsson I, Lindhe J, Berglundh T. The mucosal barrier following abutment dis/reconnection: an experimental study in dogs. *J Clin Periodontol.* 1997;24(8):568–572.

Abrahamsson I, Berglundh T, Sekino S, Lindhe J. Tissue reactions to abutment shift: an experimental study in dogs. *Clin Implant Dent Relat Res.* 2003;5:82–88.

Adell R, Eriksson B, Lekholm U, Brånemark PI, Jemt T. Long-term follow-up study of osseointegrated implants in the treatment of totally edentulous jaws. *Int J Oral Maxillofac Implants.* 1990;5(4):347.

Agar JR, Cameron SM, Hughbanks JC, Parker MH. Cement removal from restorations luted to titanium abutments with simulated subgingival margins. *J Prosthet Dent.* 1997;7: 843–847.

Ahmad I. Geometric considerations in anterior dental aesthetics: restorative principles. *Pract Periodontics Aesthet Dent.* 1998;10:813–822.

Alkhatib MN, Holt R, Dedi R. Age and perception of dental appearance in tooth color. *Gerodontology.* 2005;22:32–36.

Al-Omiri M, Abu Hammad O, Lynch E, Lamey P, Clifford T. Impacts of implant treatment on daily living. *Int J Oral Maxillofac Implants.* 2011;26:877–886.

American Academy of Periodontology. *Glossary of Periodontal Terms.* 4th ed. Chicago, IL: American Academy of Periodontology; 2001:44.

Araújo M, Lindhe J. Dimensional ridge alterations following tooth extraction: an experimental study in the dog. *J Clin Periodontol.* 2005;32:212–218.

Araújo M, Linder E, Lindhe J. Effect of a xenograft on early bone formation in extraction sockets: an experimental study in dog. *Clin Oral Implants Res.* 2009;20(1):1–6.

Araújo M, Linder E, Wennström J, Lindhe J. The influence of Bio-Oss Collagen on healing of an extraction socket: an experimental study in the dog. *Int J Periodontics Restorative Dent.* 2008;28(2):123–135.

Araújo M, Wennström J, Lindhe J. Modeling of the buccal and lingual bone of fresh extraction site following implant installation. *Clin Oral Implants Res.* 2006;17:606.

Araújo MG, Lindhe J. Ridge preservation with the use of Bio-Oss® Collagen: a 6-month study in the dog. *Clin Oral Implants Res.* 2009;20:433–440.

Araújo MG, Liljenberg B, Lindhe J. Dynamics of Bio-Oss Collagen incorporation in fresh extraction wounds: an experimental study in the dog. *Clin Oral Implants Res.* 2010;21(1):55–64.

Araújo M. Alveolar socket preservation after extraction. *Int Symp Osteol Cannes April 14-16 AO News* 2011, 142: 26–28.

Atieh M, Payne AGT, Duncan W, De Silva RK, Cullinan MP. Immediate placement or immediate restoration/loading of single implants for molar tooth replacement: a systematic review and meta-analyses. *Int J Oral Maxillofac Implants.* 2010;25(2), 401–415.

Attal JP, Tirlet G, Diagnostic du sourire gingival sur le sourire posé ou spontané? *Inf Dent.* 2011:18–21.

Barbant C, Lallam C, Tirlet G., Attal JP. Etiologies et traitements du sourire gingival. *Inf Dent.* 2011a:18–25.

Barbant C, Saint-Martin R, Tirlet G, Attal JP. Diagnostic du sourire gingival sur le sourire posé ou spontané? *Inf Dent.* 2011b:17–21.

Barros, RRM. Influence of interimplant distances and placement depth on peri-implant bone remodelling of adjacent and immediately loaded Morse cone connection implants – a histomorphometric study in dogs. *Clin Oral Implants Res.* 2010;21(4):371–378.

Barros RRM, Novaes Jr. AB, Grisi MFM, Souza SLS, Taba M Jr., Palioto DB. A 6-month comparative clinical study of a conventional and a new surgical approach for root coverage with acellular dermal matrix. *J Periodontol.* 2004;75: 1350–1356.

Bashutski JD, Wang HL. Common implant esthetic complications. *Pract Proced Aesthet Dent.* 2008;20(4):245.

Baumgarten H, Cocchetto R, Testori T, Meltzer A, Porter S. A new implant design for crestal bone preservation: initial observations and case report. *Pract Proced Aesthet Dent.* 2005;17(10):735–740.

Becker W, Goldstein M, Becker B, Sennerby L. Minimally invasive flapless implant surgery: a prospective multicenter study. *Clin Implant Dent Relat Res.* 2005; 7(Suppl.):S21–S27.

Bennani V, Vaudoin A. Success criteria for esthetic implant restoration. In: *Esthetic and Emergence Profile in Implantology.* Paris: Editions CDP; 2000:116–136.

Berglundh T, Lindhe J, Jonsson K, Ericsson I. The topography of the vascular systems in the periodontal and peri-implant tissues in dogs. *J Clin Periodontol.* 1994;21:189–193.

Bichacho N. Restauration de deux implants unilatéraux et adjacents sur une crête déficiente en zone esthétique: une solution alternative prothétique rose et blanche. *Le Fil Dentaire.* 2011;66:48–52.

Esthetic Soft Tissue Management of Teeth and Implants, First Edition. André P. Saadoun.

Bichacho N, Landsberg C. A modified surgical/prosthetic approach for an optimal single implant supported crown, part II. The cervical contouring concept. *Pract Periodontics Aesthet Dent.* 1994;6(4):35–41.

Bissada, N, Sears S. Quantitative assessment of free gingival grafts with and without periosteum and osseous perforation. *J Periodontol.* 1978;49:15.

Bitter RN. The periodontal factor in esthetic smile design-altering gingival display. *Gen Dent.* 2007;55(7):616–622.

Blanes RJ, Allen EP. The bilateral pedicle flap tunnel technique: a new approach to cover connective tissue grafts. *Int J Periodontics Restorative Dent.* 1999;19(5):471–479.

Blatz M, Hurzeler M, Strub J. Reconstruction of the lost interproximal papilla-presentation of surgical and non-surgical approaches. *Int J Periodontics Restorative Dent.* 1999;19(4): 395–406.

Botticelli D, Berglundh T, Buser D, Lindhe J. The jumping distance revisited: an experimental study in the dog. *Clin Oral Implants Res.* 2003;14:35–42.

Botticelli D, Berglundh T, Lindhe J. Hard tissue alterations following immediate implant placement in extraction sites. *J Clin Periodontol.* 2004;31:820–828.

Botticelli D, Persson L, Lindhe J, Berglundh T. Bone tissue formation adjacent to implants placed in fresh extraction sockets: an experimental study in dogs. *Clin Oral Implants Res.* 2006;17:351–358.

Bouri A, Bissada N, Al-Zahrani M, Faddoul F, Nourneh I. Width of keratinized gingiva and the health status of the supporting tissues around dental implants. *Int J Oral Maxillofac Implants.* 2008;23:323–326.

Bruchon-Schweitzer M. *Une psychologie du Corps.* Paris: PUF; 1990.

Bukhardt R, Joss A, Lang N. Soft tissue dehiscence coverage around endosseous implants: a prospective cohort study. *Clin Oral Implants Res.* 2008;19:451–457.

Buser D. Good prognosis with early implantation. *News Geistlich* 2005;1:12–14.

Buser D, Martin W, Belser UC. Optimizing esthetics for implant restorations in the anterior maxilla: anatomic and surgical considerations. *Int J Oral Maxillofac Implants.* 2004;19(Suppl.):43–61.

Buser D, Bornstein M, Weber H, Grütter L, Schmid B, Belser UC. Early implant placement with simultaneous guided bone regeneration following single-tooth extraction in the esthetic zone: a cross-sectional, retrospective study in 45 subjects with a 2- to 4-year follow-up. *J Periodontol.* 2008;79(9):1773–1781.

Butler B. Use of the Er, CR: YSGG laser to improve periodontal plastic surgery: the periodontist's perspective. *Pract Proced Aesthet Dent.* 2006;18(4 Suppl):S10–S11.

Cardaropoli G, Araújo M, Hayacibara R, Sukekava F, Lindhe J. Healing of extraction sockets and surgically produced – augmented and non-augmented – defects in the alveolar ridge: an experimental study in the dog. *J Clin Periodontol.* 2005;32:435–440.

Cachay H, Velásquez H. Rhinoplasty and facial expression. *Ann Plast Surg.* 1992;28(5):427–433.

Cairo F, Pagliaro U, Nieri M. Treatment of gingival recession with coronally advanced flap. *J Periodontol.* 2010;81(2): 616–625.

Caneva M, Salata L, de Souza S, Baffone G, Lang N, Botticelli D. Influence of implant positioning in extraction sockets on osseointegration: histomorphometric analyses in dogs. *Clin Oral Implants Res.* 2010;21:43–49.

Canullo, L, Iannello G, Götz W. The influence of individual bone patterns on peri-implant bone loss: preliminary report from a 3-year randomized clinical and histologic trial in patients treated with implants restored with matching-diameter abutments or the platform-switching concept. *Int J Oral Maxillofac Implants.* 2011:26;618–630.

Canullo L, Fedele GR, Iannello G, Jepsen S. Platform switching and marginal bone-level alterations: the results of a randomized-controlled trial. *Clin Oral Implants Res.* 2010;21: 115–121.

Canullo L, Pellegrini G, Allievi C, Trombelli L, Annibali S, Dellavia C. Soft tissues around long-term platform switching implant restorations: a histological human evaluation. Preliminary results. *J Clin Periodont.* 2010;38(1):86–94.

Caplanis N. Interpositional connective tissue graft. *Acad Osseoint News.* 2008;19(2):1–3.

Cappiello M, Luongo R, Di Iorio D, Bugea C, Cocchetto R, Celletti R. Evaluation of peri-implant bone loss around platform-switched implants. *Int J Periodontics Restorative Dent.* 2008;28(4):347–355.

Cardaropoli G, Lekholm U, Wennstrom J. Tissue alterations at implant-supported single-tooth replacements: a 1-year prospective clinical study. *Clin Oral Implants Res.* 2006;17: 165–171.

Castellanos A, De la Rosa M, De la Garza M, Caffesse RG. Enamel matrix derivative and coronal flaps to cover marginal tissue recessions. *J Periodontol.* 2006;77:7–14.

Charruel S, Perez C, Foti B, Camps J, Monnet-Corti V. Gingival contour assessment: clinical prameters useful esthetic diagnosis and treatment. *J Periodontol.* 2008;79:795–808.

Chang M, Wennstrom JL, Odman P, Andersson B. Implant supported single-tooth replacements compared to contralateral nature teeth: crown and soft tissue dimensions. *Clin Oral Implants Res.* 1999;10:185–194.

Chang M, Wennstrom JL, Odman P, Andersson B. Influence of gingival tissue thickness on marginal bone stability. *Clin Oral Implants Res.* 2003;20:827–832.

Chen S, Evans C. Immediate and conventional single implant treatment in the anterior maxilla. *J Clin Periodont.* 2009;38:385–394.

Chen S, Darby I, Reynolds E. A prospective clinical study of non-submerged immediate implants: clinical outcome and esthetic results. *Clin Oral Implants Res.* 2007;18: 552–562.

Chen S, Darby I, Buser D. Ridge preservation techniques for implant therapy. *Int J Oral Maxillofac Implants.* 2009;24(Suppl.):186–217.

Cheng-Yi Lin J, Yeh CL, Jein-Wein Liou E, Bowman SJ. Treatment of skeletal-origin gummy smiles with miniscrew anchorage. *J Clin Orthod.* 2008;42(5):285–289.

Chiche GJ, Pinault A. *Esthetics of Anterior Fixed Prosthodontics*. Chicago, IL: Quintessence; 1994:33.

Choquet V, Hermans M, Adriaenssens P, Daelemans P, Tarnow DP, Malevez C. Clinical and radiographic evaluation of the papilla level adjacent to single-tooth dental implants: a retrospective study in the maxillary anterior region. *J Periodontol.* 2001;72:1364–1371.

Chow Y, Eber R, Tsao Y, Shotwell J, Wang H. Factors associated with the appearance of gingival papillae. *J Clin Periodontol.* 2010;37:719–727.

Chu SJ. A biometric approach to predictable treatment of clinical crown discrepancies. *Pract Proced Aesthet Dent.* 2007;19(7):401–409.

Chu SJ, Hochman MN. A biometric approach to esthetic crown lengthening: part I – midfacial considerations. *Pract Proced Aesthet Dent.* 2007;19(1):17–24.

Chu SJ, Hochman M. Interdisciplinary approach for managing esthetics. *AAP Meeting*. Miami, Nov. 2011.

Chu SJ, Tarnow DP, Tan JHP, Stappert CFJ. Papilla height to crown length proportions in the maxillary anterior dentition. *Int J Periodontics Restorative Dent.* 2008. Manuscript submitted for publication.

Chu SJ, Okubo S. Range and mean discordance of individual tooth width of the mandibular anterior dentition. *Pract Proced Aesthet Dent.* 2007;19(5):313–320.

Chung D, Oh T, Shotwell J, Misch C, Wang H. Significance of keratinized mucosa in maintenance of endosseous dental implant with different surfaces. *J Periodontol.* 2006;77:1410–1420.

Claffey N, Polyzois I, Ziaka P. An overview of nonsurgical and surgical therapy. *Periodontol 2000.* 2004;36:35–44.

Coachman C, Van Doren E, Gurel G, Calamita M, Calgaro M, de Souza Neto J. Minimally invasive reconstruction in implant therapy: the prosthetic gingival restoration. *QDT*. 2010.

Cocchetto R, Traini T, Addeo F, Celletti R. Evaluation of hard tissue response around wider platform-switched implants. *Int J Periodontics Restorative Dent.* 2010;30:163–171.

Cochran D, Hermann J, Schenk R, Higginbottom F, Buser D. Biologic width around titanium implants: a histometric analysis of the implanto-gingival junction around unloaded and loaded nonsubmerged implants in the canine mandible. *J Periodontol.* 1997;68:186–198.

Cooper L, Albrektsson, T. Marginal bone reduction with AstraTech implant system. *AstraTech Implant Congress*. New York, 2008.

Cornelini R, Barone A, Covani U. Connective tissue grafts in postextraction implants with immediate restoration: a prospective controlled clinical study. *Pract Proced Aesthet Dent.* 2008;20(6):337–343.

Coslet GJ, Vanarsdall R, Weisgold A. Diagnosis and classification of delayed passive eruption of the dentogingival junction in the adult. *Alpha Omegan*. 1977;70, December: 24–28.

Covani U, Marconcini S, Gaalassini G, Cornelini R, Santini S, Barone A. Connective tissue graft used as biological barrier to cover immediate implant. *J Periodontol.* 2007;78(8): 1644–1649.

Cueva MA, Boltchi FE, Hallmon WW, Nunn ME, Rivera-Hidalgo F, Rees T. A comparative study of coronally advanced flaps with and without the addition of enamel matrix derivative in the treatment of marginal tissue recession. *J Periodontol.* 2004;75:949–956.

Dapril G, Gatto M, Checchi, L. The evolution of the buccal gingival recession in a student population: a 5-year follow up. *J Periodontol.* 2007;78(4):611–614.

Darby I, Chen ST, Buser D. Ridge preservation techniques for implant therapy. *Int J Oral Maxillofac Implants.* 2009;24(7), 260–271.

Davis LG, Ashworth PD, Spriggs LS. Psychosocial effects of esthetic dental treatment. *J Dent.* 1998;26:547–554.

De Queroz Côrtes A, Guimaraes Marins A, Nociti Jr. FH, Sallum AW, Casati MZ, Sallum EA. Coronally positioned flap with or without an acellular dermal matrix graft in the treatment of class I gingival recessions: a randomized controlled clinical study. *J Periodontol.* 2004;75:1137–1144.

Decharrière-Hamzawi H, Attal JP, Tirlet G. Peur d'une dysmorphose. *Inf Dent.* 2005;87(40):2523–2527.

Decharriere-Hamzawi H, Savard G, Tirlet G, Attal JP. Dentistrie esthétique et santé. *Inf Dent.* 2007;24:1381–1388.

Degorce T. Late peri implant gingival recession in the esthetic zone. *Inf Dent.* 2009;22:1182–1183.

Del Corso M. Soft tissue response to platelet rich fibrin clinical evidences. *Cosm Dent.* 2008;3:16–20.

Deporter D, Al-Sayyed A, Pilliar RM, Valiquette N. "Biologic width" and crestal bone remodeling with sintered porous-surfaced dental implants: a study in dogs. *Int J Oral Maxillofac Implants.* 2008;23(3):544–550.

Dersot JM. Adult orthodontics and gingival recession. *Inf Dent.* 2011;8:18–24.

Desai S, Upadhyay M, Nanda R. Dynamic smile analysis: changes with age. *Am J Orthod Dentofacial Orthop.* 2009;136:310–321.

Eckert S. Has implant dentistry become a boutique practice? *Int J Oral Maxillofac Implants.* 2008;4:583–584.

Elian N, Jalbout ZN, Classi J, Wexler A, Tarnow DP, Wallace SS. Realities and limitations in the management of interdental papilla between implants. *Int J Periodontics Restorative Dent.* 2006;26(6):543–551.

Elian N, Cho S, Froum S, Smith R, Tarnow D. A simplified socket classification and repair technique. *Pract Proced Aesthet Dent.* 2007;19(2);99–104.

Elter C, Heuer W, Demling A, Hannig M. Supra-and subgingival biofilm formation on implant abutments with different surface characteristics. *Int J Oral Maxillofac Implants.* 2008;23:327–334.

Ericsson I, Nielson H, Lindh T, Nilner K, Randow K. Immediate functional loading of Brånemark single tooth implants: an 18 month's clinical pilot follow up study. *Clin Oral Implants Res.* 2000;11:26–33.

Ericsson I, Persoon L, Berglundh T, Marineloo C, Lindhe J, Klinge B. Different types of inflammatory reactions in peri-implant soft tissues. *J Clin Periodontol.* 1995;22(3): 255–261.

Esposito M, Hirsch J, Lekholm U, Thomsen P. Measure around functioning osteointegrated dental implant. *J Periodontol.* 1993;64:1173–1186.

Estafanous E, Clark S, Huynh-Ba G. Platform switching and clinical science. *Int J Oral Maxillofac Implants.* 2011;26(2):655–658.

Evans CJD, Chen ST. Esthetic outcomes of immediate implant placements. *Clin Oral Implants Res.* 2008;19:73–80.

Ezquerra F, Berrazueta MJ, Ruiz-Capillas A, Sainz Affegui J. New approach to the gummy smile. *Plast Reconstr Surg.* 1999;104(4):1143–1152.

Fairbairn PJ. Lip repositioning surgery: a solution to the extremely high lip line. In: Romano R, ed., *The Art of Treatment Planning.* Chicago, IL: Quintessence; 2010:391–406.

Feigenbaum N. Reliable porcelain repairs. *J Esthet Restor Dent.* 1991;3:79–84.

Foley TF, Sandhu HS, Athanasopoulos C. Facteurs parodontaux esthétiques à considérer durant un traitement orthodontique: prise en charge de l'exposition excessive de gencives. *Can Sent Assoc.* 2003;69(6):368–372.

Fradeani M. *Esthetic Rehabilitation in Fixed Prosthodontics.* Chicago, IL: Quintessence; 2004.

Fradeani M, Barducci G. *Esthetic Rehabilitation in Fixed Prosthodontics: Prosthetic Treatment, a Systematic Approach to Esthetic, Biologic, and Functional Integration.* Chicago, IL: Quintessence; 2008.

Fu J, Lee A, Wang H. Influence of tissue biotype on implants esthetics. *Int J Oral Maxillofac Implants.* 2011; 26:499–508.

Fuerhauser R, Floresu D, Benesch T, Haas R, Mailath J, Watzek J. Evaluation of soft tissue around single tooth implant crown: the pink aesthetic score. *Clin Oral Implants Res.* 2005;16:639–644.

Garber DA, Salama MA. The aethestic smile: diagnostic and treatment. *Periodontol 2000.* 1996;11:18–28.

Garber D, Salama M, Salama H, Funato, Ishikawa T. Three dimensional bone and soft tissue requirements for optimizing esthetic results in compromised cases with multiple implants. *DentalXP.* October 27, 2010.

Gardner DM. Platform switching as a means to achieving implant esthetics. *N Y State Dent J.* 2005;71(3):34–37. Review.

Gargiulo AW, Wentz F, Orban B. Dimensions and relations of the dento-gingival junction in humans. *J Periodontol.* 1961;32:261–267.

Glauser R, Lundgreen A, Gottlow J, *et al.* Immediate occlusal loading of Brånemark System TiUnite implants placed predominantly in soft bone: 1-year result of a prospective clinical study. *Clin Implant Dent Relat Res.* 2003;5(Suppl. 1):47–56.

Glauser R, Ruhstaller P, Windisch S, *et al.* Immediate occlusal loading of Brånemark System TiUnite implants placed predominantly in soft bone: 4-year results of a prospective clinical study. *Clin Implant Dent Relat Res.* 2005;7 (Suppl. 1): 52–59.

Goldenberg B. Shape, color and contour of peri-implant tissue – the role of the abutment-connection complex. *DentalXP.* 9-2011.

Goldstein R, Niessen L. Issues in esthetic dentistry for older adults. *J Esthet Dent.* 1988;10:235–242.

Goldstein R, Garber D, Salama M, Salama H, Adar, P. Smile design in everyday and implant dentistry, part 3. *Dental XP.* 2010.

Goubron C, Thomasset F, De Deunynck A, Tardivo D. Eruption passive incomplète: rétablissement chirurgical d'un sourire harmonieux. *Inf Dent.* 2011;93(10):16–20.

Grunder U. Immediate functional loading of immediate implant placed in edentulous ridge. *Int. J Oral Maxillofac Implants.* 1999;1:2–16.

Grunder U. Stability of the mucosal topography around single-tooth implants and adjacent teeth: 1-year results. *Int J Periodontics Restorative Dent.* 2000;20:11–17.

Grunder U, Gracis S, Capelli M. Influence of the 3-D bone-to-implant relationship on esthetics. *Int J Periodontics Restorative Dent.* 2005;25(2):72–83.

Gürel G. Improving the esthetics of healthy teeth with porcelain laminate veneers. In: Cohen M., ed., *Interdisciplinary Treatment Planning: Principles, Designs, Implementation.* Chicago, IL: Quintessence; 2008a.

Gürel G. Permanent diagnostic provisional: predictable outcomes using porcelain laminate veneers. In: Cohen M, ed., *Interdisciplinary Treatment Planning: Principles, Designs, Implementation.* Chicago, IL: Quintessence; 2008b:30,43–55.

Hämmerle C. Augmenting bone plus soft tissue. *News Geistlich* 2005;1:10–11.

Han JS, Vanchit J, Blanchard S, Kowolik M, Eckert G. Changes in gingival dimensions following connective tissue grafts for root coverage: comparison of two procedures. *J Periodontol.* 2008;79(8):1346–1354.

Harris RJ. A comparative study of root coverage obtained with guided tissue regeneration utilising a bioabsorbable membrane versus the connective tissue with partial-thickness double pedicle graft. *J Periodontol.* 1997;68(8):779–790.

Harris RJ. A short-term and long-term comparison of root coverage with an acellular dermal matrix and a subepithelial graft. *J Periodontol.* 2004;75:734–743.

Heitz-Mayfield LJ. How effective is surgical therapy compared with nonsurgical debridement? *Periodontol 2000.* 2005; 37:72–87.

Hempton TJ, Esrason F. Crown lengthening to facilitate restorative treatment in the presence of incomplete passive eruption. *J Calif Dent Assoc.* 2000;28(4):290–291, 294–296, 298.

Heng N, N'Guessan P, Kleber B, Bernimoulin J, Pischon N. Enamel matrix derivative induces connective tissue growth factor expression in human osteoblastic cells. *J Periodontol.* 2007;78(12):2369–2379.

Hermann J, Buser D, Schenk R, Cochran D. Crestal bone change around titanium implants: a histometric evaluation of unloaded non-submerged and submerged implants in the canine mandible. *J Periodontol.* 2000;71:1412–1424.

Hirsch A, Goldstein M, Goultschin J, Boyan BD, Shwartz Z. A 2 years follow up of root coverage using subpedicle acellular dermal matrix allografts and subepithelial connective tissue autografts. *J Periodontol.* 2005;76:1323–1328.

Holbrook T, Oschenbein C. Complete coverage of denuded root surfaces with one stage gingival graft. *Int J Periodontics Restorative Dent.* 1993;3(3):8–27.

Horning GM, Vernino A, Towle HJ 3rd, Baccaglini L. Gingival grafting in periodontal practice: results of 103 consecutive surgeries in 82 patients. *Int J Periodontics Restorative Dent.* 2008;28(4):327–335.

Hu WJ, Li LS, Zhang H. Root reshaping in combination of conservative osseous resection: a modified technique for surgical crown lengthening. *Beijing Da Xue Xue Bao.* 2008;40(1):83–87.

Hürzeler MB, Zuhr O, Schupbach P, Rebele SF, Emmanouilidis N, Fickl S. The socket-shield technique: a proof-of-principle report. *J Clin Periodontol.* 2010;37(9):855–862.

Huynh-Ba G, Pjetursson BE, Sanz M, *et al.* Analysis of the socket bone wall dimensions in the upper maxilla in relation to immediate implant placement. *Clin Oral Implants Res.* 2010;21(1):37–42..

Imberman M. Gingival augmentation with an acellular dermal matrix revisited: surgical technique for gingival grafting. *Pract Proced Aesthet Dent.* 2007;19(2):123–128.

Ingber J. Forced eruption: a method of treating isolated 1 and 2 wall infra bony defects – rationale and case report. *J Periodontol.* 1974;45:199–206.

Ingber J. Forced eruption: part II. A method of treating nonrestorable teeth – periodontal and restorative considerations. *J Periodontol.* 1976;47(4):203–216.

Ingber J, Rose L, Coslet F. The "biologic width" – a concept in periodontics and restorative dentistry. *Alpha Omegan.* 1977;70(3):62–65.

Ishikawa T, Salama M, Funato A, Kitajima H, Moroi H, Salama H, Garber D. Three-dimensional bone and soft tissue requirements for optimizing esthetic results in compromised cases with multiple implants. *Int J Periodontics Restorative Dent.* 2010;30(5):503–511.

Jacques L, Coelho A, Hollweg H, Conti P. Tissue sculpturing: an alternative method for improving esthetics of anterior fixed prosthodontics. *J Prosthet Dent.* 1999;81:630–633.

Jansen CE, Weisgold A. Presurgical treatment planning for the anterior single-tooth implant restoration. *Compend Contin Educ Dent.* 1995;16:746–752.

Jemt T. The papilla index. *Int J Oral Maxillofac Implants.* 2004;10:702–711.

Jovanovic S, Paul S, Nishimura R. Anterior implant-supported reconstruction: a surgical challenge. *Pract Periodontics Aesthet Dent.* 1999;11(5):551–558.

Jung R, Sailer, I, Hammerle CH, Attin T, Schmidin P. *In vitro* color changes of the covering mucosa caused by restorative materials made of titanium and ceramic. *Int J Periodontics Restorative Dent.* 2007;27(3):251–257.

Kan JY, Rungcharassaeng K, Lozada J. Dimensions of peri-implant mucosa: an evaluation of maxillary anterior single implants in humans. *J Periodontol.* 2003a;74(4):557–562.

Kan JY, Rungcharassaeng K, Lozada J. Immediate placement and provisionalization of maxillary anterior single implants: 1-year prospective study. *Int J Oral Maxillofac Implants.* 2003b;18:31–39.

Kan J, Rungcarassaeng K, Lozada J. Bilaminar subepithelial connective tissue grafts for immediate implant placement and provisionalization in the esthetic zone. *J Calif Dent Assoc.* 2005;33:865–871.

Kan J, Rungcharassaeng K, Lozada J, Zimmerman G. Facial gingival tissue stability following immediate placement and provisionalization of maxillary anterior single implants: a 2- to 8-year follow-up. *Int J Oral Maxillofac Implants* 2011;26:179–187.

Kan JY, Rungcharassaeng K, Liddelow G, Henry P, Goodacre C. Periimplant tissue response following immediate provisional restoration of scalloped implants in the esthetic zone: a one-year pilot prospective multicenter study. *J Prosthet Dent.* 2007;97(6 Suppl.):S109–S118.

Kan JY, Roe P, Rungcharassaeng K, Patel RD, Waki T, Lozada JL, Zimmerman G. Classification of sagittal root position in relation to the anterior maxillary osseous housing for immediate implant placement: a cone bean computed tomography study. *Int J Oral Maxillofac Implants.* 2011;26:873–876.

Karkar A. Esthetic expression. *J Indian Acad Esthet Cosm Dent.* 2007;10:1.

Kao RT, Dault S, Frangadakis K, Salehieh JJ. Esthetic crown lengthening: appropriate diagnosis for achieving gingival balance. *J Calif Dent Assoc.* 2008;36(3):187–191.

Kawabata H, Zeki S. Neural correlates of beauty. *J Neurophysiol.* 2004;91(4):1699–1705.

Kehl M, Swierko K, Mengel R. Three-dimensional measurement of bone lost at implants in patients with periodontal disease. *J Periodontol.* 2011;82:689–699.

Kennedy J, Bird W, Palcanis K, Dorfman H. A longitudinal evaluation of varying widths of attached gingiva. *J Clin Periodontol.* 1985;12:667–675.

Kerner S, Monnet-Corti V, Sarfati A, Mora F, Bouchard P. Recouvrement radiculaire la technique influence-t-elle le resultat? *Inf Dent.* 2009;18:964–969.

Kim T, Cascione D, Knezevic A. Simulated tissue using a unique pontic design: a clinical report. *J Prosthet Dent.* 2009;102:205–210.

Kinsel R, Capoferri D. A simplified method to develop optimal gingival contours for the single implant-supported, metal-ceramic crown in the esthetic zone. *Pract Proced Aesthet Dent.* 2008;20(4):231–236.

Kois J. Altering gingival levels: the restorative connection, part I. Biologic variables. J Esthet Dent. 1994;6:3–9.

Kois JC. Exploring the periodontal–restorative interface. *Pract Proced Aesthet Dent.* 2006;18(4 Suppl.):S1.

Kokich V Jr., Kiyak H, Shapiro P. Comparing the perception of dentists and lay people to altered dental esthetic. *J Esthet Dent.* 1999;11:311–324.

Koszegi Stoianov V. The concept of "platform switching" in implant dentistry. *Implants.* 2010;1:20–25/2:18–22.

Kourkouta S, Dedi K, Paquette D, Mol A. Interproximal tissue dimensions in relation to adjacent implants in the anterior maxilla: clinical observations and patient esthetic evaluation. *Clin Oral Implants Res.* 2009;20:1375–1385.

Kurtzman G, Silverstein L. Dental implants: oral hygiene and maintenance. *Int Dent SA* 2008;10(1):56–62.

Kurtzman GM, Silverstein LH. Diagnosis and treatment planning for predictable gingival correction of altered passive eruption. *Pract Proced Aesthet Dent.* 2008;20(2):103–108.

Landolt M, Blatz M. The concept of platform switching. *Pract Proced Aesthet Dent.* 2008;20(1):5.

Landsberg C. Socket seal surgery combined with immediate implant placement: a novel approach for single-tooth replacement. *Int J Periodontics Restorative Dent.* 1997;17(2):140–149.

Landsberg C. Preservation of the interimplant papilla of the esthetic zone. In: Romano R, ed., *The Art of the Smile: Integrating Prosthodontics, Orthodontics, Periodontics, Dental Technology, and Plastic Surgery in Esthetic Dental Treatment.* Chicago, IL: Quintessence; 2005:297–320.

Landsberg C. Implementing socket seal surgery as a socket preservation technique for implant placement. *J Periodontol.* 2008;79(5):945–954.

Lang NP, Löe H. The relationship between the width of keratinized gingiva and gingival health. *J Periodontol.* 1972;43(10):623–627.

Langer B, Langer L. Subepithelial connective tissue graft technique for root coverage. *J Periodontol.* 1985;56:397–402.

Lazzara RJ, Porter SS. Platform switching: a new concept in implant dentistry for controlling post-restorative bone levels. *Int J Periodontics Restorative Dent.* 2006;26(1):9–17.

Lesclous, P. Prescriptions antibiotiques. Afssaps 2011. *Inf Dent.* 2011;36:3.

Levine RA, McGuire M. The diagnosis and treatment of the gummy smile. *Plast Reconstr Surg.* 1979;63(3):372–373.

Leziy S, Miller B. Developing ideal implant tissue architecture and pontic site form. *QDT* 2007;20:143–154.

Leziy S, Miller B. Prefabricated zirconia abutments: surgical advantages, indications and handling considerations. *Quintessence of Dental Technology* 2008a;1:68–80.

Leziy S, Miller B. Interdisciplinary treatment planning. Chapter 3 in: *Esthetics in Implant Therapy: A Blueprint for Success.* Chapter 3: Chicago, IL: Quintessence; 2008b.

Leziy S, Miller B. Esthetics in implant therapy: a blueprint for success. In: *Seattle Study Club Symposium Manual.* 2009: 69–80.

Liebart MF, Monnet-Corti V, Fouque-Deruelle C, Glise JM, Santoni A, Borghetti A. Sourire, l'incontournable esthétique gingivale. *Inf Dent.* 2011;93(11):14–20.

Liebart MF, Fouque-Duruelle C. Dillier FL, *et al.* Smile line and periodontium visibility. *Periodont Pract Today.* 2004;1:17–25.

Litton C, Fournier P. Simple surgical correction of the gummy smile. *Plast Reconstr Surg.* 1979:63(3):372–373.

Lindhe J, Berglundh T. The interface between the mucosa and the implant. *Periodontol 2000.* 1998:17:47–54.

Lindhe J, Berglundh T, Ericsson I, Liljenberg B, Marinello C. Experimental breakdown of peri-implant and periodontal tissues: a study in the beagle-dog. *Clin Oral Implants Res.* 1992;3:9–16.

Linkevicius T, Apse P, Med H, Grybauskas, S, Puisys A. The influence of soft tissue thickness on crestal bone changes around implants: a 1-year prospective controlled clinical trial. *Int J Oral Maxillofac Implants.* 2009;24:712–719.

Listgarten M, Buser D, Steinemann S, Donath K, Lang N, Weber H. Light and transmission electron microscopy of the intact interfaces between non-submerged titanium-coated epoxy resin implants and bone or gingiva. *J Dent Res.* 1992;71:364–371.

Livin L, Pathael S, Dolev E, Schwartz-Arad D. Esthetic versus surgical success of single dental implants: 1- to 9- year follow up. *Pract Proced Aesthet Dent.* 2005;17(8):533–538.

Lowe RA. The use of dental lasers and ridge preservation to maximize esthetic outcomes. *Contemp Esthet Rest Pract.* 2004;8(7):48–53.

Lowe RA. Clinical use of the Er, Cr: YSGG laser for osseous crown lengthening redefining the standard of care. *Pract Proced Aesthet Dent.* 2006;18(4 Suppl.):S2–S9.

Lowe, RA. Comment préserver la hauteur des bords alvéolaires osseux? *Dentoscope.* 2009;46:4–10.

Maeda Y, Miura J, Taki I, Sogo M. Biomechanical analysis on platform switching: Is there any biomechanical rationale? *Clin Oral Implants Res.* 2007;18(5):581–584.

Magne P, Belser U. *Restaurations adhésives en céramique: approche biomimétique.* Chicago, IL: Quintessence; 2003.

Mahajan A, Dixit J, Verma UP. A patient-centered clinical evaluation of acellular dermal matrix graft in the treatment of gingival recession defects. *J Periodontol.* 2007;78(12): 2348–2355.

Marincola M, Coelho PG, Morgan V, Cicconetti A. The importance of crestal bone preservation in the use of short implants. *Implants.* 2009;4:34–35.

Martins da Rosa JC, Martins da Rosa D, Zardo CM, Pértile de Oliveira Rosa AC, Canullo L. Reconstruction of damaged fresh sockets by connective-bone sliver graft from the maxillary tuberosity, to enable immediate dentoalveolar restoration (IDR) – a clinical case. *Implants.* 2009;3:12–17.

Materdomini D, Friedman MJ. The connect lens effect: enhancing porcelain veneer esthetics. *J Esthet Dent.* 1993;7(3):99–103.

Mathews D. Soft tissue management around implants in the esthetic zone. *Int J Periodontics Restorative Dent.* 2000;20:141–149.

Mattos CML, Santana RB. A quantitative evaluation of the spatial displacement of the gingival zenith in the maxillary anterior dentition. *J Periodontol.* 2008;79:1880–1885.

Mattout C, Mattout P. La greffe conjonctive. *Inf Dent.* 2008;3:68–72.

Maynard JG, Wilson RD. Physiologic dimensions of the periodontium significant to the restorative dentist. *Compend Contin Educ Dent.* 1980;1:161–173.

Maynard JG, Wilson RD. The rationale for muco gingival therapy in the child and adolescent. *Int. J Periodontics Restorative Dent* 1987;7(1):36–51.

McGuire M, Levine RA. The diagnosis and treatment of the gummy smile. *Compend Contin Educ Dent.* 1997;18(8): 757–764.

Mechanic E. 2008. Change the life of your patient. *Conference at the HAED.* March 2008.

Mellonig JT. Enamel matrix derivative for periodontal reconstructive surgery: technique and clinical and histologic case report. *Int J Periodontics Restorative Dent.* 1999; 19:8–19.

Miller PD Jr. A classification of marginal tissue recession. *Int J Periodontics Restorative Dent.* 1985;5(2):8–13.

Miara P, Touati B. De l'impact de l'esthétique en dentisterie actuelle *Inf Dent.* 2011;30:1.

Misch CE. Bone density – a key determinant for clinical success. In: Misch CE, ed., *Contemporary Implant Dentistry.* 2nd ed. St. Louis, MO: Mosby; 1999: 1009–1119.

Miskinyar S. A new method for correcting a gummy smile. *Plast Reconstr Surg.* 1983;72(3):397–400.

Mitrani R, Phillips K, Kois J. An implant-supported, screw-retained, provisional fixed partial denture for pontic site enhancement. *Pract Proced Aesthet Dent.* 1999;81:136–142.

Miyasato M, Crigger M, Egelberg J. Gingival condition in areas of minimal and appreciable width of keratinized gingiva. *J Clin Periodontol.* 1977;4(3):200–209.

Monnet-Corti V, Borghetti A. *Chirurgie plastique parodontale,* 2nd ed. Paris: Editions CDP; 2008.

Nato N. Are systemic risk factors affecting implant survival and esthetic result? *Acad Osteoint News.* 2010;13:16–18.

Nemcovsky CE, Artzi Z, Moses O. Preprosthetic clinical crown lengthening procedures in the anterior maxilla. *Pract Proced Aesthet Dent.* 2001;13(7):581–588; quiz 589.

Nevins M, Camelo M, Boyesen J, Kim D. Human histological evidence of a connective tissue attachment to a dental implant. *Int J Periodontics Restorative Dent.* 2008;28:111–119.

Nevins M, Camelo M, De Paoli S, *et al.* A study of the fate of the buccal wall of extraction sockets of teeth with prominent roots. *Int J Periodontics Restorative Dent.* 2006;26:19–29.

Neumann LM, Christensen C, Cavanaugh C. Dental esthetic satisfaction in adults. *J Am Dent Assoc.* 1989;118: 565–570.

Newton JT, Prabhu N, Robinson PG. The impact of dental appearance on the appraisal of personal characteristics. *Int J Prosthodont.* 2004;16:429–434.

Nguyen H, Tran K, Nicholls, J. Load fatigue performance of implant–ceramic abutment combination. *Int J Oral Maxillofac Implants.* 2009;24:636–646.

Nguyen HL. Are local risk factors affecting implant survival and esthetic result? *Acad Osteoint News.* 2010;13:11–15.

Nisapakultorn K, Suphanantachat S, Silkosessak O, Rattanamongkolgul S. Factors affecting soft tissue level around anterior maxillary single-tooth implants. *Clin Oral Implants Res.* 2010;21(6):662–670.

Norton MR. Multiple single-tooth implant restorations in the posterior jaws: maintenance of marginal bone levels with reference to the implant–abutment microgap. *Int J Oral Maxillofac Implants.* 2006;21(5):777–784 (Ref. No. 78773).

Nowzari H, Rich S. Hyperplasie gingivale chez les jeunes patients. *Inf Dent.* 2008;15:758–763.

Oates T. Are systemic factors affecting implants survival? *Int J Oral Maxillofac Implants.* 2011:26;469–470.

Paolantonio M, Dolci M, Scarano A. Immediate implantation in fresh extraction sockets: a controlled clinical and histological study in man. *J Periodontol.* 2001;72: 1560–1571.

Paris J-C, Faucher A. *Le guide esthétique: comment réussir le sourire de vos patients?* Chicago, IL: Quintessence; 2003.

Patel R, Richards P, Inglehart M. The smile-related quality of life and periodontal health. *J Periodontol.* 2008;79:224–231.

Patzer GI. Improving self-esteem by improving physical attractiveness. *J Esthet Dent.* 1997;9(1):41–47.

Patzer GL, Faucher AJ. Understanding the causal relationship between physical attractiveness and self-esteem. *J Esthet Dent.* 1996;8(3):144–147.

Peck S, Peck L, Kataja M. The gingival smile line. *Angle Orthod.* 1992;62(2):91–100.

Poitras Y. Reformer les limites du traitement implantaire au-delà des zones anatomiques défavorables. *Inf Dent.* 2003;5:273–274.

Pollack R. Bilateral creeping attachment using free mucosal grafts: a case report with 4-year-follow-up. *J Periodontol.* 1984;55(11):670–672.

Polo M. Botulinum toxin type A in the treatment of excessive gingival display. *Am J Orthod Dentofacial Orthop.* 2005;127(2):214–218.

Ponsi J, Lahti S, Rissanen H, *et al.* Change in subjective oral health after single dental implant treatment. *Int J Oral Maxillofac Implants.* 2011;26:571–577.

Pontoriero R, Carnevale F. Surgical crown lengthening: a 12-month clinical wound healing study. *J Periodontol.* 2001;72(7):841–848.

Pozzi, A. Nouvelles tendance en implantologie moderne. *Le Fil Dentaire.* 2011;66(5):32–37.

Prato G, Rotundo R, Cortellini P, Tinti C, Azzi R. Interdental papilla management: a review and classification of the therapeutic approaches. *Int J Periodontics Restorative Dent.* 2004;24(3):246–255.

Prichard J. Gingivoplasty, gingivectomy and osseous surgery. *J Periodontol.* 1961;32:275–282.

Puchades-Roman L, Palmer RM, Palmer PJ, Howe LC, Ide M, Wilson RF. A clinical, radiographic, and microbiologic comparison of Astra Tech and Brånemark single tooth implants. *Clin Implant Dent Relat Res.* 2000;2:78–84.

Range H. Peut-on surfacer sans faire un lambeau? *Inf Dent.* 2008;18:1931–1933.

Ravins H. Smiling on the inside and outside. *Pract Proced Aesthet Dent.* 2008;20(6):369–370.

Reddy MS. Achieving gingival esthetics. *J Am Dent Assoc.* 2003;134(3):295–304.

Rees T, La Trenta G. The long face syndrome and rhinoplasty. *Perspect Plast Surg.* 1989;3:116.

Rignon-Bret C, Fattouh J, Tchuendjo Kom N, Tezenas du Monteel S, Jonas P. La demande esthétique des seniors. *Inf Dent.* 2007;33:1965–1968.

Rimondini L, Cerroni L, Carrassi A, Toricelli P. Bacterial colonization of zirconia ceramic surfaces: an *in vitro* and *in vivo* study. *Int J Oral Maxillofac Implants.* 2002;17:793–798.

Robbins JW. Differential diagnosis and treatment of excess gingival display. *Pract Periodontics Aesthet Dent.* 1999;11(2):265–272.

Roccuzzo M, Romagnoli R. Coronally advanced flap for the treatment of buccal gingival recessions. *Int J Oral Maxillofac Implants.* 2006;21(5):696–710.

Romagna C. Dent naturelle-implant un contour gingival harmonieux. *Inf Dent.* 2009;20:1066–1070.

Rompen E, Peri implant soft tissue increase: clinical evidence and indication. In: *Int Symp Osteol Cannes, April 14-16. AO News* 2011,142:26–28.

Rompen E, Touati B, Van Dooren E. Factors influencing marginal tissue remodeling around implants. *Pract Proced Aesthet Dent.* 2003;15(10):754–776.

Rompen E, Raepsaet N, Domken O, Touati B, Van Dooren E. Soft tissue stability at the facial aspect of gingivally converging abutments in the esthetic zone: a pilot clinical study. *J Prosthet Dent.* 2007;97(6 Suppl.):S119–S125.

Rosenberg ES, Cho SC, Garber DA. Crown lengthening revisited. *Compend Contin Educ Dent.* 1999;20:527–532.

Rosenberg ES, Evian C, Garber DA. Crown lengthening procedure. *Compend Contin Educ Dent.* 1980;1:3–9.

Rosentiel SF, Rashid RG. Public preferences for anterior tooth variations: a web-based study. *J Esthet Restor Dent.* 2002;14:97–106.

Rosenblatt A, Simon Z. Lip repositioning for reduction of excessive gingival display: a clinical report. *Int J Periodontics Restorative Dent.* 2006;26(5):433–437.

Rufenacht, C. *Fundamentals of Esthetics.* Chicago, IL: Quintessence; 1990.

Ryser MR, Block MS, Mercante DE. Correlation of papilla to crestal bone levels around single tooth implants and in immediate or delayed crown protocols. *J Oral Maxillofac Surg.* 2005;63:1184–1195.

Saadoun AP. The key to peri-implant aesthetics hard and soft tissue management. *Dent Implantol Update.* 1997;8 (6):41–46.

Saadoun AP. Immediate implant placement and temporization in extraction and healing sites. *Compend Contin Educ Dent.* 2002;23(4):309–318.

Saadoun AP. All about the smile. In: Romano R, ed., *The Art of the Smile: Integrating Prosthodontics, Orthodontics, Periodontics, Dental Technology, and Plastic Surgery in Esthetic Dental Treatment.* Chicago, IL: Quintessence; 2005:265–293.

Saadoun AP. Current trends in gingival recession coverage – part I: the tunnel connective tissue graft. *Pract Proced Aesthet Dent.* 2006;18(7):433–438.

Saadoun AP. Current trends in gingival recession coverage – part II: enamel matrix derivative and platelet-rich plasma. *Pract Proced Aesthet Dent.* 2006;18(8):521–526.

Saadoun AP. Root coverage with Emdogain/AlloDerm: a new way to treat a gingival recession. *Eur J Esthet Dent.* 2008;3:46–65.

Saadoun AP. A thought on the future of implantology. *Dent Implantol Update* 2009;20(7):49–56.

Saadoun AP. Multifactorial parameters in peri-implant soft tissue management. In: Romano R, ed., *The Art of Treatment Planning.* Chicago, IL: Quintessence; 2010:75–154.

Saadoun AP, Le Gall M. Implant positioning for periodontal, functional, and esthetic results. *Pract Periodontics Aesthet Dent.* 1992;4:43–54.

Saadoun AP, Le Gall MG. Implant site preparation with osteotomes: principles and clinical application. *Pract Periodontics Aesthet Dent.* 1996;8(5):453–463.

Saadoun AP, Le Gall MG, Touati B. Selection and ideal tridimensional implant position for soft tissue esthetics. *Pract Periodontics Aesthet Dent.* 1999;11(9):1063–1074.

Saadoun AP, Le Gall MG, Touati B. Current trends in implantology, part I. *Pract Periodontics Aesthet Dent.* 2004;16(7):529–535.

Saadoun AP, Le Gall MG, Touati B. Current trends in implantology, part II. *Pract Periodontics Aesthet Dent.* 2004;16(10): 707–714.

Saadoun AP, Touati B. Soft tissue recession around implant: Is it still unavoidable? Part I. *Pract Proced Aesthet Dent.* 2007;19(1):55–64.

Saadoun AP, Touati B. Soft tissue recession around implant: Is it still unavoidable? Part II. *Pract Proced Aesthet Dent.* 2007;19(2):81–87.

Salama H, Jundslalys G. Immediate implantation and soft tissue reaction. *Clin Oral Implants Res.* 2003:14(2):144–149.

Salama H, Salama M. The role of orthodontics extrusive remodeling in the enhancement of soft and hard tissue profiles prior to implant placement: a systematic approach to the management of extraction site defects. *Int J Periodontics Restorative Dent.* 1993;13(4):312–333.

Salama H, Salama M, Garber D. The tunnel technique. *Inside Dentistry.* 2008:4(9):78–81.

Salama H, Salama M, Garber D, Adar P. The interproximal height of bone: a guidepost to predictable esthetic strategies and soft tissues contours in anterior tooth replacement. *Pract Periodontics Aesthet Dent.* 1998;10:1131–1141.

Salama M. De la chirurgie pré-implantaire à la mise en charge immediate: acquis et perspectives. *Inf Dent.* 2011;12:13.

Sallum EA. Coronally positioned flap with or without an acellular dermal matrix graft in the treatment of Class I gingival recessions: a randomized controlled clinical study. *J Periodontol.* 2004;75:1137–1144.

Savard F, Tirlet G, Attal J.P. La dentisterie esthétique: pourquoi maintenant? *Le Fil Dentaire*; April 2007.

Scarano A, Barros R, Iezzi G, Piattelli A, Novaes Jr. A. Acellular dermal matrix graft for gingival augmentation: a preliminary clinical, histologic, and ultrastructural evaluation. *J Periodontol.* 2009;80(2):253–259.

Schroeder HE. *Oral Structural Biology.* New York: Thieme; 1991:230–232.

Schroetenboer J, Tsao Y-P, Kinariwala V, Wang H-L. effect of microthreads and platform switching on crestal bone stress levels: a finite element analysis. *J Periodontol.* 2008;79: 2166–2172.

Schroop L, Isidor F, Kostopoulos, Wenzel A. Optimizing anterior aesthetics with immediate implant placement and single implant placement. *Int J Periodontics Restorative Dent.* 1999;19(1):21–29.

Schropp L, Kostopoulos L, Wenzel A, Isidor F. Clinical and radiographic performance of delayed-immediate single-tooth implant placement associated with peri-implant bone defects: a 2-year prospective, controlled, randomized follow-up report. *J Clin Periodontol.* 2005;32(5):480–487.

Schwartz-Arad D, Chaushu G. The ways and wherefores of immediate placement of implants into fresh extraction sites: a literature review. *J Periodontol.* 1997;68(10):915–923.

Schupbach P, Glauser R. The defense architecture of the human periimplant mucosa: a histological study. *J Prosthet Dent.* 2007;97(6 Suppl.):S15–S25.

Sculean A, Donos N, Blaes A, Lauermann M, Reich E, Brecx M. Comparison of enamel matrix proteins and bioabsorbable membranes in the treatment of intrabony periodontal defects: a split-mouth study. *J Periodontol.* 1999;70:255–262.

Serino G, Wennstrom J, Lindhe, Eneroth, L. The prevalence and distribution of gingival recession in subjects with a high standard of oral hygene. *J Clin Periodontol.* 1994:21(1): 57–63.

Sethi S. Staging the challenge – a single implant tissue training in the esthetic zone. *Implants.* 2008;4:30–34.

Shapoff CA, Lahey B, Wasserlauf PA, Kim DM. Radiographic analysis of crestal bone levels around Laser-Lok collar dental implants. *Int J Periodontics Restorative Dent.* 2010;30: 129–137.

Shepherd N, Greenwell H, Hill M, Vidal R, Scheetz JP. Root coverage using acellular dermal matrix and comparing a coronally positioned tunnel with and without platelet-rich plasma. *J Periodontol.* 2009;3:397–404.

Shi L, Beng M, Haiyan L. Shape optimization of dental implant. *Int J Oral Maxillofac Implants.* 2007;22:911–920.

Shin HS, Cueva MA, Kerns DG, Hallmon WW, Rivera-Hidalgo F, Nunn M. A comparative study of root coverage using acellular dermal matrix with and without enamel matrix derivative. *J Periodontol.* 2007;78:411–421.

Silderberg N, Goldstein M, Smidt A. Excessive gingival display – etiology, diagnosis, and treatment modalities. *Quintessence Int.* 2009;40(10):809–818.

Simonpieri A, Choukroun J, Del Corso M, Sammartino, G, Ehrenfest D, Dohan D. Simultaneous sinus-lift and implantation using microthreaded implants and leukocyte- and platelet-rich fibrin as sole grafting material: a six-year experience. *Implant Dentistry.* 2011;20(1):2–12.

Singh J, Mattoo SK, Sharan P, Basu D. Quality of life and its correlates in patients with dual diagnosis of bipolar affective disorder and substance dependence. *Bipolar Disord.* 2005;7:187–191.

Small P, Tarnow D. Gingival recession around implants: a 1-year longitudinal prospective study. *Int J Oral Maxillofac Implants.* 2000;15:527–532.

Small PN, Tarnow DP, Cho SC. Gingival recession around wide-diameter versus standard-diameter implants: a 3- to 5-year longitudinal prospective study. *Pract Proced Aesthet Dent.* 2001;13(2):143–146.

Socransky SS, Haffajee AD. The bacterial etiology of destructive periodontal disease: current concepts. *J Periodontol.* 1992,63:322–331.

Sonick M, Hwang D, Saadoun A. *Implant Site Development.* Chichester: Wiley-Blackwell; 2012.

Spear F. Maintenance of the interdental papilla following anterior tooth removal. *Pract Periodontics Aesthet Dent.* 1999;11(1):21–28.

Spear F. The use of implant and ovate pontiffs in the esthetic zone. *Compend Contin Educ Dent.* 2008;29(2):72–74.

Stetler K, Bissada N. Significance of the width of keratinized gingiva on the periodontal status of teeth with submarginal restorations. *J Periodontol.* 1987;58:696–702.

Tabata LF, Rocha EP, Barao VA, Assunçao WG. Platform switching: biomechanical evaluation using three-dimensional finite element analysis. *Int J Oral Maxillofac Implants.* 2011;26:482–491.

Tarnow D. Papilla management and teeth contact relation. April 2008. Hellenic Academy of Esthetic Dentistry.

Tarnow D., Cho S, Wallace S. The effect of inter-implant distance on the height of the inter-implant bone crest. *J Periodontol.* 2000;71:546–549.

Tarnow D, Elian N, Fletcher P. Vertical distance from the crest of bone to the height of the interproximal papilla between adjacent implants. *J Periodontol.* 2003;74:1785–1788.

Tarnow D, Magner AW, Fletcher P. The effect of the distance from the contact point to the crest of bone on the presence or absence of the interproximal dental papilla. *J Periodontol.* 1992;63(12):995–996.

Tawil G. Comparison between immediate and delayed implant placement. *Int J Oral Maxillofac Implants.* 2009; 24(7 Suppl.):237–259.

Terry D, Leinfelder K, Lee E. The impression: a blueprint to restorative success. *Inside Dentistry.* 2006:66–71.

Tetè S, Mastrangelo F, Bianchi A, Zizzari V, Scarano A. Collagen fiber orientation around machined titanium and zirconia dental implant necks: an animal study. *Int J Oral Maxillofac Implants* 2009;24:52–58.

Thornhill R, Gangestad S. Facial attractiveness. *Trends Cogn Sci.* 1999;3:452–460.

Tinti C, Vincenzi P, Cortellini Pini Prato G, Clauser C. Guided tissue regeneration in the treatment of human facial recession: a 12-case report. *J Periodontol.* 1992;63(6):554–560.

Tjan L, Anthony H, Miller GD, *et al.* The some esthetic factors in a smile. *J Prosthet Dent.* 1984;51(1):24–28.

Toca E, Paris J-C, Brouillet J-L. Exposition gingivale excessive: quels sourires? *Inf Dent.* 2008;11:514–519.

Tomasi C, Sanz M, Cecchinato D, *et al.* Bone dimensional variations at implants placed in fresh extraction sockets: a multilevel multivariate analysis. *Clin Oral Implants Res.* 2010;21:30–36.

Touati B. Envisioning final results. *Pract Proced Aesthet Dent.* 2008;20(5):268.

Touati B. Reussir esthetiquement un implant anterieur. *Inf Dent.* 2009;22:1164.

Touati, B. Remplacement par un implant d'une incisive centrale maxillaire fortement compromise. *Le Fil Dentaire.* 2011;66(5):42–46.

Touati B, Etienne JM, Van Dooren E. Esthetic integration of digital-ceramic restorations. Montage Media 2008.

Touati B, Rompen E, Van Dooren E. A new concept for optimizing soft tissue integration. *Pract Proced Esthetic Dent.* 2005;17(10):712–715.

Tucker L. Framing your masterpiece: guidelines for treatment planning the ideal soft tissue framework. In: *Seattle Study Club Symposium Manual.* 2009:111–126.

Valderhaug J. Periodontal conditions and carious lesions following the insertion of fixed prostheses: a 10-year follow-up study. *Int Dent J.* 1980;30(4):296–304.
Vallittu PK, Vallittu SJ, Lassila P. Dental esthetics – a survey of attitudes in different groups of patients. *J Dent.* 1996;24: 335–338.
Van der Geld P, Oosterveld P, Kuijpers-Jagtman AM. Age-related changes of the dental esthetic zone at rest and during spontaneous smiling and speech. *Eur J Orthod.* 2008;30: 366–373.
Van Dooren E. Management of soft and hard tissue surrounding dental implants: esthetic principles. *Pract Periodontics Aesthet Dent.* 2000;12:837–841.
Van Kesteren CJ, Schoolfield J, West J, Oates T. A prospective randomized clinical study of changes in soft tissue position following immediate and delayed implant placement. *Int J Oral Maxillofac Implants.* 2010;25(3):562–570.
Vela X. Immediate implant placement and immediate loading after. *Implants* 2008;1:26–29.
Vig, R, Brundo GC. The kinetics of anterior tooth display. *J Prosthet Dent.* 1978;39(5):502–504.
Vigolo P, Givani A. Platform-switched restorations on wide-diameter implants: a 5-year clinical prospective study. *Int J Oral Maxillofac Implants.* 2009;24:103–109.
Warrer K, Buser D, Lang NP, Karring T. Plaque-induced peri-implantitis in the presence or absence of keratinized mucosa: an experimental study in monkeys. *Clin Oral Implants Res.* 1995;6:131–138.
Weinstein SP. Classification of clinical attributes in tooth appearance. *Pract Proced Aesthet Dent.* 2008;20(3):143–151.
Weisgold A, Coslet G. Diagnosis and classification of periodontal type. *Alpha Omegan.* 1977;1:18–23.
Wennström J. Mucogingival therapy. *Ann Periodontol.* 1996;1:671–706.
Wennström J, Lindhe J. Some effects of enamel matrix proteins on wound healing in the dento-gingival region. *J Clin Periodontol.* 2002;29(1):9–14.
Wilson Jr. G. The positive relationship between excess cement and peri-implant disease: a prospective clinical endoscopic study. *J Periodontol.* 2009;80:1388–1392.
Wöhrle PS. Single-tooth replacement in the aesthetic zone with immediate provisionalization: fourteen consecutive case reports. *Pract Periodontics Aesthet Dent.* 1998;10(9): 1107–1114.
Wöhrle PS. Nobel Perfect esthetic scalloped implant: rationale for new design. *Clin Implant Dent Relat Res.* 2003;5: 64–73.
World Health Organization. General well-being as an important co-factor of self-assessment of dental appearance. *Int J Prosthodont.* 2006;19:449–454.
York J, Holtzman J. Facial attractiveness and the aged. *Spec Care Dentist.* 1999;19(2):84–88.
Zabalegui I, Sicilia A, Cambra J, *et al.* Treatment of multiple adjacent gingival recessions with the tunnel recession sub-epithelial connective tissue graft: a clinical report. *Int J Periodontics Restorative Dent.* 1999;19(2):199–206.
Zaidel D, Cohen J. The face, beauty, and symmetry: perceiving asymmetry in beautiful faces. *Int J Neurosci.* 2005;115: 1165–1173.
Zaidel D, Aarde S, Baig K. Appearance of symmetry, beauty, and health in human faces. *Brain Cogn.* 2005;57: 261–263.
Zipprich H, Weigl P, Lange B, Lauer HC. Micro-movements at the implant–abutment interface: measurement, causes and consequences. *Implantologie.* 2007;15(1):31–46.
Zlowodzki A, Tirlet G, Attal JP. Autour de l'ésthétique. *Inf Dent.* 2008;42:2534–2538.
Zuchelli G. A method to predetermine the line of gingival root coverage. *J Periodontol.* 2006;77(4):714–721.
Zuchelli G, De Sanctis M. Treatment of multiple recession-type defects in patients with esthetic demands. *J Periodontol.* 2000;71:1506–1514.
Zuchelli G, Testori T. De Sanctis, *et al.* A method to predetermine the line of root coverage in the esthetic zone. *J Periodontol.* 2006;4:714–721.
Zuhr O. Implantology: esthetic in question. *Inf Dent.* 2011: 15–16.

Index

Note: Page numbers in *italics* refer to Figures; those in **bold** to Tables.

Printed in the United States
By Bookmasters